DNA REPLICATION AND RELATED CELLULAR PROCESSES

Edited by **Jelena Kušić - Tišma**

DNA Replication and Related Cellular Processes
Edited by Jelena Kušić - Tišma

Published by InTech
Janeza Trdine 9, 51000 Rijeka, Croatia

Publishing Process Manager Iva Simcic

Technical Editor Teodora Smiljanic

Cover Designer InTech Design Team

Additional hard copies can be obtained from orders@intechopen.com

DNA Replication and Related Cellular Processes, Edited by Jelena Kušić - Tišma
p. cm.
ISBN 978-953-307-775-8

For EU product safety concerns:
IN TECH d.o.o., Prolaz Marije Krucifikse Kozulić 3, 51000 Rijeka, Croatia,
info@intechopen.com or visit our website at intechopen.com.

Meet the editor

Dr. Jelena Kušić-Tišma is currently a research associate at the Institute of Molecular Genetics and Genetic Engineering, Belgrade. She received her PhD in Molecular Biology from Belgrade University in 2005. Her main research interest includes origin recognition mechanisms during initiation step of DNA replication in higher eukaryotes. She published several articles in peer review journals and is presently a visiting lecturer at the postgraduate studies of the Belgrade University.

Contents

Preface

Since the discovery of the DNA structure, researchers have been highly interested in the molecular basis of genome inheritance. This book covers a wide range of aspects and issues related to the field of DNA replication. The basic process of DNA replication is highly conserved among all domains of life. To sustain genetic stability the cell has to ensure that entire genome is replicated exactly once and only once per cell cycle. However, modifications of the cell cycle leading to genome multiplication occur in the animal cells during polyploidization of trophoblast cells in mammalian placenta (reviewed by Zybina and Zybina). On the other hand, meiotic DNA replication reduces a diploid cell to four haploid gametes. Stuart in his chapter describes numerous features that distinguish regulation and progression of meiotic DNA replication from DNA replication during mitotic proliferation, connecting DNA replication and homologous recombination.

Several chapters are dealing with viral DNA replication. Isomura points to regulation of expression of human cytomegalovirus DNA polymerase processivity factor as a link of viral DNA replication and transcription. Successful development of new approaches for antiviral therapy necessitates better comprehension of molecular mechanisms that regulate viral DNA replication fidelity (chapters by Matamoros et al., Hwang).

The DNA repair is one of the most important genome surveillance systems of the cell and DNA replication is an integral part of all mechanisms for the repair of DNA damage. Members of repair family of proteins are emerging as essential components linking DNA damage recognition to cell-cycle checkpoints (Her, Xu and Wu). In his chapter, author McCabe summarized mechanisms of DNA repair with focus on biochemical activity of polymerases, while relationship between the processes of DNA synthesis and recombination is discussed in chapter by Zavec.

Insights into the process of the protein-primed replication mechanism as one of the strategies for management the end-replication problem of linear genomes is describedin chapter by Salas and de Vega.

Two chapters are addressing tissue-specific regulation of DNA replication. Current molecular understanding of DNA replication with a focus on developmental-stage and tissue-specific regulation in the animal model *Caenorhabditis elegans* is presented in chapter by Ruijtenberg and Heuvel and The, whereas Czaja and coworkers discuss possibility of DNA replication in the adult mammalian neural tissue.

Presence of proteins implicated in formation of prereplication complex could be the first sign of cells intention to proliferate and their use as novel proliferative markers is reviewed in chapter by Karimi.

DNA replication is tightly coordinate with other cellular processes and it's not surprising that proteins involved in chromosome replication also has additional role in cell life, like SeqA regulation of transcription (Amine et al.).

This volume outlines our current understanding of DNA replication and related cellular processes, and gives insights into their potential for clinical application.

Dr. Jelena Kušić - Tišma
Laboratory for Molecular Biology,
Institute of Molecular Genetics and Genetic Engineering,
Belgrade,
Serbia

1

Mini-Chromosome Maintenance Protein Family: Novel Proliferative Markers - The Pathophysiologic Role and Clinical Application

Shirin Karimi[1] and Makan Sadr[2]
[1]Shahid Beheshti University of Medical Science
[2]Faculty of Medicine, Tehran University of Medical Science, Tehran, Iran

1. Introduction

Proliferation markers are among the most important biologic markers in the pathogenesis of many benign and malignant tumoral lesions and also some non-neoplastic diseases. Extensive studies have been conducted on this matter shedding light on the role of these markers in the pathogenesis of many of these lesions and their contribution to standard diagnostic protocols, determination of prognosis and even treatment monitoring of diseased cases.

Cancer is among the major causes of morbidity and mortality worldwide. Determination and recognition of biomarkers that detect cancer in its early stages, monitor the disease progression or work as a specific marker for disease prognosis can boost our ability in confronting such conditions and improve cancer patients' care by creating a personalized medicine for them. Assessment of the cell growth or proliferative signature of tumoral lesions is among the main parameters in recognition of the biologic course of cancer, prognosis and evaluation of the treatment course.

At present, we focus on recently introduced proliferative markers; MCM protein family, their basic biologic role and short review of the clinical application.

2. Cell cycle and proliferative markers

Cell proliferation is a precisely supervised process initiated and controlled by a large number of molecules and interrelated pathways. Cell proliferation is induced and started by the act of growth factors. A controlled sequence of events take place sequentially for duplication and division of cell DNA during a process called cell cycle. The cell cycle consists of four distinct phases: G_1 phase (pre-synthetic), S phase (DNA synthesis), G_2 phase (premyotic) and M phase (mitosis). Quiescent phase or G0 is a resting phase where the cell has left the cycle and has stopped dividing (1). Replication of the genomic DNA should be completed before the onset of mitosis and is performed once in every cell cycle.

Diagram of the cell cycle:

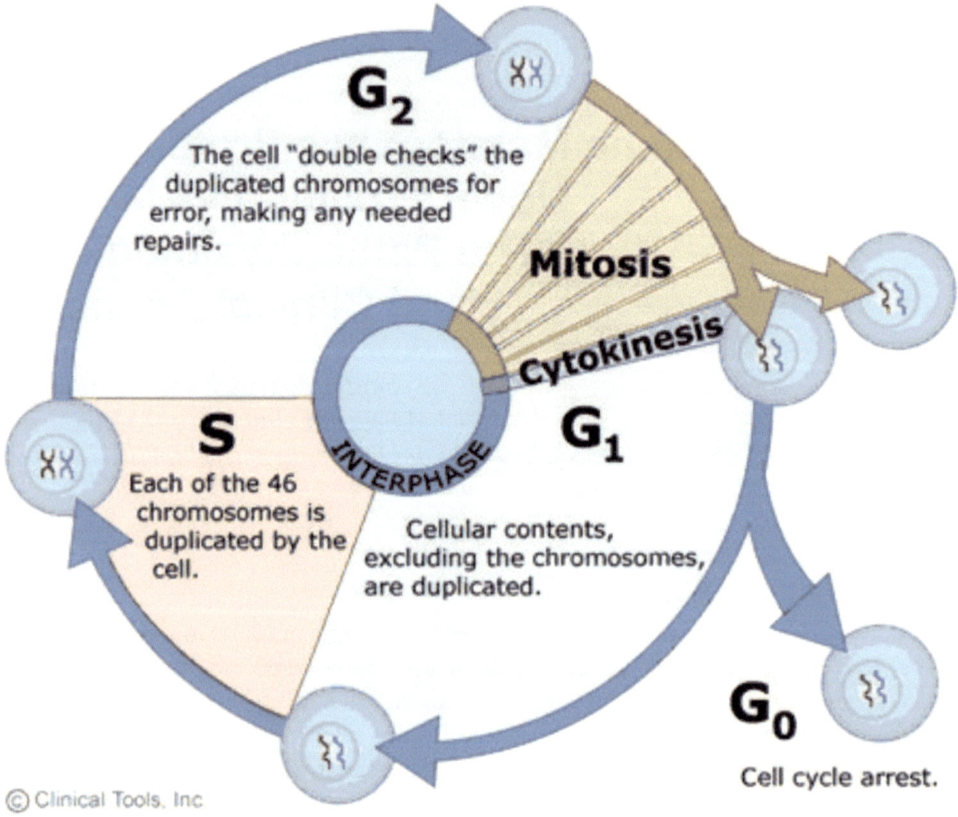

Several antigens are expressed during a cell cycle the oldest of which being Ki67 antigen. Some important antigens related to cell cycle were discovered later including PCNA, KiS2 and MCM.

Ki67 antigen was discovered by a German group of scientists (2) in early 1980s and identified by using mice monoclonal antibodies against a nuclear antigen from Hodgkin's lymphoma cell line. This antigen is a non-histone protein. The name is derived from the city of origin (Kiel, Germany) and the number of the original clone in the 96-well plate (2). Ki67 antigen has different expressions during various phases of cell cycle. Cells express this antigen in G1, S, G2 and M phases but they lack it in G0 phase. Concentration of Ki67 is low in G1 phase and reaches its peak during S phase. Ki67 is down-regulated during anaphase and telophase. Various studies on cell cycle analysis have shown that Ki67 antigen is not expressed in early G1 phase. Several antibodies are routinely being used for detection of Ki67 in paraffin embedded tissue samples using immunohistochemistry. At present, Ki67 index score is routinely employed showing tumoral cells exhibiting nuclear staining. Use of Ki67 as a diagnostic and prognostic marker in many neoplasms has been extensively studied and its role in standard biological evaluation of the clinical course and management of cancers among them Lymphomas and breast cancers has been well recognized (3-6).

MCM and cell cycle:

Numerous proteins have been recognized to play a role in initiation of DNA replication which mainly include Origin Recognition Complex (ORC) and MCMs (7). Prokaryotes lack

MCM proteins and only eukaryotes possess this special type of molecules. However, some related proteins have been found in some prokaryotes like Archaea (8-10).

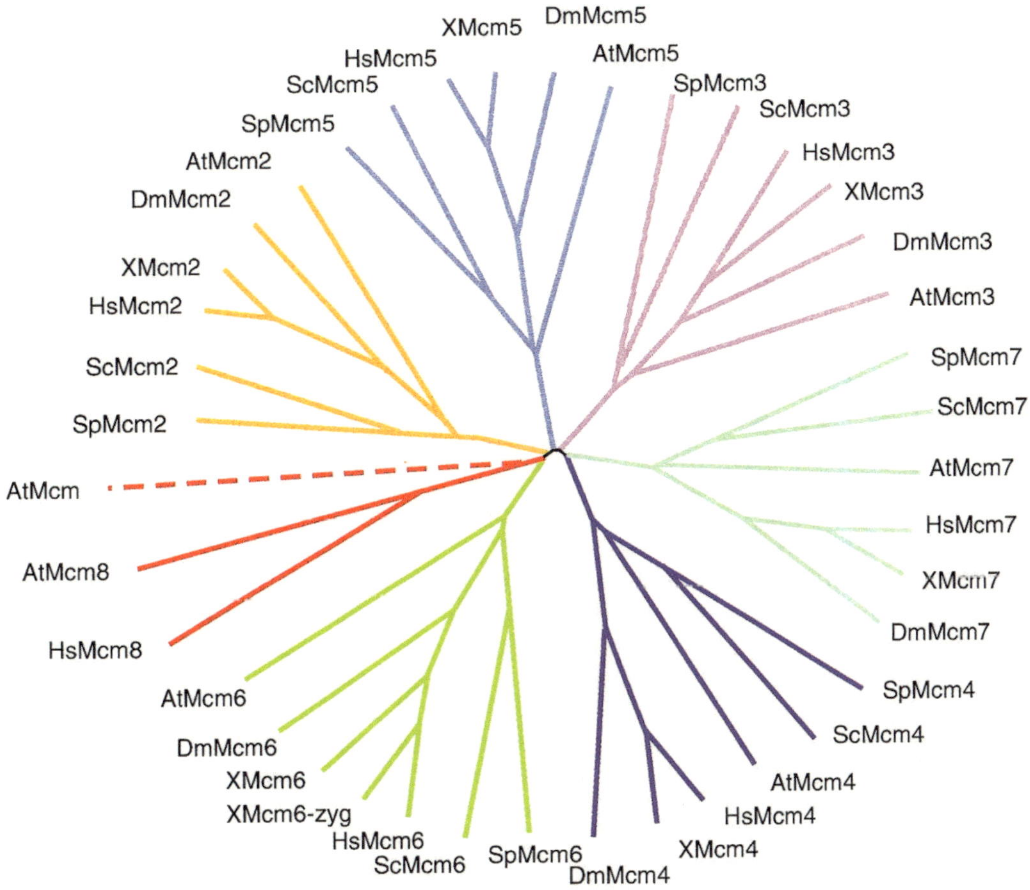

Fig. 1. Phylogenetic tree of eukaryotic MCMs, assembled using ClustalX (ftp://ftp-igbmc.u-strasbg.fr/pub/ClustalX/) and Phylip 3.6 (http://evolution.genetics.washington.edu/phylip.html) for Macintosh. Colors correspond to the seven MCM subfamilies. Dashed line, loose relationship. Accession numbers are as follows. *S. pombe*: SpMcm2, CAB58403; SpMcm3, P30666; SpMcm4, P29458, SpMcm5, CAA93299 and CAB61472; SpMcm6, CAB75412; SpMcm7, O75001. *S. cerevisiae*: ScMcm2, NP_009530; ScMcm3, NP_010882; ScMcm4, S56050; ScMcm5, A39631; ScMcm6, NP_011314; ScMcm7, S34027. Human: HsMcm2, P49736; HsMcm3, P25205; HsMcm4, NP_005905; HsMcm5, AAH03656; HsMcm6, NP_005906; HsMcm7, P33993; HsMcm8, NP_115874. *Xenopus*: Xmcm2, JC5085; Xmcm3, I51685; Xmcm4, T47223; Xmcm5, PC4225; Xmcm6Z, AAC41267; Xmcm6, T47222; Xmcm7, T47221. *Arabidopsis*: AtMcm2, NP_175112.1; AtMcm3, NP_199440.1; AtMcm4, NP_179236.2; AtMcm5, NP_178812.1; AtMcm6, NP_680393.1; AtMcm7, NP_192115.1; AtMcm8?, NP_187577.1; unknown Mcm, NP_179021.1. *Drosophila*: DmMcm2, AAF54207; DmMcm3, NP_511048.2; DmMcm4, S59872; DmMcm5, NP_524308.2; DmMcm6, NP_511065.1; DmMcm7, NP_523984.1. [11]

MCM proteins were first recognized in early 1980's in Bik-Kwoon laboratory because of their role in maintenance of plasmids and mini chromosomes in Saccharomycess Cervisiae proliferative cells (11).

The MCM protein family is named for the genetic screen in budding yeast from which the founding members were originally isolated. They were defective in minichromosome maintenance, showing a high rate of loss of plasmids that contained a cloned centromere and replication origin [12, 13].

These proteins play a role in the formation of prereplicative complex in G1 phase. By doing so, they license the chromatin for replication in the next phase of S (14).

The MCM family of proteins is considered the key factor for initiation of replication regulation through cyclical DNA unwinding (14). Also, they play a role in condensation, cohesion, transcription and recombination (11). These proteins mainly include 6 major groups of MCM2 to MCM7 (11). In addition, 4 proteins of this family have been recognized to have independent function from the previously mentioned group including MCM1, MCM10, MCM8 and MCM9. It seems that the latter group of proteins only exists in multi-cellular organisms and higher eukaryotes.

Although MCM1 and MCM10 belong to this family name wise, they do not have much in common with MCM2-MCM7. MCM1 is a transcription factor and does not have a direct role in DNA replication (15, 16).

MCM10 associates with MCM2-7 hexamer in the active replisome and helps to stabilize DNA polymerase α-primase [Reviewed in 17].

MCM8 has been reported in vertebrates and Drosophila, but not in fungi and nematodes, and although it retains some sequence similarities in the Walker B and R-finger, its Walker A ATPase motif contains sequences more like the canonical ATPases. [18] Intriguingly, while human MCM8 shares all the classic MCM features including a putative zinc finger and the IDEKFM and arginine finger motifs, it is the only MCM that has a classic GKS motif in its Walker A sequence. It is widely expressed in a variety of tissues and may not be restricted to proliferating cells [19, 20]. The protein is found in the nucleus, apparently chromatin associated during S phase [19].

MCM9 is also found in similar organisms with the exception that it is missing in Drosophila, and it is unique to the family in that it lacks the carboxy-terminal ATPase domain including the Walker B motif. [18] *MCM9* mRNA was up-regulated by transcription factor E2E1 and serum stimulation in NIH3T3 cells [21].

Various members of this family have been studied in all eukaryotes by genetic and biochemical methods and it has been demonstrated that MCM2-MCM7 proteins have been present in the genome of all the studied eukaryotes and have not been subject to gene loss or functional replacement during evolutionary diversification of eukaryotes.

In *Drosophila*, MCM4 corresponds to the gene *disc proliferation abnormal* [22], while in *Arabidopsis*, MCM7 is *PROLIFERA* [23], stressing their role in cell division. Human MCM2 (BM28) was first identified as a nuclear protein [24], and human MCM3 (P1) was isolated as a DNA polymerase alpha-associated protein [25].

Unusual MCMs

Unusual MCMs have been recognized during the course of various studies. For example, at present it has been found that some yeasts possess MCM6. However, some variants i.e. the zygotic form of MCM6 have been detected in Xenopus. Also, some variants of MCM4 have also been found (26). It seems that these variants are a substitute for normal MCM when adequate growth conditions are met.

3. DNA replication and MCM2-7 family proteins

Prior to DNA replication and during late M and G1 phases of the cell cycle, MCM2-7 form the pre-replication complex (pre-RC) by being loaded on to the origin recognition complex (ORC) at the origin of replication. This is activated at the G1-S transition of the cell cycle by the assembly of further protein components. [27] Only MCM2 and MCM3 have identifiable nuclear localization sequences (NLS), leading to an early suggestion that these MCMs provide nuclear targeting to the other members of the family [28]. In nearly all species, the bulk of MCMs are constitutively located in the nucleus throughout the entire cell cycle, with their chromatin association, rather than nuclear localization, subject to cell cycle regulation [24, 29-37]. However, there is still a role for the nuclear envelope in MCM complex assembly. This has been molecularly characterized using mutational analysis with the yeasts.

MCM core is a trimeric complex that forms during purification in result of binding MCM4, MCM6, and MCM7 subunits tightly together. MCM2 binds to the core, but with decreased affinity. MCM3 and MCM5 form a dimer together and bind most weakly to the other MCMs, probably through MCM7 (Figure 2). [11] In the absence of other MCMs during in vitro reconstitution experiments, the MCM4,6,7 core will itself dimerize to form a dimer-trimer $(MCM4,6,7)_2$, which is disrupted by addition of MCM2 [38-40].

All MCM members belong to the AAA+ ATPase family, which has a distinct ATPase domain that spans ~200 bases. This domain, referred to as the MCM box, consists of a Walker A ATPase motif, a Walker B ATPase motif, and an arginine finger motif (R-finger). Conserved sequences within the Walker B motif (IDEFDKM) and R-finger (SRDF) define the MCM family. Six of these members are conserved in all eukaryotes and form a heterohexameric complex known as MCM2-7, which has been studied extensively for its role in DNA replication. MCM2-7 is required for licensing and initiating origins of replication, and it acts during elongation as a helicase at the replication forks. Because of this function and studies in yeast, Arabidopsis and Drosophila, members of the MCM2-7 complex, are thought to be essential [41].

The assessment of other multiple functions is consistent with studies in yeast, which showed that MCM proteins are far more abundant than would likely be required for the number of replication origins that exist, and this abundance cannot explain the fact that slight decreases in amounts of MCM proteins lead to the inability to complete S-phase and progress through the cell cycle [41].

Early data led to the identification of MCMs as central players in the initiation of DNA replication. More recent studies have shown that MCM proteins also function in replication elongation, probably as a DNA helicase. This is consistent with structural analysis showing that the proteins interact together in a heterohexameric ring. However, MCMs are strikingly abundant and far exceed the stoichiometry of replication origins; they are widely distributed on unreplicated chromatin. Analysis of *MCM* mutant phenotypes and interactions with other factors has now implicated the MCM proteins in other chromosome transactions including damage response, transcription, and chromatin structure. These experiments indicate that the MCMs are central players in many aspects of genome stability [11].

This family of proteins has been studied for interaction with other genes like Rb gene.

4. MCM gene expression, DNA replication and Retinoblastoma gene

Model showing RBR3 role in the RBR/E2F pathway controlling the expression of MCM2–7 genes, DNA replication, and cell transformation. RepA inhibits RBR1; thus, stimulating the pathway leading to S-phase gene expression, DNA synthesis, and cell transformation through up-regulation of RBR3. The transgenic approaches to down- or up-regulate RBR3 are indicated in italics. The dotted line illustrates a potential inhibitory effect of RepA on RBR3 ruled out by Sabelli et al work[42].

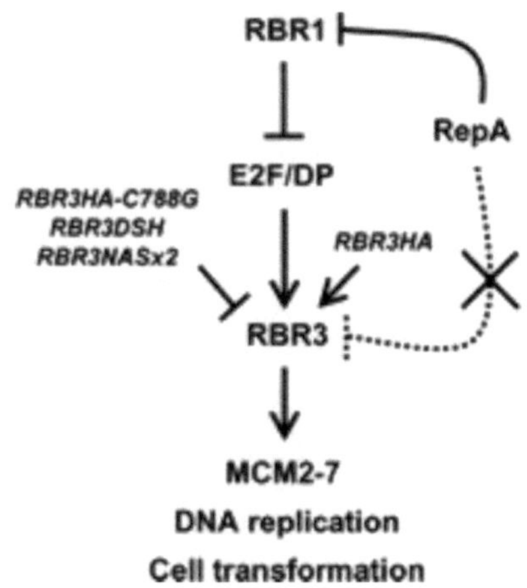

Fig. 3.

5. Expression of MCM protein family as a biological marker of proliferation in various diseases

Genome of the MCM family is necessary for DNA replication and its role has been studied in various diseases and cancers. After the conduction of aforementioned basic studies, it was quickly revealed that this family of proteins not only can be considered as a cell proliferation marker but also can out-power previous classic factors of proliferation such as Ki67 because MCM expression in all phases of cell cycle.

Parvaresh and colleagues (7) through cytometer analysis showed that number of cells expressing MCM6 in the proliferation phase was higher than those expressing Ki67 which was due to the expression of MCM6 at early G1 phase, a phase of cell cycle which does not express Ki67 antigen. This study suggested that MCM6 may be a unique marker of cell cycle and might be employed as a novel prognostic marker for management of cancers.

The following is the summary of studies on different members of this family:

6. Clinicopathologic studies on expression of MCM family proteins as proliferative markers

6.1 Expression of MCM family proteins in non neoplastic diseases

DNA synthesis disorders and DNA damage response can also be important in pathogenesis of many non-neoplastic diseases. Since MCM family proteins play a major role in initiation of DNA synthesis and DNA damage response, evaluation of MCM subunits can be effective in recognizing the cause of various non neoplastic diseases.

Cortez and colleagues showed that 2 MCM subunits namely MCM2-3 and MCM7 can be used as a check point for S phase considering their correlation with Ataxia-telangiectasia mutated (ATM) and ATM- and Rad3-related (ATR) and ATR-interacting protein (ATRIP)-interacting subunit (43).

Evaluation of these factors has also helped in pathogenesis of Diabetes and some viral diseases.

Willcox and coworkers (45) demonstrated that in type I diabetes Alpha and Beta cells undergo an increase in proliferation during progression. These cells show a high level of co-expression of Ki67 and MCM which are indicative of a proliferative response in an autoimmune attack during the course of diabetes type I.

Qian and colleagues (44) showed that MCM complex can be effective in understanding the pathogenesis of many viral diseases. Targeting MCM complex is one mechanism pUL117 employs to help block cellular DNA synthesis during HCMV infection. Their finding substantiates an emerging picture that deregulation of MCM is a conserved strategy for many viruses to prevent host DNA synthesis and helps to elucidate the complex strategy used by a large DNA virus to moderate cellular processes to promote infection and pathogenesis.

6.2 Role of MCM family proteins in neoplastic lesions

Since classically proliferative biomarkers like Ki67 and proliferating cell nuclear antigen (PCNA) are known as the indices of proliferation phase, they are extensively used as diagnostic biomarkers in many types of cancers.

Recently, MCM family proteins are a group of proteins that has been described in DNA replication in both benign and malignant tumors. As MCM proteins are only recognizable in cells which are in the cell cycle, therefore, it seems that they could be a better indicator of proliferative cells, cancer cells or malignant tissues compared to conventional biomarkers. Numerous studies has been suggested that their expression in some of the preneoplastic lesions and malignancies is often associated with a higher degree of cell atypia and poor prognosis.

Up to our knowledge, expression of MCM family proteins has been extensively studied in neoplastic disorders including skin tumors, meningioma, non-small cell lung cancer, Hodgkin's lymphoma [47], prostate cancer, oral tongue squamous cell carcinoma [48], chondrosarcoma, oligodendroglial tumors, esophageal neoplasm, renal cell carcinoma, colonic cancer, breast cancer, endometrial carcinoma, thyroid carcinoma, gastric adenocarcinoma, merckle cell carcinoma, cervical carcinoma and bladder carcinoma. A summary of these studies is as follows:

- Among skin tumors, squamous cell carcinoma, Bowen disease, basal cell carcinoma, malignant melanoma, and nevus have been studied (46). Also, Shin et al. reported a significant positive correlation between MCM2 immunoactivity and grade of actinic keratosis. They declared MCM2 as a reliable marker for diagnosis and grading and suggested further investigation on its prognostic value.
- Shahjahan and associates [49] studied ProEx C, a biomarker reagent containing antibodies to minichromosome maintenance protein 2 (MCM2) and topoisomerase II A (TOP2A) used to detect aberrant S-phase induction in cells. The authors studied 289 non-small cell lung cancers using immunohistochemistry and found ProEx C expression in more than two-thirds of the cancers and an association between strong expression and a longer 5-year survival in certain cellular subtypes. The findings suggested a role in tumor progression of these cancer cells and might be a potential basis for targeted therapy.

- Histomorphology and immunohistochemistry studies also showed increased expression of MCM2 in areas of malignant transformation in recurrent pleomorphic adenoma (50).
- Nuclear expression of MCM2 has been demonstrated in a large number of breast cancer patients. Its expression in dysplastic, malignant and cancer cells can be predictive of potential malignancy and can help in determining the grade of breast cancer (51, 52).
- Expression of MCM3 has been evaluated in astrocytic tumors and cervical carcinoma (53).
- High expression of MCM4 has been reported in meningioma and cervical carcinoma (52, 54).
- Also, MCM4 may play an essential role in the proliferation of some NSCLC cells. Taken together with higher expression in NSCLCs and its correlation with clinicopathologic characteristics such as non-adenocarcinoma histology, MCM4 may have potential as a therapeutic target in certain population with NSCLCs [55, 56].
- Increased expression of MCM4 might be associated with pathological staging of esophageal cancer [57].
- MCM5 expression has been shown in hepatitis induced carcinogenesis (58), adenocarcinoma of the stomach (59), and meningioma (60). Co-expression of MCM2 and MCM5 as a marker of proliferation and differentiation has been evaluated in colon cancer. High expression of these two in mild and moderate cutaneous dysplasia in proliferative lesions of verrucous leukoplakia can help in studying the prognosis of their malignant transformation. Despite the expression of MCM4 and MCM5, increased expression of MCM6 and MCM7 has also been studied in meningioma (54).
- A study showed that expression of MCM7 in esophageal squamous cell carcinoma was associated with a more invasive nature (61).
- Aberrant over-expression of proteins called minichromosome maintenance (MCM) proteins at the mucosal surface of dysplastic esophageal squamous epithelium and Barrett's mucosa may indicate proliferation potential. [62]
- MCM7 detected more cells in the cycle than Ki67 and PCNA and all cases of SC glioblastoma, the most aggressive subset, displayed a significant increase of MCM7-stained nuclei versus those stained with Ki67. [63] These studies implicate MCM7, and the DNA replication licensing gene family, in prostate cancer progression, growth and invasion. [64] MCM-7 also has been studied in gestational trophoblastic disease [65] and metastatic colon carcinoma [66].
- In previous studies such as in Fujioka et al [67] study they demonstrated that higher levels of MCM 7 expression were correlated with poor differentiation of tumors, non-bronchioloalveolar carcinomas of lung, large tumor size and poor prognosis. Li et al [68] also showed that MCM 7 expression was significantly correlated with poor histologic grade, old age, and poor survival in cases of endometrial carcinoma. Padmanabhan et al [69] revealed that MCM 7 was associated with tumor stage and perineural invasion in prostatic intraepithelial neoplasia and invasive adenocarcinoma.

6.3 The role of MCM protein family in cancer treatment

Because of MCM family proteins' vital role in genome duplication in proliferating cells, deregulation of the MCM function results in chromosomal defects that may contribute to tumorigenesis. As we already reviewed, the MCM proteins are highly expressed in malignant human cancers cell and pre-cancerous cells undergoing malignant transformation. They are not expressed in differentiated somatic cells that have been withdrawn from the cell cycle. Therefore, these proteins are ideal diagnostic markers for cancer and promising targets for anti-cancer drug development. [70)

In this respect, medications targeting some members of the MCM family are considered novel anticancer drugs.

Two studies evaluated the role of medications in management of the tumor in prostate cancer patients by measuring the expression of MCMs. In one of these studies due to the high level of MCM expression in these lesions Genistein and Trichostatin (TSA) were administered resulting in down-regulation of all MCM genes and subsequently decreasing the S phase in tumoral cells of the prostate cancer (54).

Iljin et al, (71) in their study indicated that three novel cancer selective growth inhibitory compounds can result in decreased DNA synthesis. This reduction can be evaluated via MCM expression.

7. Conclusion

Members of the MCM family play a key role as the initiator of DNA replication working as DNA helicase. They are also involved in the process of transcription, cohesion, condensation, and recombination in both the nucleus and the cytoplasm. These markers have been extensively evaluated in basic and clinical studies. Aforementioned clinical studies showed the expression of these proteins specially MCM 2, 3,4,5,6,7 specially in preneoplastic and cancers and also in some viral and endocrine diseases eg Diabetes . They have been suggested as standard diagnostic and prognostic biomarkers in some tumoral lesions.

Many of these proteins can be employed as a target for anti-cancer medications currently present in the market or those under development.

Further studies on various members of this family in all the pathologic diseases specially precancerous lesions and malignant processes can illuminate their pathogenesis and biologic behavior . In tumoral lesions, these markers can be easily evaluated through immunohistochemistry. Therefore, it is recommended that research projects focus on studying not only one of them but evaluation co expression of some of the various members of this family in tumoral, pre-neoplastic and neoplastic lesions in all organs.In this way, these proliferative markers can gradually substitute the standard proliferative index markers like Ki67 which was the main objective of the present review.

8. References

[1] Kumar V, Abbas A, Fausto N, Aster J C. Pathologic Basis of Disease 8th ed. Philadelphia, PA: Saunders/Elsevier, 2010; p266-267.

[2] Gerdes J, Schwab U, Lemke H, Stein H. Production of a mouse monoclonal antibody reactive with a human nuclear antigen associated with cell proliferation. Int J Cancer 1983;31:13-20.

[3] Dai H, vant Veer L, Lamb J et al. A cell proliferation signature is a marker of extremely poor outcome in a subpopulation of breast cancer patients. Cancer Res 2005; 65: 4059-66.

[4] Bonnefoi H, Underhill C, Iggo R, Cameron D. Predictive signatures for chemotherapy sensitivity in breast cancer: are they ready for use in the clinic? Eur J Cancer 2009; 45: 1733-43.

[5] Whitfield ML, George LK, Grant GD et al. Common markers of proliferation. Nat Rev Cancer 2006; 6: 99-106.

[6] Kreipe H, Wacker H H, Heidebrecht H J, Haas K, Hauberg M, Tiemann M, Parwaresch R. Determination of the growth fraction in non-Hodgkin's lymphomas by monoclonal antibody Ki-S5 directed against a formalin-resistant epitope of the Ki-67 antigen. Am J Pathol 1993;142(6): 1689-94.

[7] Heidebrecht H J, Buck F, Endl E, Kruse M L, Adam-Klages S, Andersen K, Frahm S O, Schulte C, Wacker H H, Parwaresch R. Ki-Mcm6, a new monoclonal antibody specific to MCM6: Comparison of the distribution profile of MCM6 and the Ki67 antigen. Laboratory Investigation 2001; 81: 1163-65.

[8] Kearsey, S. E., and K. Labib. MCM proteins: evolution, properties, and role in DNA replication. Biochim. Biophys. Acta 1998;1398:113-136.

[9] Kelman, Z., and J. Hurwitz. Structural lessons in DNA replication from the third domain of life. Nat. Struct. Biol. 2003;10:148-150.

[10] Tye, B. K. Insights into DNA replication from the third domain of life. Proc. Natl. Acad. Sci. USA 2000; 97:2399-2401.

[11] Forsburg S L. Eukaryotic MCM proteins: Beyond Replication Initiation. Molecular & Cell Biology Laboratory, The Salk Institute for Biological Studies, La Jolla, California 92037.

[12] Maine, G. T., P. Sinha, and B.-K. Tye. Mutants of *S. cerevisiae* defective in the maintenance of minichromosomes. Genetics 1984; 106:365-385.

[13] Sinha, P., V. Chang, and B.-K. Tye. A mutant that affects the function of autonomously replicating sequences in yeast. J. Mol. Biol. 1986; 192:805-814.

[14] Burger M. MCM2 and MCM5 as Prognostic Markers in Colon Cancer: A Worthwhile Approach. Dig Dis Sci 2009; 54: 197-8.

[15] Passmore S, Elble R, Tye BK. A protein involved in minichromosome maintenance in yeast binds a transcriptional enhancer conserved in eukaryotes. Genes Dev 1989; 3: 921-35.

[16] Christ C, Tye BK. Functional domains of the yeast transcription/replication factor MCM1. Genes Dev 1991; 5: 751-63.

[17] Moore K, Aves SJ. MCM10 and DNA replication in fission yeast. In: The Eukaryotic cell cycle. Edited by: Bryant JA, Francis D. Abingdon: Taylor and Francis; 2008: 45-69.

[18] Lake C. M., Teeter K., Page S. L., Nielsen R. and Hawley R. S. A genetic analysis of the Drosophila mcm5 gene defines a domain specifically required for meiotic recombination. Genetics 2007; 176(4): 2151-63.

[19] Gozuacik, D., M. Chami, D. Lagorce, J. Faivre, Y. Murakami, O. Poch, E. Biermann, R. Knippers, C. Brechot, and P. Paterlini-Brechot. Identification and functional characterization of a new member of the human Mcm protein family: hMcm8. Nucleic Acids Res. 2003; 31:570-579.

[20] Johnson, E. M., Y. Kinoshita, and D. C. Daniel. A new member of the MCM protein family encoded by the human MCM8 gene, located contrapodal to GCD10 at chromosome band 20p12.3-13. Nucleic Acids Res. 2003; 31:2915-2925.

[21] Yoshida K. Identification of a novel cell-cycle-induced MCM family protein MCM9. Biochemical and Biophysical Research Communications 2005; 331(2): 669-74.

[22] Feger, G., H. Vaessin, T. T. Su, E. Wolff, L. Y. Jan, and Y. N. Jan. *dpa,* a member of the MCM family, is required for mitotic DNA replication but not endoreplication in *Drosophila*. EMBO J. 1995; 14:5387-5398.

[23] Springer, P. S., W. R. McCombie, V. Sundaresan, and R. A. Martienssen. Gene trap tagging of PROLIFERA, and essential MCM2-3-5 like gene in *Arabidopsis*. Science 1995; 268:877-880.

[24] Todorov, I. T., R. Pepperkok, R. Philipova, S. E. Kearsey, W. Ansorge, and D. Werner. A human nuclear protein with sequence homology to a family of early S phase proteins is required for entry into S phase and for cell division. J. Cell Sci. 1994; 107:253-265.

[25] Thömmes, P., R. Fett, B. Schray, R. Burkhart, M. Barnes, C. Kennedy, N. C. Brown, and R. Knippers. Properties of the nuclear P1 protein, a mammalian homologue of the yeast *MCM3* replication protein. Nucleic Acids Res. 1992; 20:1069-1074.

[26] Sible, J. C., E. Erikson, M. Hendrickson, J. L. Maller, and J. Gautier. Developmental regulation of MCM replication factors in *Xenopus laevis*. Curr. Biol. 1998; 8:347-350.

[27] Liu Y, Richards T A, Aves S J. Ancient diversification of eukaryotic MCM DNA replication proteins. BMC Evolutionary Biology 2009; 9:60. doi:10.1186/1471-2148-9-60.

[28] Kimura, H., T. Ohtomo, M. Yamaguchi, A. Ishii, and K. Sugimoto. Mouse MCM proteins: complex formation and transportation into the nucleus. Genes Cells 1996; 1:977-993.

[29] Fujita, M., T. Kiyono, Y. Hayashi, and M. Ishibashi. Hcdc47, a human member of the MCM family—dissociation of the nucleus-bound form during S phase. J. Biol. Chem. 1996; 271:4349-4354.

[30] Hu, B., R. Burkhart, D. Schulte, C. Musahl, and R. Knippers. The P1 family—a new class of nuclear mammalian proteins related to the yeast MCM replication proteins. Nucleic Acids Res. 1993; 21:5289-5293.

[31] Kearsey, S. E., S. Montgomery, K. Labib, and K. Linder. Chromatin binding of the fission yeast replication factor Mcm4 occurs during anaphase and requires ORC and Cdc18. EMBO J. 2000; 19:1681-1690.

[32] Kimura, H., N. Nozaki, and K. Sugimoto. DNA polymerase alpha associated protein P1, a murine homolog of yeast *MCM3*, changes its intranuclear distribution during the DNA synthetic period. EMBO J. 1994; 13:4311-4320.

[33] Madine, M. A., C. Y. Khoo, A. D. Mills, C. Musahl, and R. A. Laskey. The nuclear envelope prevents reinitiation of replication by regulating the binding of Mcm3 to chromatin in *Xenopus* egg extracts. Curr. Biol. 1995; 5:1270-1279.

[34] Okishio, N., Y. Adachi, and M. Yanagida. Fission yeast nda1 and nda4, MCM homologs required for DNA replication, are constitutive nuclear proteins. J. Cell Sci. 1996; 109:319-326.

[35] Pasion, S. G., and S. L. Forsburg. Nuclear localization of *Schizosaccharomyces pombe* Mcm2/Cdc19p requires MCM complex assembly. Mol. Biol. Cell 1999; 10:4043-4057.

[36] Schulte, D., R. Burkhart, C. Musahl, B. Hu, C. Schlatterer, H. Hameister, and R. Knippers. Expression, phosphorylation and nuclear localization of the human P1

protein, a homoogue of the yeast Mcm 3 replication protein. J Cell Sci. 1995; 108:1381-1389.

[37] Su, T. T., and P. H. O'Farrell. Chromosome association of minichromosome maintenance proteins in *Drosophila* mitotic cycles. J. Cell Biol. 1997; 139:13- 21.

[38] Ishimi, Y. A DNA helicase activity is associated with an MCM4, -6, and -7 protein complex. J. Biol. Chem 1997;272:24508-24513.

[39] Lee J K and Hurwitz J. Isolation and characterization of various complexes of the minichromosome maintenance proteins of *Schizosaccharomyces pombe*. J. Biol. Chem. 2000; 275:18871-18878.

[40] Prokhorova, T. A., and J. J. Blow. Sequential MCM/P1 subcomplex assembly is required to form a heterohexamer with replication licensing activity. J. Biol. Chem. 2000; 275:2491-2498.

[41] Minichromosome maintenance 5. Biological overview. http://www.sdbonline.org/fly/genebrief/mcm5.htm

[42] Sabelli P A, Hoerster G, Lizarraga L E, Brown S W, Gordon-Kamm W J, Larkins B A. Positive regulation of minichromosome maintenance gene expression, DNA replication, and cell transformation by a plant retinoblastoma gene. PNAS 2009; 106(10):4042-47.

[43] Shechter D, Gautier J. MCM proteins and checkpoint kinases get together at the fork. http://www.pnas.org/content/101/30/10845.full

[44] Qian Zh, Leung-Pineda V, Xuan B, Piwnica-Worms H, Yu D. Human cytomegalovirus protein pUL117 targets the mini-chromosome maintenance complex and suppresses cellular DNA synthesis. PLoS Pathogens 2010;6(3):1-14 (e1000814).

[45] Willcox A, Richardson SJ, Bone AJ, Foulis AK, Morgan NG. Evidence of increased islet cell proliferation in patients with recent-onset type 1 diabetes.Diabetologia 2010;53(9):2020-8.

[46] Shin JW, Kim Y K, Cho K H. Minichromosome maintenance protein expression according to the grade of atypism in actinic keratosis. Am J Dermatopathology 2010;32:794-8.

[47] Karimi Sh, Mohammadi F, Khodadad K, Emami H, Seyfollahi L. High Expression of Minichromosome Maintenance Protein 6 in Classic Hodgkin's Lymphoma Points to a Cell Cycle Arrest in G1 Phase. *Archives of Iranian Medicin 2008*; 11(5): 532 – 538.

[48] Gueiros LA, Coletta RD, Kowalski LP, Lopes MA. Clinicopathological features and proliferation markers in tongue squamous cell carcinomas. Int J Oral Maxillofacial Sur 2011.

[49] DABS D. Diagnostic immunohistochemistry: theranostic and genomic applications. 3rd ed. Philadelphia, PA: Saunders/Elsevier,2010;p412.

[50] Soares A B, Atemani A, De Araujo V C. Study of histopathological, morphological and immunohistochemical features of recurrent pleomorphic adenoma: an attempt to predict recurrence of pleomorphic adenoma. J Oral Pathol Med 2011;40:352-358.

[51] Wojnar A, Kobierzycki C, Krolicka A, Pula B, Podhorska-Okolow M, Dziegiel P. Correlation of Ki-67 and MCM-2 proliferative marker expression with grade of histological malignancy (G) in ductal breast cancers. Folia Histochemica et Cytobiologica 2010;48(3):442-446.

[52] Cobanoglu U, Mungan S, Gundogdu C, Ersoz S, Ozoran Y, Aydin F. The expression of MCM-2 in invasive breast carcinoma: a stereologic approach. Bratisl Lek Listy 2010; 111(1): 45-49.

[53] Söling A, Sackewitz M, Volkmar M, Schaarschmidt D, Jacob R, Holzhausen H R, Rainov N G. Minichromosome Maintenance Protein 3 Elicits a Cancer-Restricted Immune Response in Patients with Brain Malignancies and Is Strong Independent Predictor of Survival in Patients with Anaplastic Astrocytoma. *Clinical Cancer Research* 2005;11:249.

[54] Majid S, Dar AA, Saini S, Chen Y, Shahryari V, Liu J, Zaman MS, Hirata H, Yamamura S, Ueno K, Tanaka Y, Dahiya R. Regulation of Minichromosome Maintenance Gene Family by MicroRNA-1296 and Genistein in Prostate Cancer. *Cancer Res 2010;* 70(7): 2809-18.

[55] Kikuchi J, Kinoshita I, Shimizu Y, Kikuchi E, Takeda K, Aburatani H, Oizumi S, Konishi J, Kaga K, Matsuno Y, Birrer MJ, Nishimura M, Dosaka-Akita H. Minichromosome maintenance (MCM) protein 4 as a marker for proliferation and its clinical and clinicopathological significance in non-small cell lung cancer. *Lung Cancer,* Sep 2010.

[56] Kikuchia J, Kinoshitab I, Shimizub Y, Kikuchia E, Takedab K, Aburatanie H, Oizumia S, et al. Proliferation marker and its clinical and clinicopathological significance in non small cell lung cancer. ??? 2011;72(2):229-237.

[57] Huang X P. Mcm4 Expression in Esophageal Cancer from Southern China and Its Clinical Significance. UICC World Cancer Congress 2006. Bridging the Gap: Transforming Knowledge into Action.July 8-12, 2006, Washington, DC, USAhttp://2006.confex.com/uicc/uicc/techprogram/P1872.HTM

[58] Qu A, Shah YM, Matsubara T, Yang Q, Gonzalez FJ. Pdent activation of cell cycle control and DNA repair genes in hepatic nonparenchymal cells. Toxicol Sci 2010;118(2):404-10.

[59] Giaginis C, Giagini A, Tsourouflis G, Gatzidou E, Agapitos E, Kouraklis G, Theocharis S. MCM-2 and MCM-5 expression in gastric adenocarcinoma: clinical significance and comparison with Ki-67 proliferative marker. Dig Dis Sci 2011;56(3):777-85.

[60] Saydam O, Senol O, Schaaij-Visser T B. M., Pham T V, Piersma S R, Stemmer-Rachamimov A O, Wurdinger T, Saskia M. Peerdeman S M, and Jimenez C R. Comparative Protein Profiling Reveals Minichromosome Maintenance (MCM) Proteins As Novel Potential Tumor Markers for Meningiomas. *J. Proteome Res* 2010; 9(1): 485–494.

[61] Ahn J H & Chang H K. (2010) Expression of Minichromosome Maintenance Protein 7 and Smad 4 in Squamous Cell Carcinoma of the Esophagus. *Korean J Pathol* 2010;44(4):346-353.

[62] Alison MR, Hunt T, Forbes SJ. Minichromosome maintenance (MCM) proteins may be pre-cancer markers. *Gut* 2002;50:290-291.

[63] Facoetti A, Ranza E, Benericetti E, Ceroni M, Tedeschi F & Nano R. Minichromosome Maintenance Protein 7: A Reliable Tool for Glioblastoma Proliferation Index. *Anticancer Research* 2006; 26(2A): 1071-1075.

[64] Baoguo R, Guoying Y, George C. T, Kathleen C, George K. M, Joel N, Yan P. Y and Jian-Hua L. MCM7 amplification and overexpression are associated with prostate cancer progression. Amer Assoc Cancer Res 2006; 47.

[65] Evrin C, Clarke P, Zech J, Lurz R, Sun J, Uhle S, Li H, Stillman B, Speck C. A double-hexameric MCM2-7 complex is loaded onto origin DNA during licensing of eukaryotic DNA replication. Proc Natl Acad Sci U S A. 2009;106(48):20240-5.

[66] Brewster AS, Slaymaker IM, Afif SA, Chen XS. Mutational analysis of an archaeal minichromosome maintenance protein exterior hairpin reveals critical residues for helicase activity and DNA binding. BMC Molecular Biology 2010, 11:62doi:10.1186/1471-2199-11-62

[67] Fujioka S, Shomori K, Nishihara K, et al. Expression of minichromosome maintenance 7 (MCM7) in small lung adenocarcinoma (pT1): prognostic implication. Lung Cancer 2009; 65: 223-9.

[68] Li SS, Xue WC, Khoo US, et al. Replicative MCM7 protein as a proliferation marker in endometrial carcinoma: a tissue microarray and clinicopathological analysis. Histopathology 2005; 46: 307-13.

[69] Padmanabhan V, Callas P, Philips G, Trainer TD, Beatty BG. DNA replication regulation protein Mcm7 as a marker of proliferation in prostatic cancer. J Clin Pathol 2004; 57: 1057-62.

[70] Lei M. The MCM complex: its role in DNA replication and implications for cancer therapy. Curr Cancer Drug Targets 2005;5(5):365-80.

[71] Iljin K, Ketola K, Vainio P, Halonen P, Kohonen P, Fey V et al. High-throughput cell-based screening of 4910 known drugs and drug-like small molecules identifies disulfiram as an inhibitor of prostate cancer cell growth.

2

Regulation of DNA Synthesis and Replication Checkpoint Activation During *C. elegans* Development

Suzan Ruijtenberg,
Sander van den Heuvel and Inge The
Developmental Biology, Utrecht University
The Netherlands

1. Introduction

Replication of the DNA during the synthesis (S) phase of the cell cycle is one of the most critical aspects of cell division. DNA replication must be highly accurate and tightly controlled to maintain genomic integrity over many rounds of cell division. This is particularly important during animal development, since genetic instability can lead to cell death, birth defects, developmental abnormalities and diseases such as cancer. The developmental context also adds specific constraints to S-phase regulation. For instance, variations in DNA replication control are needed to accommodate the rapid embryonic divisions in early embryos, the production of haploid germ cells, and the generation of polyploid tissues. A comprehensive understanding of DNA replication requires insight in these developmental aspects of S phase control. Here, we review the initiation of DNA replication in the genetic animal model *Caenorhabditis elegans* (*C. elegans*), with a focus on developmental-stage and tissue-specific regulation.

2. *Caenorhabditis elegans*

Caenorhabditis elegans (*C. elegans*) was introduced as a model organism in the 1960s by Sydney Brenner and became, in a relative short time, one of the leading model organisms in biological research (Ankeny 2001). One of the appealing aspects of this nematode is its rapid and reproducible development from the one-cell embryo to the adult stage (Sulston & Horvitz 1977). The invariance, combined with the fact that the animals are transparent and contain a relatively low number of cells (adult hermaphrodites contain only 959 somatic cell nuclei), has made it possible to record the entire somatic cell lineage of *C. elegans* (Horvitz & Sulston 1980; Sulston & Horvitz 1977; Sulston & Horvitz 1981). Knowing when each cell normally divides is a major benefit for studies of the cell cycle. Efficient genetics has allowed identification of mutations that alter the normal cell lineage (*lin* mutants), some of which affect DNA replication or DNA content (Horvitz & Sulston 1980; Sulston & Horvitz 1981). As an additional advantage, many cell cycle regulators that exist in gene families in higher eukaryotes are represented by single genes in *C. elegans*, which helps identification of gene function and determination of the hierarchy of gene functions in regulatory pathways.

While these aspects make *C. elegans* suitable for cell cycle studies, there are additional reasons for adding this animal to the repertoire of cell cycle models. Studies of DNA replication in the context of a developing organism may identify regulatory mechanisms that are not important for single cell eukaryotes and cells in tissue culture. The developmental context adds an extra layer of S-phase regulation. For instance, in meiosis, two rounds of chromosome segregation follow each other without intervening S phase, while in endoreplication cycles, rounds of DNA replication continue in the absence of M phases. In addition, a broad range of models also increases the potential for uncovering important aspects of DNA replication control. For example, studies in *C. elegans* identified a CUL-4/DDB-1 E3 ubiquitin ligase complex as an important inhibitor of DNA re-replication, which is functionally conserved in mammals (Arias & Walter 2007; Kim & Kipreos 2007a; Zhong, et al. 2003). In addition, defects in DNA synthesis were found to cause lineage-specific delays in cell division in *C. elegans*, through a checkpoint mechanism that also contributes to the difference in timing of founder cell division in the early embryo (Brauchle, et al. 2003; Encalada, et al. 2000). Furthermore, our recent results support tissue specific contributions of a conserved general regulator of DNA replication, MCM-4 (Korzelius, et al. 2011). Below, we describe the currently known factors that control DNA replication in *C. elegans*, as well as their functions in particular stages of development and specific cell types. Several techniques used for analysis of DNA replication in *C. elegans* are summarized in BOX 1.

3. The factors that regulate DNA replication

The regulation of DNA replication in eukaryotes involves two discrete steps. First, pre-replication complexes assemble at sites of replication initiation ("origin licensing"), and subsequently, the actual initiation of DNA synthesis can be triggered ("origin firing"). Comprehensive studies aimed at identifying all components involved in DNA replication have not been reported for *C. elegans*. However, functional annotations by the *C. elegans* genome sequence consortium have revealed orthologs of many DNA replication components (www.wormbase.org). In addition, some DNA replication genes have been identified through mutations, and genome-wide RNA interference (RNAi) has confirmed that most putative replication components exert critical functions (Encalada, et al. 2000; Korzelius, et al. 2011; Sonnichsen, et al. 2005). Despite their clear conservation, certain well-known replication genes currently appear to lack *C. elegans* counterparts (see Table 1). For instance, in eukaryotes ranging from yeast to human, the origin recognition complex (ORC) has been found to consists of 6 subunits, ORC1 to ORC6. At present, ORC-2 is the only ORC protein identified in *C. elegans*, and its function has not been characterized in detail.

Recruitment of the ORC is normally the first step in pre-replication complex assembly, which is followed by association of the CDC6 and CDT1 proteins. *C. elegans* does contain legitimate CDC-6 and CDT-1 orthologs, which are essential for DNA replication and required for embryonic as well as larval viability (Kim, et al. 2007; Kim & Kipreos 2008; Kim & Kipreos 2007a; Kim & Kipreos 2007b). Simultaneous overactivation of CDC-6 and CDT-1 leads to extensive re-replication, which underscores the role of CDC-6 and CDT-1 as critical regulators of origin licensing.

BOX1: *C. elegans* DNA replication analysis

One of the advantages of the use of *C. elegans* as a model system is that the animal is fully transparent, which allows the use of Differential Interference Contrast (DIC, also known as Nomarski) microscopy for live observations of cell division. Moreover, expression and localization of the green fluorescent protein (GFP) and other fluorophores can be followed by time-lapse microscopy. Introduction of transgenes with tissue or cell type-specific promoters that drive expression of GFP or GFP-tagged fusion proteins is a routine procedure in *C. elegans* (Mello & Fire 1995). However, transgenes are usually silenced in the germline and in early embryos, which can be avoided by integrating a single copy transgene through DNA particle bombardment or the MosSCI technique (Frokjaer-Jensen, et al. 2008; Praitis, et al. 2001). We have recently applied the MosSCI strategy for integration of a single copy transgene expressing an MCM-4::mCherry protein fusion, which rescues *mcm-4* null mutants and shows a similar expression pattern and subcellular localizations as the endogenous MCM-4 protein (Korzelius, et al. 2011, and our unpublished results).

In addition to gene expression studies, DNA replication itself can be visualized in multiple different ways. The most quantitative method makes use of determination of the DNA content. The DNA content of a cell correlates with the cell cycle phase: cells in G1 have a ploidy of 2n; S phase cells between 2n and 4n; and cells in the G2 and M phases 4n. To measure the DNA content, animals are fixed and stained with a dye that fluoresces when bound to DNA, such as propidium iodide, Hoechst 33258, or DAPI (4′6′- diamidino-2-phenylindole dihydrochloride). The most accurate method, but also the most time consuming, for *in situ* quantification is analysis of the fluorescence signal in confocal serial sections of propidium iodide-stained nuclei (Boxem, et al. 1999; Feng, et al. 1999; Zhong, et al. 2003). The accuracy of this method makes it ideal for experiments in which small differences in DNA content must be distinguished, e.g. when comparing cells in G1 vs. S phase.

In order to investigate if cells go through the process of DNA replication, or whether DNA replication takes place at specific times of development, incorporation of the thymidine analogues 5-bromo-2′-deoxyuridine (BrdU) or 5-ethynyl-2′-deoxyuridine (EdU) can be used. BrdU incorporation can be detected by immunostaining with specific anti-BrdU antibodies. EdU detection is based on a copper (Cu^{1+}) catalyzed covalent "click" reaction between an azide attached to a fluorescent dye and the alkyne group of EdU (Salic & Mitchison 2008). While BrdU detection in *C. elegans* has been possible for some time (Boxem, et al. 1999), the EdU method is new and has been applied only in a few recent studies (Fig.1) (Cinquin, et al. 2010; Korzelius, et al. 2011). The EdU method has a major advantage over BrdU staining: while BrdU detection requires DNA denaturation, this step is not needed in the EdU procedure. As a result, EdU incorporation can be combined with immunostaining with antibodies, which can be a great help in visualizing cells of interest.

Flow cytometry is commonly used for DNA quantification in other systems. Although this technique is not widespread, flow cytometry has been used to produce accurate measurements of DNA content for freshly dissociated *C. elegans* cells (Bennett, et al. 2003). The dissociated *C. elegans* cells represented multiple cell types, which reduces the utility of the DNA distribution information. This limitation can be avoided by using strains in which cells of interest are marked with transgenes that express GFP (or other fluorescent tags). GFP expression can be used to gate cells of interest in the flow cytometry analysis so that the DNA distribution of only the GFP expressing cells is analyzed. In future studies, this coupling of selective GFP expression with propidium iodide staining will probably be applied more broadly in the analysis of the DNA distribution of specific tissues and cells of interest.

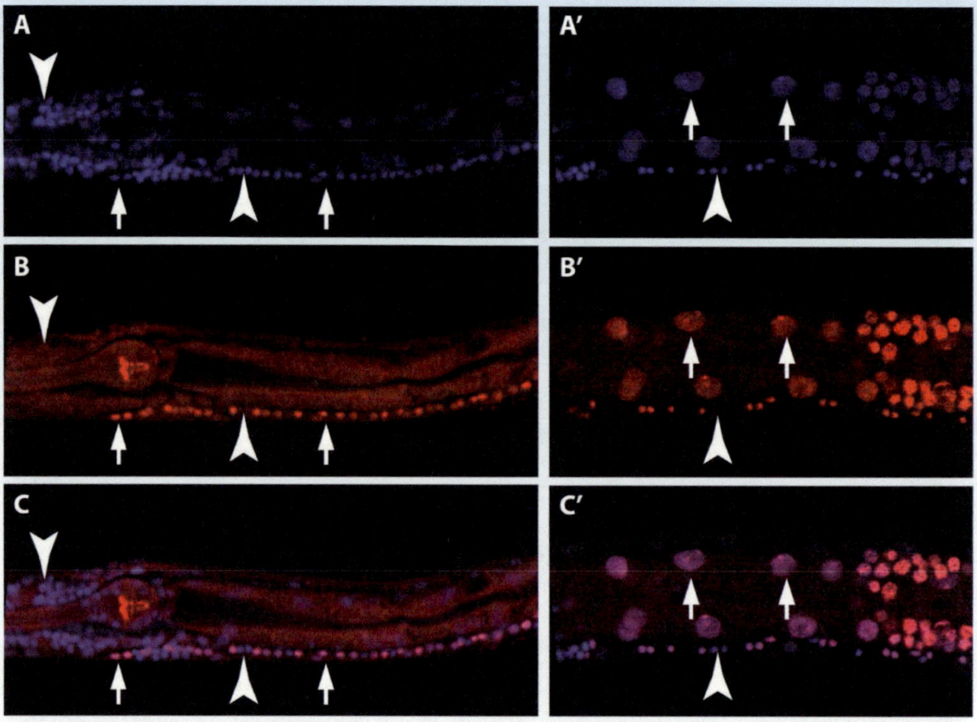

Fig. 1. EdU incorporation and staining visualizes DNA replication in *C. elegans* larvae. EdU incorporation in cells of the ventral nerve cord in a first stage larva (A, B, and C) and nuclei in the intestine of an early L4 larva (A′, B′, and C′) are indicated by arrows. Panels show DNA staining by DAPI (A and A′), EdU staining (B and B′) and merged images (C and C′). Note that cells that completed S phase prior to EdU addition stain with DAPI but do not incorporate EdU, such as the neurons indicated by arrowheads. One arm of the developing gonad is visible at the right (A′, B′, C′).

Studies in other systems have shown that CDC-6 and CDT-1 are needed to load the minichromosome maintenance (MCM) protein complex onto the replication origins. The MCM complex consists of 6 proteins, MCM2 to MCM7, which is thought to act as the helicase that unwinds the DNA at the replication origins. *C. elegans* contains orthologs of all six MCM genes, which are known as *mcm-2* to *mcm-7* and cause similar embryonic lethal phenotypes when inactivated by RNAi (Sonnichsen, et al. 2005). MCM-4 was initially identified through a mutation in the *lin-6* gene, and is the only *C. elegans* MCM protein studied in detail (Korzelius, et al. 2011). MCM-4 is expressed in all dividing cells during embryonic and postembryonic development. It is strongly induced just prior to the G1/S transition in somatic cells and disappears when cells exit the cell cycle. MCM-4 localizes to the cell nucleus in interphase, while in mitosis MCM-4 localization becomes diffuse throughout the cell upon nuclear envelope breakdown. In late anaphase, MCM-4 starts to colocalize with the DNA, presumably licensing the DNA for the next round of S-phase (Fig. 2).

Protein Name	*S. cerevisiae*	*S. pombe*	*Drosophila melanogaster*	Mammals	*C. elegans*
Prereplication complex					
Orc1-6	Orc1-6	Orc1-6	Orc1-6	Orc1-6	ORC-2
Cdc6	Cdc6	Cdc18	Cdc6	Cdc6	CDC-6
Cdt1	Cdt1/Tah11/ Sid2	Cdt1	Dup	Cdt1	CDT-1
Mcm2	Mcm2	Mcm2/Cdc19/Nda1	Mcm2	Mcm2	MCM-2
Mcm3	Mcm3	Mcm3	Mcm3	Mcm3	MCM-3
Mcm4	Cdc54/ Mcm4	Cdc21	Dpa	Mcm4	MCM-4
Mcm5	Cdc46/ Mcm5	Mcm5/Nda4	Mcm5	Mcm5	MCM-5
Mcm6	Mcm6	Mcm6/Mis5	Mcm6	Mcm6	MCM-6
Mcm7	Cdc47/ Mcm7	Mcm7	Mcm7	Mcm7	MCM-7
Preinitiation complex					
Mcm10	Mcm10/Dna43	Cdc23	Mcm10	Mcm10	Y47D3a.28
Cdc45	Cdc45/Sld4	Sna41/Cdc45	Cdc45	Cdc45	F34D10.2
Sld3	Sld3	Sld3	-	-	-
Dbp11	Dbp11	Cut5/Rad4	Mus101	TopBP1	MUS-101
Sld2	Sld2/Drc1	Drc1	-	-	-
Sld5	Sld5	Sld5	Sld5	Sld5	Y113G7B.24
Psf1	Psf1	Psf1	Psf1	Psf1	R53.6*
Psf2	Psf2	Psf2	Psf2	Psf2	F31C3.5*
Psf3	Psf3	Psf3	Psf3	Psf3	-
Kinases					
Cdc7	Cdc7	Hsk1	Cdc7	Cdc7	C34G6.5
Dbf4	Dbf4	Dfp1	Chiffon	Dbf4/Ask/Drf1	-

Table 1. Homologues of DNA replication components. *Based on homology searches only.

The absence of DNA replication, as observed in *mcm-4* mutants, might be expected to trigger a checkpoint that delays mitotic entry. However, *mcm-4* mutants enter mitosis in the absence of DNA replication and, initially, with normal timing, suggesting that *mcm-4* is not only required for DNA replication but also activates a checkpoint that monitors completion of DNA replication (Korzelius, et al. 2011). This second function corresponds to the results obtained in studies with other organisms, which clarified the requirement of the MCM complex in activation of the DNA damage and replication checkpoints (Labib, et al. 2001; Zou & Elledge 2003). In addition to these well conserved functions, *mcm-4* also displays a tissue-specific requirement in *C. elegans*, which will be discussed below (Korzelius, et al. 2011).

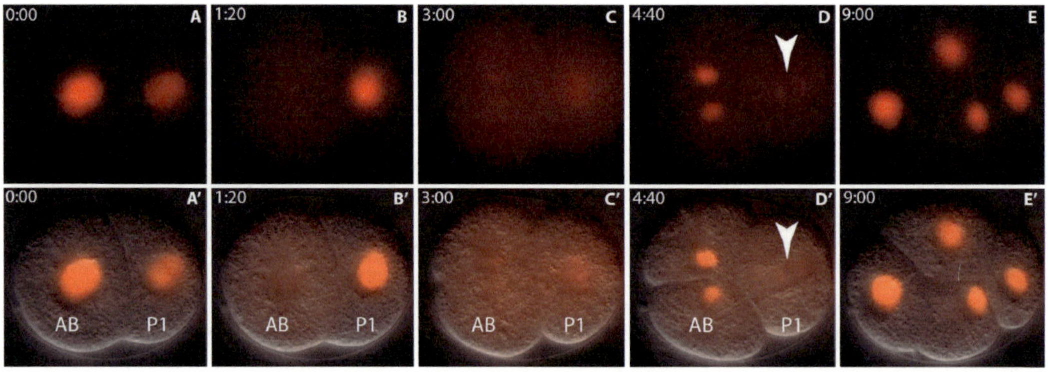

Fig. 2. Time-lapse fluorescence microscopy shows expression and localization of MCM-4 in an early embryo. MCM-4 is fused to mCherry and expressed from the *mcm-4* promoter (A-E). Merged images of the DIC and fluorescence channels are shown in the bottom panels (A'-E'). The red MCM-4::mCherry fluorescence is visible in the anterior AB and posterior P1 cell in the two stage embryo (A and A'). Note that the AB cell enters mitosis before the P1 cell (B and B'). MCM-4 can be detected on the chromosomes in late anaphase (arrowhead in P1 cell, D and D").

Activation of the MCM2-7 complex is needed for opening the DNA helix and allowing the DNA polymerases to start DNA replication. This activation marks the end of origin licensing and the start of origin firing (Labib & Diffley 2001). Studies in several organisms have shown that the onset of S-phase requires CDK (cyclin dependent kinase) and DDK (Dbf-4 dependent Cdc7 kinase) activity to promote activation of the MCM2-7 helicase, while at the same time the recruitment of pre-replication complexes is inhibited (Bousset & Diffley 1998; Nguyen, et al. 2001; Remus, et al. 2005). CDKs and DDK4 are not only required for the activation of the MCM complex, they also trigger the assembly of additional factors. This results in the formation of a "preinitiation complex" that contains a large and still growing group of proteins, such as Cdc45, Mcm10, RPA and the DNA polymerases α and ε (Bell & Dutta 2002; McGarry & Kirschner 1998; Mechali 2010; van Leuken, et al. 2008). Most of these factors have not been identified or investigated in *C. elegans*, and the formation and function of the preinitiation complex in *C. elegans* therefore remains elusive (Table 1). In animal systems, Geminin acts as an inhibitor of CDT-1, which is degraded in mitosis in an APC/C-dependent fashion (McGarry & Kirschner 1998; van Leuken, et al. 2008). *C. elegans* Geminin GMN-1 also associates with CDT-1 and inhibits origin licensing when added to frog egg extracts (Yanagi, et al. 2005). GMN-1 inhibition results in germline defects and intestinal abnormalities with chromatin bridges. Thus, Geminin may be an example of a metazoan-specific regulator of DNA replication initiation.

4. Preventing re-replication

When DNA replication is initiated, origin licensing should be prevented, as re-firing of only a single origin may lead to gene amplification and could have dramatic consequences. Hence, all eukaryotes use multiple levels of control to prevent more than one round of DNA synthesis within a single S-phase, although the exact players and mechanisms differ somewhat between species. In general, there are two mechanisms used to prevent re-replication: firstly, formation of the pre-replication complex (prior to S-phase) and the activation of the origins (during S phase) are temporally separated, and secondly, proteins required for the formation of the pre-replication complex are inactivated as soon as DNA replication starts (Arias & Walter 2007; Blow & Dutta 2005; Machida, et al. 2005). Surprisingly, despite the importance of a single round of DNA replication and the redundant levels of control, certain single gene mutations cause substantial re-replication. As an important example, *C. elegans cul-4* displays such a re-replication phenotype (Zhong, et al. 2003).

cul-4 encodes the core subunit of a cullin based E3 ubiquitin ligase that targets substrate proteins for ubiquitylation and degradation. Kipreos and coworkers studied the effects of *cul-4* inhibition by RNAi in the epithelial stem-cell like "seam" cells in the *C. elegans* skin. Interestingly, they observed that *cul-4* RNAi resulted in seam cells with up to a 100n DNA content and showed that this results from extensive re-replication rather than failed mitosis (Zhong, et al. 2003). As mentioned above, a key mechanism of preventing re-replication is inactivation of the components that form the pre-replication complex. Indeed, it was shown that *cul-4* is required for the degradation of one of these components. When *cul-4* is inhibited, CDT-1 levels do not drop at the end of G1 but remain constant throughout S-phase, indicating that CUL-4 is required for S-phase degradation of CDT-1. Subsequent studies in *C. elegans* and other systems demonstrated that CUL-4 in association with the DNA damage binding protein 1 (DDB-1) recognizes CDT-1 as a substrate (Arias & Walter 2007; Blow & Dutta 2005; Kim & Kipreos 2007a; Kim & Kipreos 2007b). However, degradation of CDT-1 by CUL-4 is not the whole story, since expression of stable CDT-1 alone does not cause noticeable re-replication. CUL-4 was also found to be responsible for the localization of CDC-6, another member of the pre-replication complex. CDC-6 normally accumulates in the nucleus during G1 phase, and is exported from the nucleus to the cytoplasm during S-phase. The activity of CUL-4 turned out to be needed for nuclear export of CDC-6. Thus, CUL-4 inactivation deregulates two essential factors of the pre-replication complex. High nuclear levels of both CDT-1 and CDC-6 in S-phase allow continued origin licensing and promote re-replication (Kim, et al. 2007; Kim & Kipreos 2007a).

Although intriguing, the mechanism by which CUL-4 regulates nuclear export of CDC-6 in S-phase was not immediately apparent. However, two clues were available: CDC6 nuclear export is regulated by Cyclin-CDKs in other systems, and, similar to the human homolog, the amino terminus of *C. elegans* CDC-6 contains multiple nuclear localization signals flanked by potential CDK phosphorylation sites (Kim, et al. 2007; Kim & Kipreos 2007b; Kim, et al. 2008). Phosphorylation at these sites coincides with nuclear export, as demonstrated by phosphospecific-antibody staining, and mutation of all six CDK sites prevented nuclear export. Thus, CUL-4 could promote nuclear export by stimulating CDK phosphorylation of the CDC-6 N-terminus. This is likely accomplished by degradation of a CDK inhibitor of the Cip/Kip family, known as CKI-1 in worms, Dacapo in flies and $p21^{Cip1}$ in vertebrates (Fig. 3) (Bondar, et al. 2006; Higa, et al. 2006; Kim & Kipreos 2007a; Kim & Kipreos 2007b; Kim & Kipreos 2007b; Kim, et al. 2008; Korzelius, et al. 2011).

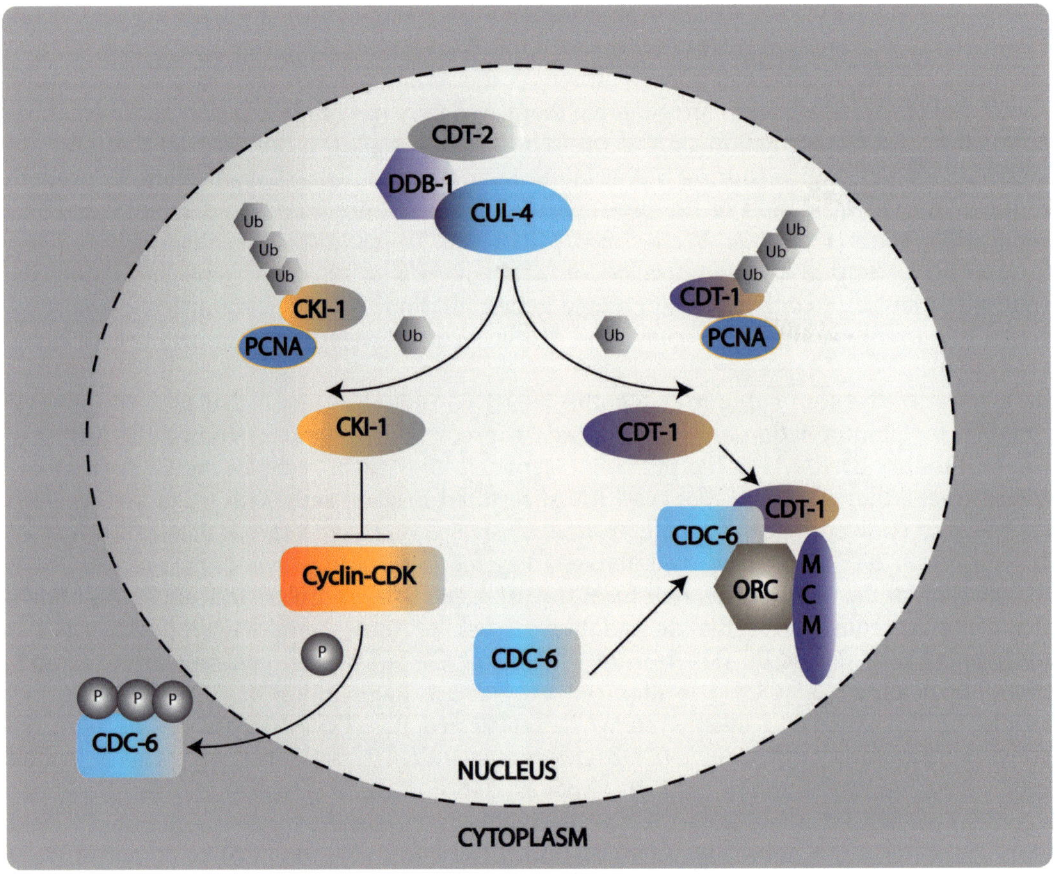

Fig. 3. Preventing re-replication. Inactivation of CDT-1 and CDC-6 in S phase provides a key mechanism for preventing re-replication. The cullin RING ubiquitin E3 ligase (CRL) complex $CRL4^{Cdt2}$ is critical in the inactivation of CDT-1 as well as CDC-6. $CRL4^{Cdt2}$ contains the cullin protein CUL-4, adaptor DDB-1 and substrate recognition unit CDT-2. This complex recognizes its substrates in association with PCNA. CDT-1 and a CDK inhibitor of the Cip/Kip family, CKI-1, contain a PCNA interacting protein (PIP) motif in the N-terminus and are degraded by $CRL4^{Cdt2}$. As PCNA is an auxiliary factor of DNA polymerases, the degradation of CDT-1 and CKI-1 can be coupled to DNA replication. Inactivation of CKI-1 allows activation of S phase CDK/Cyclin kinases. CDK phosphorylation of the CDC-6 N-terminus promotes nuclear export of CDC-6. Because of its control of two critical pre-replication complex components, CUL-4 inactivation leads to extensive re-replication in *C. elegans* (see text for further details).

In each of these models, a cullin RING ubiquitin E3 ligase (CRL) has been identified that contains CUL-4, DDB-1 and a substrate recognition unit CDT-2. This $CRL4^{Cdt2}$ complex recognizes its substrates in an unusual manner. CKI-1, $p21^{Cip1}$ and CDT-1 all contain a PCNA interacting protein (PIP) motif in the N-terminus (Havens & Walter 2009). PCNA is an auxiliary factor of DNA polymerases, which forms a ring around the DNA and acts as a sliding clamp. Because interaction with PCNA is a prerequisite for $CRL4^{Cdt2}$ substrate ubiquitylation, degradation of the CKI and CDT-1 substrates is coupled to DNA replication.
In summary, upon association with PCNA, the CDK-inhibitor CKI-1 is recognized by $CRL4^{Cdt2}$ and targeted for degradation. This allows S-phase Cyclin-CDKs to phosphorylate CDC-6, which triggers CDC-6 export from the nucleus. In addition to CKI-1, $CRL4^{Cdt2}$ also targets PCNA-bound CDT-1 for ubiquitin-dependent proteolysis. In *C. elegans*, CDC-6 nuclear export and CDT-1 degradation are two redundant mechanisms that prevent re-replication (Fig. 3) (Kim & Kipreos 2007b; Korzelius & van den Heuvel 2007). Because *C. elegans* does not show redundancy for the $CRL4^{Cdt2}$ E3 ligase in CDT-1 degradation, the function of this complex has been more obvious in *C. elegans*.

5. Activation of the DNA replication checkpoint in early embryos

Incomplete DNA replication activates an S-phase checkpoint, which delays progression through the cell cycle to create time for repair (Branzei & Foiani 2010). Central in this checkpoint is the ATR-Chk1 protein kinase pathway, which is activated by lesions created by stalled replication forks. Active Chk1 phosphorylates downstream cell cycle regulators such as the CDC25 phosphatase that controls the activity of CDK1. This S-phase checkpoint is generally not functional in early embryos. For example, inhibition of DNA replication with a low concentration of hydroxyurea (HU) does not affect cell cycle progression in embryos of *Drosophila*, *Xenopus* or Zebrafish (Hartwell & Weinert 1989). However, the situation is quite different in early *C. elegans* embryos, which not only contain an active S-phase checkpoint, but also activate the ATR-1/Chk-1 pathway as part of normal development (Brauchle, et al. 2003; Encalada, et al. 2000).
The first division of the *C. elegans* zygote is unequal and generates a larger anterior blastomere, AB, and smaller posterior blastomere, P1. These cells give rise to different daughter cell lineages. For instance, P1 continues an additional three asymmetric divisions to produce the germline precursor P4 (Sulston, et al. 1983). In addition to the different fates, cell division in the AB and P1 lineages also occurs with a different timing, with the AB cell dividing approximately 2 minutes earlier than the P1 cell (visible in Fig. 2). Interestingly, *atl-1* ATR and *chk-1* function contributes to this asynchrony of cell division in normal embryos (Brauchle, et al. 2003). Double inactivation of *atl-1* and *chk-1* reduced the time between mitotic entry (nuclear envelope breakdown) of AB and P1 from 125 sec in the wild-type to 75 sec after *atl-1/chk-1* RNAi. Thus, somehow the P1 blastomere might preferentially and highly reproducibly activate the S phase checkpoint. Asymmetric division of the zygote is needed for this distinction between AB and P1 (Brauchle, et al. 2003).
Preferred checkpoint activation in P1 is also visible in mutants with defects in DNA replication, or embryos treated with HU, which inhibits ribonucleotide reductase (Brauchle, et al. 2003; Encalada, et al. 2000; Encalada, et al. 2005; Korzelius, et al. 2011). Both the zygote (P0) and P1 daughter are able to delay mitosis by about 12 minutes when replication is compromised, while the AB daughter halts for only a few minutes. Inactivation of *atl-1* and/or *chk-1* prevents these delays, indicating that this is a legitimate, though limited, S-

phase checkpoint response. The different response of the P1 versus AB lineage has been interpreted as protection of the germline against replication errors. Surprisingly, however, the checkpoint response to DNA damage (rather than replication arrest) appears actively repressed in the P1 lineage (Holway, et al. 2006). Bypassing the checkpoint could serve to maintain the relative timing of blastomere divisions, which is an essential part of development.

6. The MCM helicase is needed for activation of the replication checkpoint

Defects in some replication components trigger a checkpoint arrest, while others do not. For instance, partial loss of function of *div-1*, which encodes a DNA polymerase α-subunit, gives rise to substantial cell cycle delays (Encalada, et al. 2000). The same is true for inhibition of ribonucleotide reductase by HU treatment or *rnr-1* RNAi (Brauchle, et al. 2003). However, *mcm-4* inactivation interferes with DNA synthesis without the induction of a checkpoint response (Korzelius, et al. 2011). Cells in *mcm-4(RNAi)* embryos and *mcm-4* mutant larvae enter mitosis at the appropriate time and continue chromosome segregation as well as cell division. Moreover, RNAi of *mcm-4* suppressed the checkpoint delay induced by *rnr-1* inhibition. These data indicate that MCM-4 is not only required for DNA replication but also for activation of the S phase checkpoint. Genome fragmentation has also been reported for *cdt-1(RNAi)* and *cdc-6(RNAi)* embryos. Thus, the assembly of a pre-replication complex appears to be needed to trigger the S-phase checkpoint.

Studies in other organisms support these observations and have demonstrated that activation of the DNA damage and replication checkpoints requires MCM helicase activity. Recruitment of Replication Protein A (RPA) to single-stranded DNA is probably the actual checkpoint trigger (Zou & Elledge 2003). The helicase activity of MCM proteins generates ssDNA, through unwinding the DNA at the replication fork. Stalling of replication forks, e.g. after HU treatment, causes uncoupling of the MCM helicase from DNA polymerase activity (Byun, et al. 2005). Consequently, fork stalling leads to an accumulation of ssDNA, which recruits additional RPA and causes activation of the checkpoint kinases ATR and Chk1. The formation of replication forks and the generation of ssDNA both require MCM function. This explains why *C. elegans mcm-4* loss of function prevents DNA synthesis without activation of the replication checkpoint.

7. Endoreplication: polyploidy required for growth

Endoreplication cycles bypass mitosis while DNA replication continues, which results in a doubling of the ploidy during each endocycle. Endoreplication commonly occurs in specific cell types during metazoan development. In *C. elegans,* only two tissues become polyploid as a result of endoreplication: the intestine and the epidermis (formally known as hypodermis). Intestinal cells endoreplicate during each larval stage, increasing the ploidy to 4n at the transition from first to second larval stage and leading to intestinal nuclei with 32n DNA in adult animals (Hedgecock & White 1985).

The situation in the epidermis is more complex. Epidermal nuclei reside in syncytia, sharing a common cytoplasm without separating membranes. The largest epidermal syncytium is hyp7, which covers most of the body except for regions of the head and tail (Hedgecock & White 1985). In each larval stage, stem-cell like precursors in the epidermis, known as "seam cells", divide to create novel seam cells and daughter cells that fuse with the hyp7 syncytium (Sulston & Horvitz 1977). Ultimately, this creates a syncytium with 133 nuclei. The newly created epidermal cells duplicate their genomic DNA prior to fusion, so that they enter the syncytium as 4n nuclei (Hedgecock & White 1985). Endoreplication has been reported to occur in adult stage hyp7 nuclei, although the level varies between nuclei, with an average ploidy of 10n to 12n in older adults (Fig. 4) (Flemming, et al. 2000; Morita, et al. 2002; Nystrom, et al. 2002).

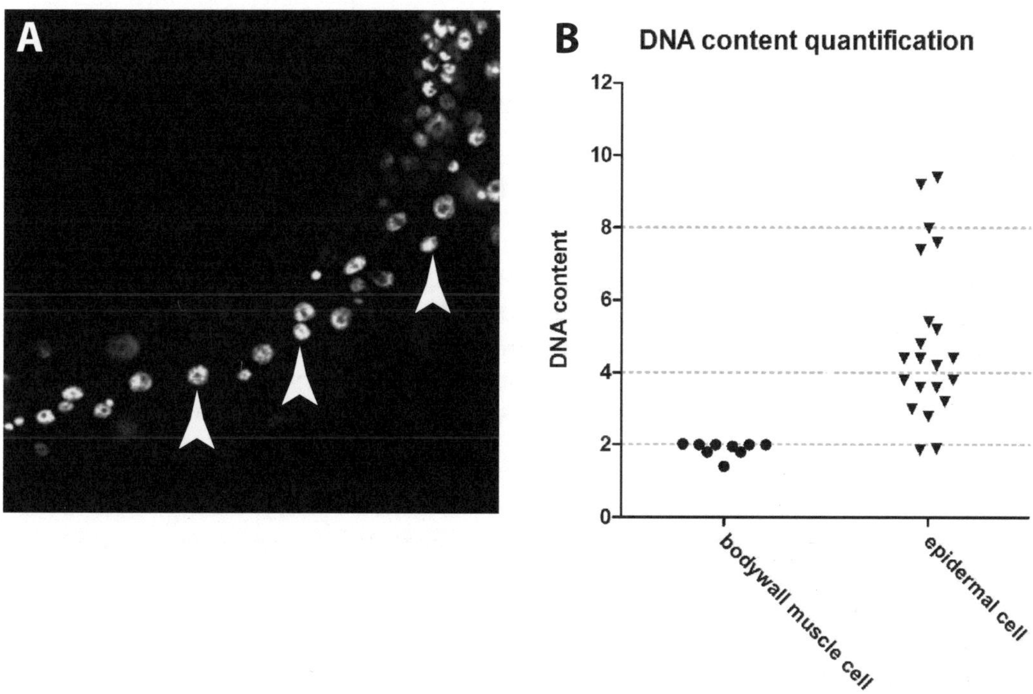

Fig. 4. DNA endoreplication in the epidermis. A. Propidium iodide staining of a young *C. elegans* adult is shown, arrowhead indicate polyploid nuclei of the epidermis. B. Quantification of DNA content based on propidium iodide staining. Nuclei of the body wall muscles are used as a reference for 2n DNA content. The epidermal nuclei show increased ploidy with up to 8n DNA content. The DNA content of epidermal nuclei further increases in concert with growth of late stage adults. Each dot represents a single nucleus.

Why these two cell types, the skin and intestine, undergo endoreplication is not fully understood. It has been speculated that endoreplication is used to maintain the integrity of these tissues, while allowing increased genome ploidy to support increases in cell volume and metabolic activity (Kipreos 2005). In many organisms however, endoreplication has been correlated with growth. Indeed, the *C. elegans* epidermis and intestine grow extensively during larval development, and endoreplication in the epidermis has been correlated with the size of the entire animal.

Several observations support this conclusion. Hydroxyurea (HU) treatment of adult animals, in which somatic cell proliferation has been completed, prevents endoreplication in the epidermis as well as growth of the animals. (Lozano, et al. 2006). In contrast, tetraploid animals are 40% larger in volume than wild type worms, which closely corresponds to the increase in epidermal polyploidy (from average 11.2n to 16.7n, in adults at 148 hrs.). Furthermore, the first generation homozygous *cye-1* cyclin E mutants survive till adulthood because of maternal CYE-1 supplies and these animals show reduced endoreplication in the epidermis and a corresponding reduction in body size (Lozano, et al. 2006). Finally, *mcm-4* mutants fail DNA replication and are severely growth retarded and larval lethal. Specific expression of MCM-4 in the epidermis of such mutants is sufficient to rescue larval growth and lethality (Korzelius, et al. 2011). Thus, the polyploidy of the epidermis contributes to the body size of the adult animal.

8. Tissue-specific regulation of DNA replication

Interestingly, endoreplication in the epidermis is regulated by a TGF-β signal transduction pathway. *C. elegans* uses several different TGF-β pathways to control a variety of developmental processes, including growth. Mutations in components of this pathway lead to smaller and thinner adult animals (small phenotype: Sma). The ligand for the growth pathway is DBL-1, which is homologous to DPP/BMP-4 (Morita, et al. 2002; Suzuki, et al. 1999). DBL-1 signals through the Type I and II TGF-β serine/threonine kinase receptors SMA-6 and DAF-4, respectively, to the downstream SMAD transcriptional regulators SMA-2, SMA-3 and SMA-4 (Savage-Dunn 2005). Notably, *daf-4* and *sma-2* mutants are not only small and thin, but also show reduced ploidy of epidermal nuclei (Flemming, et al. 2000; Nystrom, et al. 2002).

A critical downstream target of the DBL-1 pathway has also been identified: *lon-1* (Maduzia, et al. 2002; Morita, et al. 2002). Homozygous *lon-1* mutant animals are longer than normal (Lon phenotype), while overexpression of *lon-1* leads to a small phenotype. Several observations indicate that *lon-1* acts downstream of the SMA-6 TGF-β type I receptor: double *sma-6; lon-1* mutants are still somewhat long, and *lon-1* mRNA levels are increased in *sma-6* mutants. Surprisingly, *lon-1* encodes a putative transmembrane protein, related to the plant pathogenesis-related protein 1 (PR-1) and human glioma-pathogenesis related protein (GliPR-1). This LON-1 protein is expressed and required in the epidermis, and anti-LON-1 antibodies showed localization to apical junctions (Morita, et al. 2002). LON-1 is claimed to repress endoreplication, based on the increased epidermal ploidy in *lon-1(e185)* and *lon-1(RNAi)* adults. However, two other *lon-1* mutations show somewhat reduced ploidy compared to wild-type (Morita, et al. 2002). Thus, although further research is needed, there is strong evidence that the DBL-1 ligand, produced in a set of neurons, activates a TGF-β/SMA pathway, which inhibits *lon-1* expression in the epidermis, and thereby allows endoreplication and growth of the adults.

The TGF-β/SMA/LON-1 pathway should somehow connect to the cell cycle in order to regulate endoreplication. Based on the Sma phenotype of *cye-1* mutants, it has been proposed that Cyclin E is the key regulator (Lozano, et al. 2006). Cyclin E mutant mice also show defects in trophoblast endoreplication (Parisi, et al. 2003), and the fluctuating activity of Cyclin E with its kinase partner CDK-2 drives endoreplication in *Drosophila* (Claycomb & Orr-Weaver 2005; Lilly & Duronio 2005). However, TGF-β/SMA/LON-1 signaling could also act more upstream of *cye-1, e.g.,* in the regulation of *cyd-1* Cyclin D. *cyd-1* mutants are also small, and *C. elegans* Cyclin D is needed for endoreplication, at least in the intestine (Boxem & van den Heuvel 2001). At least in *C. elegans,* Cyclin D is essential for G1/S

progression and induction of S phase genes such as MCM proteins (Boxem & van den Heuvel 2001; Boxem & van den Heuvel 2002; Korzelius, et al. 2011).
The *cyd-1* and *mcm-4* mutants show an interesting phenotypic difference. Homozygous mutants of either *cyd-1* or *mcm-4* complete embryogenesis, because of maternal supplies, fail DNA replication from the first larval stage onward, and show severe growth retardation. However, only *mcm-4* mutants show larval lethality, which is fully suppressed by expression of *mcm-4* from an epidermis specific promoter (Korzelius, et al. 2011). The ability to arrest the cell cycle probably underlies the difference between *cyd-1* and *mcm-4* mutants: post-embryonic blast cells in *cyd-1* mutants arrest prior to S phase entry, while they continue abnormal mitosis in *mcm-4* mutants. As a result, the structural integrity of the epidermis is lost only in *mcm-4* mutants, which often causes larval death. Thus, not absence of DNA replication but lack of an S-phase checkpoint response may lead to death of the animal.

9. In conclusion

Studies of DNA replication in *C. elegans* have thus far been limited. Given the variation of well-established models for replication studies, which include budding and fission yeast, *Xenopus* egg extracts, cells in culture, *in vitro* systems and even flies, one could question the need for studying S phase in the worm. However, several important mechanistic insights have been obtained from observations of DNA replication-defective phenotypes in the worm. Moreover, such analyses have emphasized the variation in regulatory mechanisms between different developmental stages and in different cell types, underscoring the need for studies of replication control in a developmental context. The combination of its large embryonic cells, strong cell biology, genetic tractability and highly reproducible lineage now allows for a detailed analysis of the assembly of pre-replication and replication initiation complexes in real time in *C. elegans*. High-throughput studies have already defined RNAi phenotypes for many known DNA replication components, and have identified currently uncharacterized genes with similar phenotypes. Thus, *C. elegans* increasingly adds an attractive developmental animal system for gene discovery, functional characterizations *in vivo,* and live imaging of replication component localizations.

10. References

Ankeny, R.A. (2001). The natural history of *Caenorhabditis elegans* research. *Nature reviews.Genetics,* Vol.2, No.6, pp. 474-479, ISSN 1471-0056

Arias, E.E.&Walter, J.C. (2007). Strength in numbers: preventing rereplication via multiple mechanisms in eukaryotic cells. *Genes & development,* Vol.21, No.5, pp. 497-518, , ISSN 0890-9369

Bell, S.P.&Dutta, A. (2002). DNA replication in eukaryotic cells. *Annual Review of Biochemistry,* Vol.71, pp. 333-374, ISSN 0066-4154

Bennett, M.D.; Leitch, I.J.; Price, H.J. & Johnston, J.S. (2003). Comparisons with *Caenorhabditis* (approximately 100 Mb) and *Drosophila* (approximately 175 Mb) using flow cytometry show genome size in *Arabidopsis* to be approximately 157 Mb and thus approximately 25% larger than the *Arabidopsis* genome initiative estimate of approximately 125 Mb. *Annals of botany,* Vol.91, No.5, pp. 547-557, ISSN 0305-7364

Blow, J.J.&Dutta, A. (2005). Preventing re-replication of chromosomal DNA. *Nature reviews.Molecular cell biology,* Vol.6, No.6, pp. 476-486, ISSN 1471-0072

Bondar, T.; Kalinina, A.; Khair, L.; Kopanja, D.; Nag, A.; Bagchi, S. & Raychaudhuri, P. (2006). Cul4A and DDB1 associate with Skp2 to target p27Kip1 for proteolysis involving the COP9 signalosome. *Molecular and cellular biology,* Vol.26, No.7, pp. 2531-2539, ISSN 0270-7306

Bousset, K.&Diffley, J.F. (1998). The Cdc7 protein kinase is required for origin firing during S phase. *Genes & development,* Vol.12, No.4, pp. 480-490, ISSN 0890-9369

Boxem, M.; Srinivasan, D.G. & van den Heuvel, S. (1999). The *Caenorhabditis elegans* gene *ncc-1* encodes a cdc2-related kinase required for M phase in meiotic and mitotic cell divisions, but not for S phase. *Development (Cambridge, England),* Vol.126, No.10, pp. 2227-2239, ISSN 0950-1991

Boxem, M.&van den Heuvel, S. (2002). *C. elegans* class B synthetic multivulva genes act in G(1) regulation. *Current biology : CB,* Vol.12, No.11, pp. 906-911, ISSN 0960-9822

Boxem, M.&van den Heuvel, S. (2001). *lin-35* Rb and *cki-1* Cip/Kip cooperate in developmental regulation of G1 progression in *C. elegans*. *Development (Cambridge, England),* Vol.128, No.21, pp. 4349-4359, ISSN 0950-1991

Branzei, D.&Foiani, M. (2010). Maintaining genome stability at the replication fork. *Nature reviews. Molecular cell biology,* Vol.11, No.3, pp. 208-219, ISSN 1471-0080

Brauchle, M.; Baumer, K. & Gonczy, P. (2003). Differential activation of the DNA replication checkpoint contributes to asynchrony of cell division in *C. elegans* embryos. *Current biology : CB,* Vol.13, No.10, pp. 819-827, ISSN 0960-9822

Byun, T.S.; Pacek, M.; Yee, M.C.; Walter, J.C. & Cimprich, K.A. (2005). Functional uncoupling of MCM helicase and DNA polymerase activities activates the ATR-dependent checkpoint. *Genes & development,* Vol.19, No.9, pp. 1040-1052, ISSN 0890-9369

Cinquin, O.; Crittenden, S.L.; Morgan, D.E. & Kimble, J. (2010). Progression from a stem cell-like state to early differentiation in the *C. elegans* germ line. *Proceedings of the National Academy of Sciences of the United States of America,* Vol.107, No.5, pp. 2048-2053, ISSN 1091-6490

Claycomb, J.M.&Orr-Weaver, T.L. (2005). Developmental gene amplification: insights into DNA replication and gene expression. *Trends in genetics : TIG,* Vol.21, No.3, pp. 149-162, ISSN 0168-9525

Encalada, S.E.; Martin, P.R.; Phillips, J.B.; Lyczak, R.; Hamill, D.R.; Swan, K.A. & Bowerman, B. (2000). DNA replication defects delay cell division and disrupt cell polarity in early *Caenorhabditis elegans* embryos. *Developmental biology,* Vol.228, No.2, pp. 225-238, ISSN 0012-1606

Encalada, S.E.; Willis, J.; Lyczak, R. & Bowerman, B. (2005). A spindle checkpoint functions during mitosis in the early *Caenorhabditis elegans* embryo. *Molecular biology of the cell,* Vol.16, No.3, pp. 1056-1070, ISSN 1059-1524

Feng, H.; Zhong, W.; Punkosdy, G.; Gu, S.; Zhou, L.; Seabolt, E.K. & Kipreos, E.T. (1999). CUL-2 is required for the G1-to-S-phase transition and mitotic chromosome condensation in *Caenorhabditis elegans*. *Nature cell biology*, Vol.1, No.8, pp. 486-492, ISSN 1465-7392

Flemming, A.J.; Shen, Z.Z.; Cunha, A.; Emmons, S.W. & Leroi, A.M. (2000). Somatic polyploidization and cellular proliferation drive body size evolution in nematodes. *Proceedings of the National Academy of Sciences of the United States of America*, Vol.97, No.10, pp. 5285-5290, ISSN 0027-8424

Frokjaer-Jensen, C.; Davis, M.W.; Hopkins, C.E.; Newman, B.J.; Thummel, J.M.; Olesen, S.P.; Grunnet, M. & Jorgensen, E.M. (2008). Single-copy insertion of transgenes in *Caenorhabditis elegans*. *Nature genetics*, Vol.40, No.11, pp. 1375-1383, ISSN 1546-1718

Hartwell, L.H.&Weinert, T.A. (1989). Checkpoints: controls that ensure the order of cell cycle events. *Science (New York, N.Y.)*, Vol.246, No.4930, pp. 629-634, ISSN 0036-8075

Havens, C.G.&Walter, J.C. (2009). Docking of a specialized PIP Box onto chromatin-bound PCNA creates a degron for the ubiquitin ligase CRL4Cdt2. *Molecular cell*, Vol.35, No.1, pp. 93-104, ISSN 1097-4164

Hedgecock, E.M.&White, J.G. (1985). Polyploid tissues in the nematode *Caenorhabditis elegans*. *Developmental biology*, Vol.107, No.1, pp. 128-133, ISSN 0012-1606

Higa, L.A.; Yang, X.; Zheng, J.; Banks, D.; Wu, M.; Ghosh, P.; Sun, H. & Zhang, H. (2006). Involvement of CUL4 ubiquitin E3 ligases in regulating CDK inhibitors Dacapo/p27Kip1 and cyclin E degradation. *Cell cycle (Georgetown, Tex.)*, Vol.5, No.1, pp. 71-77, ISSN 1551-4005

Holway, A.H.; Kim, S.H.; La Volpe, A. & Michael, W.M. (2006). Checkpoint silencing during the DNA damage response in *Caenorhabditis elegans* embryos. *The Journal of cell biology*, Vol.172, No.7, pp. 999-1008, ISSN 0021-9525

Horvitz, H.R.&Sulston, J.E. (1980). Isolation and genetic characterization of cell-lineage mutants of the nematode *Caenorhabditis elegans*. *Genetics*, Vol.96, No.2, pp. 435-454, ISSN 0016-6731

Kim, J.; Feng, H. & Kipreos, E.T. (2007). *C. elegans* CUL-4 prevents rereplication by promoting the nuclear export of CDC-6 via a CKI-1-dependent pathway. *Current biology : CB*, Vol.17, No.11, pp. 966-972, ISSN 0960-9822

Kim, J.&Kipreos, E.T. (2008). Control of the Cdc6 replication licensing factor in metazoa: the role of nuclear export and the CUL4 ubiquitin ligase. *Cell cycle (Georgetown, Tex.)*, Vol.7, No.2, pp. 146-150, ISSN 1551-4005

Kim, Y.&Kipreos, E.T. (2007a). The *Caenorhabditis elegans* replication licensing factor CDT-1 is targeted for degradation by the CUL-4/DDB-1 complex. *Molecular and cellular biology*, Vol.27, No.4, pp. 1394-1406, ISSN 0270-7306

Kim, Y.&Kipreos, E.T. (2007b). Cdt1 degradation to prevent DNA re-replication: conserved and non-conserved pathways. *Cell division*, Vol.2, pp. 18, ISSN 1747-1028

Kim, Y.; Starostina, N.G. & Kipreos, E.T. (2008). The CRL4Cdt2 ubiquitin ligase targets the degradation of p21Cip1 to control replication licensing. *Genes & development*, Vol.22, No.18, pp. 2507-2519, ISSN 0890-9369

Kipreos, E.T. (2005). *C. elegans* cell cycles: invariance and stem cell divisions. *Nature reviews.Molecular cell biology*, Vol.6, No.10, pp. 766-776, ISSN 1471-0072

Korzelius, J.; The, I.; Ruijtenberg, S.; Portegijs, V.; Xu, H.; Horvitz, H.R. & van den Heuvel, S. (2011). *C. elegans* MCM-4 is a general DNA replication and checkpoint component with an epidermis-specific requirement for growth and viability. *Developmental biology,* Vol.350, No.2, pp. 358-369, ISSN 1095-564X

Korzelius, J.&van den Heuvel, S. (2007). Replication licensing: oops! ... I did it again. *Current biology : CB,* Vol.17, No.16, pp. R630-2, ISSN 0960-9822

Labib, K.&Diffley, J.F. (2001). Is the MCM2-7 complex the eukaryotic DNA replication fork helicase? *Current opinion in genetics & development,* Vol.11, No.1, pp. 64-70, ISSN 0959-437X

Labib, K.; Kearsey, S.E. & Diffley, J.F. (2001). MCM2-7 proteins are essential components of prereplicative complexes that accumulate cooperatively in the nucleus during G1-phase and are required to establish, but not maintain, the S-phase checkpoint. *Molecular biology of the cell,* Vol.12, No.11, pp. 3658-3667, ISSN 1059-1524

Lilly, M.A.&Duronio, R.J. (2005). New insights into cell cycle control from the *Drosophila* endocycle. *Oncogene,* Vol.24, No.17, pp. 2765-2775, ISSN 0950-9232

Lozano, E.; Saez, A.G.; Flemming, A.J.; Cunha, A. & Leroi, A.M. (2006). Regulation of growth by ploidy in *Caenorhabditis elegans. Current biology : CB,* Vol.16, No.5, pp. 493-498, ISSN 0960-9822

Machida, Y.J.; Hamlin, J.L. & Dutta, A. (2005). Right place, right time, and only once: replication initiation in metazoans. *Cell,* Vol.123, No.1, pp. 13-24, ISSN 0092-8674

Maduzia, L.L.; Gumienny, T.L.; Zimmerman, C.M.; Wang, H.; Shetgiri, P.; Krishna, S.; Roberts, A.F. & Padgett, R.W. (2002). *lon-1* regulates *Caenorhabditis elegans* body size downstream of the dbl-1 TGF beta signaling pathway. *Developmental biology,* Vol.246, No.2, pp. 418-428, ISSN 0012-1606

McGarry, T.J.&Kirschner, M.W. (1998). Geminin, an inhibitor of DNA replication, is degraded during mitosis. *Cell,* Vol.93, No.6, pp. 1043-1053, ISSN 0092-8674

Mechali, M. (2010). Eukaryotic DNA replication origins: many choices for appropriate answers. *Nature reviews.Molecular cell biology,* Vol.11, No.10, pp. 728-738, ISSN 1471-0080

Mello, C.&Fire, A. (1995). DNA transformation. *Methods in cell biology,* Vol.48, pp. 451-482, ISSN 0091-679X

Morita, K.; Flemming, A.J.; Sugihara, Y.; Mochii, M.; Suzuki, Y.; Yoshida, S.; Wood, W.B.; Kohara, Y.; Leroi, A.M. & Ueno, N. (2002). A *Caenorhabditis elegans* TGF-beta, DBL-1, controls the expression of LON-1, a PR-related protein, that regulates polyploidization and body length. *The EMBO journal,* Vol.21, No.5, pp. 1063-1073, ISSN 0261-4189

Nguyen, V.Q.; Co, C. & Li, J.J. (2001). Cyclin-dependent kinases prevent DNA re-replication through multiple mechanisms. *Nature,* Vol.411, No.6841, pp. 1068-1073, ISSN 0028-0836

Nystrom, J.; Shen, Z.Z.; Aili, M.; Flemming, A.J.; Leroi, A. & Tuck, S. (2002). Increased or decreased levels of *Caenorhabditis elegans lon-3,* a gene encoding a collagen, cause reciprocal changes in body length. *Genetics,* Vol.161, No.1, pp. 83-97, ISSN 0016-6731

Parisi, T.; Beck, A.R.; Rougier, N.; McNeil, T.; Lucian, L.; Werb, Z. & Amati, B. (2003). Cyclins E1 and E2 are required for endoreplication in placental trophoblast giant cells. *The EMBO journal,* Vol.22, No.18, pp. 4794-4803, ISSN 0261-4189

Praitis, V.; Casey, E.; Collar, D. & Austin, J. (2001). Creation of low-copy integrated transgenic lines in *Caenorhabditis elegans*. *Genetics,* Vol.157, No.3, pp. 1217-1226, ISSN 0016-6731

Remus, D.; Blanchette, M.; Rio, D.C. & Botchan, M.R. (2005). CDK phosphorylation inhibits the DNA-binding and ATP-hydrolysis activities of the *Drosophila* origin recognition complex. *The Journal of biological chemistry,* Vol.280, No.48, pp. 39740-39751, ISSN 0021-9258

Salic, A.&Mitchison, T.J. (2008). A chemical method for fast and sensitive detection of DNA synthesis in vivo. *Proceedings of the National Academy of Sciences of the United States of America,* Vol.105, No.7, pp. 2415-2420, ISSN 1091-6490

Savage-Dunn, C. (2005). TGF-beta signaling, In: *Wormbook,* The *C. elegans* Research Community. Retrieved from
<http://www.wormbook.org>

Sonnichsen, B.; Koski, L.B.; Walsh, A.; Marschall, P.; Neumann, B.; Brehm, M.; Alleaume, A.M.; Artelt, J.; Bettencourt, P.; Cassin, E.; Hewitson, M.; Holz, C.; Khan, M.; Lazik, S.; Martin, C.; Nitzsche, B.; Ruer, M.; Stamford, J.; Winzi, M.; Heinkel, R.; Roder, M.; Finell, J.; Hantsch, H.; Jones, S.J.; Jones, M.; Piano, F.; Gunsalus, K.C.; Oegema, K.; Gonczy, P.; Coulson, A.; Hyman, A.A. & Echeverri, C.J. (2005). Full-genome RNAi profiling of early embryogenesis in *Caenorhabditis elegans*. *Nature,* Vol.434, No.7032, pp. 462-469, ISSN 1476-4687

Sulston, J.E.&Horvitz, H.R. (1981). Abnormal cell lineages in mutants of the nematode *Caenorhabditis elegans*. *Developmental biology,* Vol.82, No.1, pp. 41-55, ISSN 0012-1606

Sulston, J.E.&Horvitz, H.R. (1977). Post-embryonic cell lineages of the nematode, *Caenorhabditis elegans*. *Developmental biology,* Vol.56, No.1, pp. 110-156, 0012-1606; 0012-1606

Sulston, J.E.; Schierenberg, E.; White, J.G. & Thomson, J.N. (1983). The embryonic cell lineage of the nematode *Caenorhabditis elegans*. *Developmental biology,* Vol.100, No.1, pp. 64-119, ISSN 0012-1606

Suzuki, Y.; Yandell, M.D.; Roy, P.J.; Krishna, S.; Savage-Dunn, C.; Ross, R.M.; Padgett, R.W. & Wood, W.B. (1999). A BMP homolog acts as a dose-dependent regulator of body size and male tail patterning in *Caenorhabditis elegans*. *Development (Cambridge, England),* Vol.126, No.2, pp. 241-250, ISSN 0950-1991

van Leuken, R.; Clijsters, L. & Wolthuis, R. (2008). To cell cycle, swing the APC/C. *Biochimica et biophysica acta,* Vol.1786, No.1, pp. 49-59, ISSN 0006-3002

Yanagi, K.; Mizuno, T.; Tsuyama, T.; Tada, S.; Iida, Y.; Sugimoto, A.; Eki, T.; Enomoto, T. & Hanaoka, F. (2005). *Caenorhabditis elegans* geminin homologue participates in cell cycle regulation and germ line development. *The Journal of biological chemistry,* Vol.280, No.20, pp. 19689-19694, ISSN 0021-9258

Zhong, W.; Feng, H.; Santiago, F.E. & Kipreos, E.T. (2003). CUL-4 ubiquitin ligase maintains genome stability by restraining DNA-replication licensing. *Nature,* Vol.423, No.6942, pp. 885-889, ISSN 0028-0836

Zou, L.&Elledge, S.J. (2003). Sensing DNA damage through ATRIP recognition of RPA-ssDNA complexes. *Science (New York, N.Y.),* Vol.300, No.5625, pp. 1542-1548, ISSN 1095-9203

3

The Relationship Between Replication and Recombination

Apolonija Bedina Zavec
National Institute of Chemistry
Slovenia

1. Inroduction

DNA replication, the process of copying double-stranded DNA, and DNA recombination, the process of breaking DNA strand and joined to a different strand, are central characteristics of life. The aim of this chapter is to discuss the relationship between replication and recombination. Understanding the intimate links between these processes gives us a more holistic approach to understanding the functioning of a cell.
Replication and recombination machineries cooperate to maintain biological inheritance and genomic integrity. While replication enables the formation of two identical DNA molecules from a single double-stranded DNA, recombination enables accurate repair of errors that occur on both strands of DNA as well as the formation of new combinations of genes. Recombination can occur between similar molecules of DNA (homologous recombination), or dissimilar molecules (non-homologous end joining). Homologous recombination predominantly occurs during and shortly after DNA replication (late S and G2), while non-homologous end joining is predominant in the G1 and early S phase of the cell cycle.
What is the relationship between DNA replication and recombination processes? Mutations in some genes with a role in DNA replication cause hyper-recombination phenotypes. These mutations require recombination protein Rad52 for their viability, suggesting that the replication errors caused by mutations are repaired by recombination mechanisms (Merrill & Holm, 1998). Furthermore, many recombination genes have S phase defects when deleted. Obviously, replication and recombination processes are tightly intertwined. In this chapter I will try to present the close coupling between these processes from a different point of view (Fig. 1): recombination is part of DNA replication and, vice versa, DNA synthesis is part of the recombination process; both processes are connected via checkpoints; both processes are regulated by common posttranslational modifications; both processes take advantage of double helix DNA and both have a common problem with DNA unfolding.
The recombination system plays a crucial role in DNA replication ensuring that replication machines can complete their task of genome duplication. DNA replication forks stall or collapse at DNA lesions or problematic genomic regions. When a fork becomes stalled, the replisome often remains firmly associated with the fork. But, when replication forks are removed, recombination is the most important rescue mechanism. The recombination mechanism forms substrates for the assembly of a new replication fork thus allowing continued DNA replication.

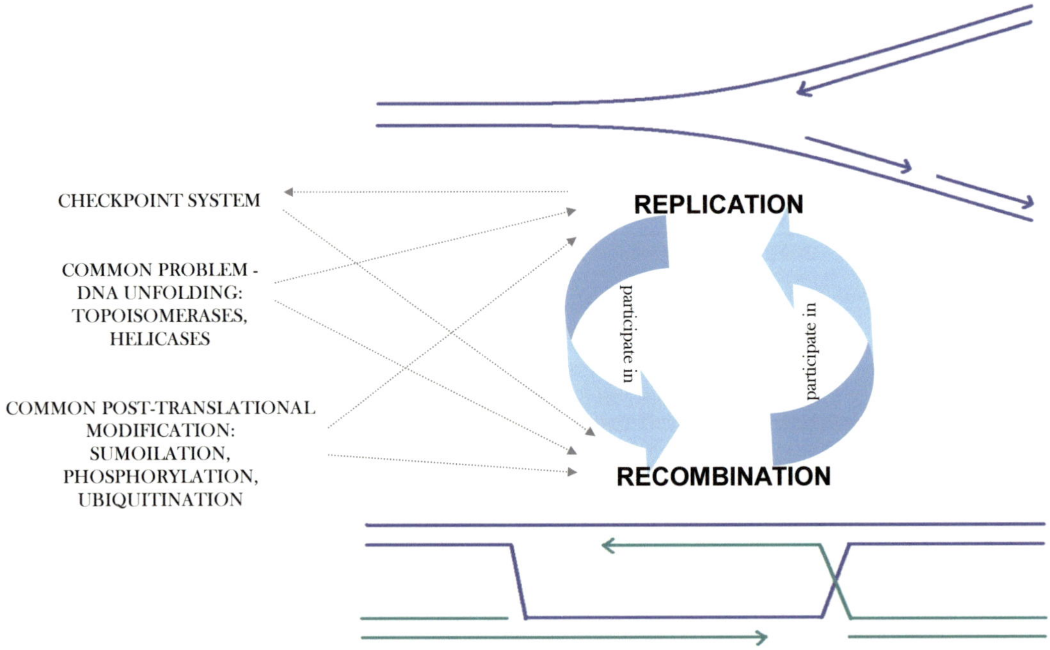

Fig. 1. Replication and recombination processes are tightly intertwined: recombination is part of DNA replication and, vice versa, DNA synthesis is part of the recombination process. They are affected by the common factors: checkpoint, DNA unfolding and post-translational modifications.

DNA synthesis is a crucial step during the recombination process. After Rad51-mediated DNA strand invasion, DNA synthesis is the next step in recombination to restore the integrity of the chromosome. After DNA strand invasion, dissociation of Rad51 is required to allow access for DNA polymerases to prime DNA synthesis at the invading 3' OH end. Repair DNA synthesis during the recombination process is similar to normal S-phase replication, but has specific properties.

A close coupling between replication and recombination is also demonstrated in the checkpoint system. In addition to sensing DNA damage, the role of the DNA damage checkpoint is also to coordinate cell cycle progression, DNA replication, and DNA repair mechanisms. When forks collapse during replication and generate single-stranded DNA ends, these ends activate the replication checkpoint. Activated replication checkpoint proteins further activate the recombination machinery.

A close coupling between replication and recombination is also demonstrated in common posttranslational modifications. Posttranslational modifications, with their key role in controlling protein function, play an important role in the maintenance of genome integrity. Sumoylation, phosphorylation, and ubiquitination are especially important for the functioning of replication and recombination proteins, allowing them to execute their functions in a rapid and efficient manner.

Replication and recombination mechanisms both take advantage of double helix DNA and have a common problem with DNA unfolding. Both processes take advantage of the complementary base pairing between the strands to undertake their tasks. Each strand of the duplex provides a template for generating the other strand. When one strand of DNA is damaged, the complementary sister strand can be used as a template to regenerate the damaged strand and recover information encoded in its sequence. However, the organization of DNA sequences into a chromatin structure represents a barrier to replication and recombination processes. Because replication and recombination require access to the sequence in the interior of the double helix DNA, the chromatin structure has to be remodeled during these processes. Both processes require DNA topoisomerase to unwind the DNA helix and DNA helicase to open the DNA helix.

This chapter mostly refers to the basic mechanisms applicable to eukaryotes that have been studied in budding yeast *Saccharomyces cerevisiae*. *S.cerevisiae* is the best studied eukaryotic model organism that providing the most integrated view of replication and recombination processes. At the end of this chapter, a lesser known yeast protein Ecm11 is discussed, which affects both replication and recombination processes.

2. Recombination during DNA replication

DNA replication represents a sensitive period in the cell cycle because the stretched chromatids and the stability of the replicating forks are highly susceptible to damage. Failure to restart replication accurately would result in serious consequences for organism: accumulation of mutations, enhanced genome instability, or even cell death. Recombination plays a crucial role in DNA replication by ensuring that replication machines can complete their task of genome duplication. DNA replication forks can stall or collapse at DNA lesions or problematic genomic regions. At problematic replication regions, e.g. inverted repeats (Ty elements) and tRNA genes, the replication fork progression is slowed down and fork stalling is a frequent event. When forks are stalled, the replisome often remains stably associated with the fork; Rad53 stabilizes stalled forks by gluing the replisome onto the replicating molecule (Lucca et al., 2004). Resumption of DNA replication can occur when the block is relieved. In other situations, like DNA breaks or unremoved protein-DNA complexes, the replisome dissociates and the fork collapses (Lambert et al., 2005). When replication forks are removed, recombination is the most important rescue mechanism. The recombination process forms substrates for the assembly of a new replication fork. There are also alternatives to a replication restart. Specialized DNA polymerases, translesion polymerases, are able to replicate across sites of DNA damage and allow re-initiation of replication by normal replicative polymerases beyond the lesion (Friedberg et al., 2002). As translesion polymerases are mutagenic, their activation is tightly controlled. It has been shown that translesion synthesis is used only when a recombination mechanism is not available (Berdichevsky et al., 2002).

Replication restart by recombination mechanisms is required when stalled replication forks are processed up to DSBs or at sub-telomeric regions where there are no converging forks that could complete DNA duplication. Cells take advantage of homologous recombination (HR) to create substrates for assembly of a new replication fork. Holliday junctions enable the site of the original lesion to be returned to a duplex formation and become accessible to repair systems. It has been shown that specific nuclear foci of Rad52 are formed during S phase and that each Rad52 focus represents a center of recombinational repair capable of processing DNA lesions (Lisby et al., 2001). Sister chromatids are the preferred partner for DSB repair in mitotic diploid yeast cells. It was confirmed that cohesion between sister chromatids is essential for efficient DSB repair in mitotic cells (Uhlmann, 2001). A major damage tolerance pathway involving recombination is the template switch, which uses the information on the sister chromatid in the proximity of replication forks. Homologous recombination factors and DNA polymerase δ promote the formation of template switch intermediates. These intermediates are dissolved by the action of the Sgs1 helicase in association with the Top3 topoisomerase rather than by Holliday Junction nucleases (Vanoli et al., 2010). Another recombination mechanism, which has been implicated in the restart of collapsed forks, is break-induced replication (BIR). BIR is an efficient homologous recombination pathway repairing a DNA double-strand break when only one of two ends of the DSB succeeds in strand invasion of a homologous sequence. This recombination pathway includes the synthesis of a long tract of DNA that can be attributed to recombination-directed DNA replication and is discussed in the section about replication during the recombination process (section 3.3.).

2.1 Replication checkpoint is linked to recombination machinery

DNA damage is constantly being sensed by sophisticated cellular networks - DNA damage checkpoints. This is because genome integrity is continuously challenged by DNA lesions, DNA single-strand breaks (SSBs) and double-strand breaks (DSBs). DNA damage and replication checkpoint proteins monitor genome integrity, recognize different forms of DNA damage, transduce appropriate signals, initiate DNA repair, and slow the progression of the cell cycle to allow DNA repair to occur (Boddy & Russell, 2001). At critical stages before or during DNA replication (G1/S and intra-S checkpoints) and before cell division (G2/M checkpoint), the checkpoint proteins delay or stop the cell cycle if DNA damage is unrepaired to prevent duplication and segregation of damaged DNA. A network of checkpoint proteins is tightly coordinated with cell cycle progression. Besides its acting in cell cycle arrest, the checkpoint response is linked to activation of the repair and recombination machinery (Zhou & Elledge, 2000). Thus, the role of the checkpoint system is very complex, in that it senses the DNA damage while also coordinating cell cycle progression, DNA replication and DNA repair mechanisms. The functioning of replication proteins, recombination proteins, and checkpoint proteins is closely intertwined.

During DNA replication, stalled forks generate single-stranded DNA ends coated with replication protein A (RPA), which activates the replication checkpoint. It has been shown that a significant amount of ssDNA must be exposed in order to activate the checkpoint response (Shimada et al., 2002). Activated replication checkpoint proteins further protect the stability of stalled replication forks (Lopes et al., 2001) or activate recombination machinery when forks collapse.

A central transducer of checkpoint proteins is the kinase Mec1 (hATR), which is recruited to stalled forks and probably activated in response to signals generated by the clamp-sensor in the presence of DNA damage (Boddy & Russell, 2001). Activated Mec1 phosphorylates Mrc1, a protein required for replisome stabilization and checkpoint activation (Katou et al., 2003). Kinase Tel1 (hATM) is also a component of the common signalling pathway and has a role similar to Mec1. Mec1 and Tel1 both phosphorylate serines and threonines on numerous target proteins, e.g. H2A, in response to DNA damage (Downs et al., 2000). Downstream from Mec1, the Rad53 kinase responds to DNA replication arrest. Rad53 is a conserved protein directly affecting replication fork stability. Mec1 and Tel1 phosphorylate Rad53 and Mrc1. Phosphorylated Mrc1 binds the fork-associated hyperphosphorylated Rad53, leading to its activation (Alcasabas et al., 2001). Kinase Rad53 phosphorylates and activates other protein kinases that induce other processes that enable repair of the damage.

The similarity between checkpoint sensors and replication proteins has been pointed out (Forsburg, 2002). One of the checkpoint complexes is a specialized version of the replication clamp-loader RFC, with the large subunit replaced by a checkpoint-specific protein Rad24. There is also a checkpoint version of the clamp related to PCNA (processivity clamp of DNA polymerases), Mec3-Rad17-Ddc1. Those proteins act as checkpoint sensors of damage and as effectors of DNA repair.

2.2 Sister chromatid cohesion is coupled to DNA replication

Cohesins are ring-shaped complexes made up of Scc1, Scc3, Smc1, Smc3, and Pds5 subunits. Smc1 and Smc3 are structural maintenance of chromosome (SMC) proteins with ATPase domains. Cohesins keep the sister chromatids connected with each other, they facilitate spindle attachment onto chromosomes during metaphase, and their presence is essential for the proper transmission of sister chromatids to dividing daughter cells.

Cohesins between sister chromatids, recombination, and replication are closely intertwined processes. The sister chromatid cohesion complex plays a crucial role in DNA damage repair by recombination mechanisms, however sister chromatid cohesion is also coupled to DNA replication. Cohesins are loaded onto chromatin before DNA replication. Establishment of cohesion between sister chromatids is coupled to DNA replication and requires the active participation of replication fork and other replication-related activities (Carson & Christman, 2001). It has been shown that proper cohesion require PCNA - a processivity clamp for DNA polymerases, Pol σ - an essential DNA polymerase, Replication Factor C (RFC) - a clamp-loader complex, and cohesion establishment factors. It has also been shown that fork progression itself is tied to cohesin acetylation (Sherwood et al., 2010). The most important cohesion establishment factor is Eco1/Ctf7 acetyltransferase. The mutation of cohesion factor *eco1* can be suppressed by overexpression of PCNA (processivity factor for some DNA polymerases), suggesting that cohesion during the S-phase might actually be mediated by replication fork components (Skibbens et al., 1999). It has also been shown that Eco1 physically interacts with all RFC complexes (Kenna & Skibbens, 2003). As Eco1 is essential for cohesion establishment and the RFC complex is a replication clamp loader that loads PCNA onto dsDNA and promote processive DNA replication, these interactions provide new evidence regarding linkage between cohesion establishment and DNA replication. Other links between the replication machinery and the cohesion machinery are DNA polymerase Trf4/Polσ and components of the replisome progression complex (RPC). Because defects in *trf4* mutants result in a failure of cohesion between the replicated sister chromatids, it was concluded that Trf4/Polσ is required to establish cohesion during S-phase (Wang et al., 2000).

While the multiprotein cohesion complexes depend on loading and establishment factors that are intimately connected to DNA replication, it has also been shown that cohesion establishment factors are implicated in maintaining the processivity and stability of replication forks (Branzei & Foiani, 2010). Interaction between replication forks and cohesin rings stabilize replication forks and/or enable sister chromatid-dependent restart pathways. Some of the components, such as the Tof1–Csm3 complex and Mrc1, appear to be involved in maintaining fork integrity and are recognized as components of the replication checkpoint (Katou et al., 2003). On the other hand, Tof1–Csm3 complex and Mrc1 are implicated in sister chromatid cohesion (Mayer et al., 2004; Xu et al., 2004).

In conclusion, DNA replication and cohesion establishment are intimately coordinated (Sherwood et al., 2010): replication forks, travelling along the DNA, modify cohesin's architecture and association with chromatin, and on the other hand, cohesion in turn affects the dynamics of DNA replication and keeps the sister chromatids connected to each other.

3. DNA synthesis during recombination

3.1 Recombination process

For the cell, it is essential that DNA breaks are repaired promptly to prevent chromosomal aberrations or cell death. Recombination is a key pathway to preserve genomic stability by repairing DNA breaks, gaps, and interstrand crosslinks. Recombination is an essential DNA repair process, particularly for the repair of DNA-double strand breaks (DSBs). The potentially, very dangerous DSBs are repaired by different recombination pathways: non-homologous end joining (NHEJ), single-strand annealing (SSA), break-induced replication (BIR; outcome is half-crossover), synthesis-dependent strand annealing (SDSA; outcome is noncrossover), and double Holliday junction pathways (dHJ; outcome is crossover or noncrossover). In yeast cells, DSBs are generally repaired by noncrossover/gene conversion pathways. The first two pathways, NHEJ and SSA, can occur within one molecule of DNA. DSB resection is a required step in SSA as in HR, but not in NHEJ where DNA end-binding factors Ku70-Ku80 inhibit DSB resection (Tomita et al., 2003). NHEJ is favoured over SSA and HR in G1 phase.

The last three pathways (dHJ pathways, SDSA, BIR) are template dependent processes involving another molecule of DNA, a sister chromatid or a chromosome. They are assigned to homologous recombination pathways (HR) that require Rad52 and Rad51. In the first phase of HR, DNA damage is processed to form a single-strand DNA (ssDNA) region that is bound by ssDNA-binding replication protein A (RPA). RPA has an important role during recombination. Its primary role is to antagonize secondary structures in the ssDNA and favor formation of the active Rad51-ssDNA filament. Besides that function, RPA is able to bind the displaced strand in the D-loop and stabilize the invasion intermediate (Eggler et al., 2002). In the second phase, the Rad51-ssDNA filament performs a homology search and invades the donor DNA strand. The displacement loop (D-loop) is formed and within the D-loop the invading strand primes DNA synthesis. Motor protein Rad54 enhances D-loop formation by Rad51. In the third phase, the pathways of HR are distinguished. Subpathways of HR require specific protein cascades that have been only partially defined to date (Heyer et al., 2010):

- When only one homologous DNA strand is found, the D-loop is converted to a replication fork and cell choose the BIR pathway of repair. This process enables the repair of the chromosome, but leads to loss of heterozygosity of genetic information distal to the DSB.
- When both ends of the break interact with homologous sequences that are used as a template for repair, the predominant pathway for DSB repair is SDSA. The D-loop is reversed and allows the annealing of the newly synthesized strand with the resected strand of the donor end. This pathway avoids crossovers and reduces potential genomic rearrangements.
- Double Holliday junction pathways with crossover or noncrossover outcome are prone to noncrossover products in the vegetative cell cycle. Crossovers are primarily intended for meiotic formation of new combinations of genes. In vegetative cells, DNA repair is infrequently associated with crossovers, because crossovers can lead to deletions, inversions, or translocations when non-allelic or repeated sequences are present.

3.2 Chromatid cohesion and recombination mechanisms

Recombination mechanisms use a genetically similar DNA molecule, usually the sister chromatid, to repair damaged DNA and maintain the original sequence information. The sister chromatid cohesion complex plays an important role in DNA damage repair by recombination mechanisms, because cohesin holds the broken chromatid in close proximity to its intact sister chromatid, thereby supporting efficient repair. On formation of DSBs, cohesin even accumulates and forms new cohesive structures on chromatin that surrounds the break site. The ability of cohesin to establish new cohesion structures is essential for its role in DNA damage repair, possibly by physically stabilizing fragmented parts of the chromosome. Accumulation of cohesin is controlled by the DNA damage response and cohesin-regulating factors. Cohesion formation is limited to the S phase of the cell cycle, but DSBs can also trigger cohesion after DNA replication has been completed (Strom et al., 2007). It has been shown that damage-induced cohesion is also essential for recombinational repair in postreplicative cells. Cohesion is established genome-wide after induction of a single DSB. Thus, a cohesion establishment pathway exists that is independent of DNA duplication but required for DNA repair. Cohesin may act as a platform for the recruitment of checkpoint and DNA repair proteins and helps to translate checkpoint signals into DNA repair.

3.3 DNA synthesis during the recombination process

DNA synthesis is a part of the recombination process. After Rad51-mediated DNA strand invasion, DNA synthesis is a crucial step in recombination to restore the integrity of the chromosome. Motor protein Rad54, which stimulates D-loop formation, also promotes the dissociation of Rad51 from the heteroduplex after DNA strand invasion (Kiianitsa et al., 2006). Dissociation of Rad51 is required to allow access for DNA polymerases to prime DNA synthesis at the invading 3′ OH end. Repair DNA synthesis during the recombination process is similar to normal S-phase replication, but has specific properties:

- The DNA polymerases required for DNA synthesis in homologous recombination remain to be defined; DNA polymerases Pol δ (Lydeard et al., 2007; Maloisel et al., 2008) and Pol η (McIlwraith et al., 2005) have been proposed.
- Recently it was shown that PCNA, the sliding clamp that locks DNA polymerase onto dsDNA and promotes processive DNA replication, has a specific role in the initiation of recombination-associated DNA synthesis (Li et al., 2009). It was shown that PCNA is required for Pol δ recruiting to a D-loop and the extension of the 3'-end of the invading strand. PCNA and RFC are essential even to synthesize as little as 30 nucleotides following strand invasion (Holmes & Haber, 1999).
- DSB-induced gene conversion does not require lagging-strand components like Polα-primase complex and Cdc45, which is responsible for loading the Polα-primase complex onto chromatin during DNA replication (Wang et al., 2004). It has been proposed that new DNA synthesis is initiated through the leading-strand, using the 3′ end that was generated by resection, and that Rad51-mediated strand invasion is used as the primer end with primase activity. On the other hand, BIR do require lagging-strand components and major replicative DNA polymerases.
- Recombination mediated replication does not require initiation replication proteins or additional MCM (Minichromosome Maintenance complex) loading. Normal DNA replication requires formation of a pre-RC (pre-replicative complex) in early G_1. Cdc6

and Cdt1 bind to the chromatin binding ORC (origin recognition complex) and enable the recruitment of Mcm2-7. Cdc6 accumulates at the end of mitosis and disappears after the initiation of DNA replication, and Cdt1 accumulates in the nucleus during G_1 and is excluded from the nucleus for the rest of the cell cycle to prevent second-round replication. Furthermore, Mcm proteins are largely excluded from the nucleus in G_2 phase. Thus, ORC and pre-RC should not be required for DSB repair. This hypothesis was confirmed in DSB-induced gene conversion during *MAT* switching (Wang et al., 2004).

- DNA repair synthesis is not as efficient and processive as normal replication. The explanation for this reduced efficiency could be the lack of processive Mcm helicase.

3.4 Break induced replication

DSB repair by homologous recombination most often involves only a short section of new DNA synthesis. On the other hand, the BIR homologous recombination pathway includes the synthesis of very long tract of DNA; therefore, this pathway can be attributed to recombination-directed DNA replication. Break induced replication (BIR) is a homologous recombination pathway that is able to repair a DNA double strand break (DSB) when homology is restricted to one end. Recombination enables the formation of a unidirectional replication fork that leads to extensive replication and copies the donor chromatid to the end of the chromosome.

BIR requires leading and lagging strand replication machinery, all three major replicative DNA polymerases, including the otherwise nonessential Pol3 (subunit of Polδ), and recombination proteins Rad51 and Rad52. In contrast to other HR pathways, BIR also requires Cdc45, GINS, and Mcm2-7 that form the functional replicative DNA helicase; and initiation factor Cdt1 that recruits Mcm2-7 to the pre-RC (Lydeard et al., 2010). The origin recognition complex (ORC) and Cdc6, parts of the pre-replication complex (pre-RC) are not required, while initiation replication protein Cdc7 is required for BIR. BIR is an effective repair mechanism, characterized by origin-independent and recombination-dependent replication. The posttranslational modifications sumoylation and ubiquitination, have a special role in BIR. Siz1 mediated sumoylation and Rad18-mediated ubiquitination of the processivity clamp PCNA are involved in BIR, but not in gene conversion.

BIR can occur outside of the S phase (Bosco & Haber, 1998), but it is not yet known how replication machinery is then formed. In BIR, Mcm2-7 and Cdt1 have to cope with a single recombination fork, while outside of the S phase they are exported from the nucleus or degraded to prevent reinitiation of replication.

3.5 Replication and recombination in a radiation-resistant organism

Bacteria *Deinococcus radiodurans* is one of the most radiation-resistant organisms yet discovered. It is capable of surviving extremely high doses of acute (10,000 Gy) and chronic (60 Gy/hour) ionizing radiation and it is resistant to other DNA damaging conditions including exposure to desiccation, ultraviolet (UV) light, and hydrogen peroxide. It has been shown that the extraordinary robustness of *D.radiodurans* depends on efficient proteome protection (Krisko & Radman, 2010). Beside manganese accumulation and specific protein protection, survival depends on the efficient and rapid reconstitution of a functional genome from numerous DNA fragments. Recombinational repair with extensive DNA synthesis is used (Slade et al., 2009). DNA repair is primed by recombination proteins RecA and RadA, while the elongation step is performed by Pol III and PolI. Pol III activity appears to be a prerequisite for initiating DNA repair synthesis, whereas Pol I enables its continuation. Deinococcus radiodurans has more complementary or homologous DNA fragments to engage as repair partners, but otherwise the steps of repair are conspicuously normal (Galhardo & Rosenberg, 2009). The key repair mechanism is the combination of long tracts of newly synthesized DNA and homologous recombination.

4. Meiosis

The meiotic cell cycle in nature does not happen as often as vegetative cell cycle, but is even more special, difficult, and controlled. Meiosis is a complex developmental program that leads to the generation of haploid spores (gametes) from diploid cells. The central feature of meiosis is homologue pairing and meiotic interhomologue recombination that is enabled by meiosis-specific factors. After chromosome pairing and recombination, two successive segregations occur: MI is a reductional division, in which homologous chromosomes segregate and MII is an equational division, in which sister chromatid segregate. Meiotic recombination is essential for proper chromosome segregation at MI where homologous chromosomes are synapsed and then distributed to opposite poles.

4.1 Meiotic replication

It has been known for a long time that cohesion between homologs, which is essential for crossing over, is established during meiotic replication and that the length of meiotic replication is modified by recombination factors like Spo11 and Rec8. Recombination initiation is directly linked to meiotic replication. It has been shown that delaying meiotic replication also delays specific meiotic break formation and it has been suggested that DSB formation occurs as part of the process initiated by DNA replication (Borde et al., 2000). These facts lead to the conclusion that meiotic replication plays a fundamental role in the meiotic recombination process.

The meiotic replication program is generally quite similar to that of the vegetative cell cycle: the same origins of replication and the same replicative machinery are used (Budd et al., 1989). But there are specific features that distinguish mitotic and meiotic replication. The most noticeable feature is a protracted meiotic replication that is universally several times longer than mitotic replication in the same organisms. The difference has been proposed to be related to the process of laying down specialized chromosome features utilized at later stages for interhomolog interactions; the progression of the S-phase might be directly coupled to this (Cha et al., 2000). Pairing of homologues is a complex process that is essential in meiosis but not required in mitosis; thus, it is not surprising that DNA replication and preparing for the next phase in meiosis takes more time.

4.1.1 Mum2 in meiosis

The study of the Mum2 protein reveals a direct correlation between the level of meiotic DSBs and DNA replication (Davis et al., 2001), which was suggested on the basis of the observation that a delay in replication results in a similar delay in DSB formation (Borde et al., 2000). Mum2 is essential for meiotic replication, but it is not required for mitotic DNA replication. Its role in meiotic replication is not clear; however, synthetic interactions with the ORC complex and polymerase α-primase suggest that it is involved in the functioning of the replication machinery. It was shown that in *mum2* mutants, chromosome pairing and synapsis occur, although at reduced levels compared to wild type, but meiotic recombination is greatly impaired. Meiotic gene expression, pairing, and synapsis were only partly reduced in *mum2* mutants, thus it was suggested that the reduction in DNA replication is directly responsible for the reduced level of DSBs and meiotic recombination (Davis et al., 2001).

4.1.2 Ime2 in meiotic replication

Ime2 is an essential meiotic protein that links DNA replication with the following phases of the meiotic cell cycle that follow it. IME2 belongs to early meiotic genes that are regulated by Ime1, while Ime2 is the key protein for the transcription of the middle genes. The transcription of the late genes is indirectly dependent on Ime1, Ime2, and Ndt80. The early genes are those which encode proteins involved in DNA replication, synapsis of homologs and meiotic recombination, whereas the middle genes encode proteins required for nuclear division and spore formation. Correlation between meiotic DNA replication and nuclear division is regulated by an early meiosis-specific gene. Ime2, which controls both initiation of premeiotic DNA replication and the transcription of *NDT80*, has a key role in the correlation between premeiotic DNA replication and nuclear division. It was also demonstrated that Ime2 functions as a negative regulator of Clb-Cdc28 (Gurevich & Kassir, 2010).

4.1.3 Clb5,Clb6–Cdc28 in meiotic replication

Many proteins with a role in meiotic replication and recombination are phosphorylated suggesting that kinases could play an important role in coordinating both processes. Kinases Clb5,6-Cdc28 and Cdc7-Dbf4, which initiate meiotic replication and DSB formation could have a key coordination role (Wan et al., 2008).

Clb5,Clb6–cyclin-dependent kinase (Clb5,6-Cdc28) is the principal activator of the S phase in the vegetative cell cycle, but the absence of Clb5 and Clb6 confers only a delay in the initiation of replication. They are replaced by functionally related B-type cyclins Clb1 and Clb4 (Schwob et al., 1994). In contrast, Clb5 and Clb6 are essential for the initiation of meiotic replication; in the *clb5clb6* double mutant, meiotic replication is not detectable (Stuart & Wittenberg, 1998). Beside its role in initiating DNA replication, Clb5,6-Cdc28 also has a crucial role in the promotion of DSB formation in meiosis. Mutants *clb5* and *clb5clb6* but not *clb6* are defective in DSB induction and SC formation (Smith et al., 2001). DSBs are formed by Spo11 protein and accessory factors like Mer2. It has been shown that Clb5,6-Cdc28 phosphorylate Mer2 and that this phosphorylation modulates interactions of Mer2 with other DSB proteins and is critical for DSB formation (Henderson et al., 2006).

4.1.4 Cdc7 kinase in meiosis

Cdc7 is an essential kinase that forms complexes with the regulator Dbf4, the levels of which fluctuate during the cell cycle. Cdc7 is a key regulator of meiosis, because it is required for the initiation of DNA replication, for meiotic recombination, for regulation of the *NDT80* promoter, and for proper recruitment to kinetochores.

In the vegetative cell cycle, phosphorylation of the MCM complex by Cdc7p-Dbf4 activates DNA replication. Loss of Cdc7 function affects initiation at all origins, even at late origins (Bousset & Diffley, 1998). An allosteric model has been proposed in which phosphorylation of Mcm2 by Cdc7p-Dbf4 confers an allosteric change on Mcm5p and produces an active, 'rolling' MCM helicase that can move with the replication fork (Sclafani, 2000). As in mitosis, the Cdc7-Dbf4 complex is essential for initiation of DNA replication during meiosis (Valentin et al., 2006).

Besides the role in initiation of meiotic replication, Cdc7 kinase also has a role in the meiotic recombination. It has been shown that Cdc7 is essential for meiotic DSBs and meiosis I progression. Cdc7 enables phosphorylation of the DSB protein, Mer2. It has been proposed that Cdc7 regulates Spo11 loading to DSBs by Mer2 phosphorylation (Sasanuma et al., 2008). In meosis, Cdc7 kinase also provides the link between replication and chromosome segregation. It has been shown that Cdc7 promotes meiotic progression by enabling transcription of *NDT80*; in addition it is required for mono-orientation of sister kinetochores in MI by allowing recruitment of the monopolin subunit, Mam1, onto kinetochores (Lo et al., 2008).

4.2 Recombination in meiosis

The unique features of meiosis are homologue pairing and inter-homologue recombination that is initiated by double-strand breaks. The specific feature of meiotic recombination is the presence of meiosis specific factors that influence the mitotic recombination machinery to use the homologous chromosome instead of a sister-chromatid as the recombination template and to counteract mitotic favorization of non-crossover outcomes.

Meiotic recombination occurs during the extended prophase. In contrast to mitotic recombination, meiotic recombination is genetically programmed and induced by Spo11-catalyzed DSBs. Therefore, in meiosis there is an additional source of DSBs that requires active recombination to be resolved. DSBs are resected to expose 3' single strand overhangs by the Mre11-Rad50-Xrs2 complex and endonuclease Sae2. Overhangs of ssDNA can load Rad51 and meiosis-specific recombinase Dmc1 to form nucleoprotein filaments that catalyze strand invasion on the homologous chromosome (Hayase et al., 2004). In contrast to mitotic cells, meiosis-initiated DSBs are repaired using the homologous chromosome, not the sister chromatid, as a template for repair. Strand invasion generates DNA synthesis and ligation that result in the formation of double Holliday junction structures (dHJ). dHJ generated between homologs are resolved by structure-specific endonucleases. Homologous recombination products (crossovers and non-crossovers) are formed. While crossovers (Cos) absolutely require double a Holliday junction (dHJ) intermediate, non-crossovers (NCOs) can occur by synthesis-dependent strand annealing (SDS) or by special cleavage of dHJ. The resolution of dHJ depends on structure-specific endonucleases. COs preferentially occur at hot spots that are influenced by DNA sequence and higher order chromosome structures, but are strongly suppressed in large chromosomal regions near the telomeres, centromeres, rRNA genes, and Ty elements (Petes, 2001). COs are associated with reciprocal exchanges of chromosome arms and promote accurate chromosome segregation in MI, while non-crossovers are not. Because of its key role in meiosis, crossover outcome is tightly controlled. At least one CO is formed per chromosome pair and a crossover in one region makes it less likely that another will be found nearby (crossover interference). The COs/NCOs ratio can change to maintain COs. It has been shown that COs tend to be maintained in *spo11* mutants with reduced DSBs at the expense of NCOs (Martini et al., 2006). Spo11 is loaded to DNA after homolog pairing; therefore, crossover control is likely based in earlier processes.

It has been shown that noncrossover products are formed at the same time as dHJ intermediates, while crossovers appear later, when dHJ intermediates are resolved (Allers &

Lichten, 2001). *ndt80* mutants arrest with unresolved dHJ intermediates and very few crossovers, while noncrossover heteroduplex products are formed at normal levels and with normal timing. These results suggest that crossovers are formed by resolution of dHJ intermediates, while most noncrossover recombinants arise by a different, earlier pathway and that dHJ resolution is under control of meiosis-specific transcription factor Ndt80. Noncrossover recombinants are most probably formed by SDSA, where the invading strand is not captured but is instead displaced. The other possibility is that dHJ intermediates are differentiated at an early stage and intermediates of noncrossovers are resolved very rapidly. The latter pathway of noncrossover formation through dHJ is less possible and cells probably use it only as an alternative pathway when crossovers could not be carried out.

4.2.1 ZMM proteins

ZMM proteins are components of SC (Zip1, Zip2, Zip3, Zip4), mutS homologues (Msh4, Msh5), and meoisis specific DNA helicase Mer3 (Borner et al., 2004). ZMM proteins play a crucial role in crossover formation; despite efficient initiation of recombination, crossovers are reduced or absent in *zmm* mutants. Elimination of crossovers is not due to reduced DSBs formation, because DSBs accumulate to wild-type levels in *zmm* mutants. The formation of NCOc is independent of ZMM proteins. Thus, ZMM are specifically required for formation of COs. ZMM proteins interact with recombination proteins, e.g. Mre11, Rad51, and Rad57 (Agarwal & Roeder, 2000). In meiosis there are two types of COs: one type of CO that is dependent on the activities of ZMM proteins and a second type of CO that is ZMM-independent. COs are not randomly assigned, but mostly they do not occur in adjacent chromosomal regions; this property is called CO-interference. The ZMM-dependent COs represent the majority of COs in yeast and are subject to interference, while ZMM-independent COs do not exhibit interference.

ZMM proteins are essential for the assembly of SC formation; Zip1 is an integral component of the SC. They play an important role in coordination between molecular recombination events and assembly of the SC.

The exact function of ZMM proteins in meiosis still remains to be clarified; although they probably affect strand invasion.

4.2.2 Synaptonemal complex

Meiotic recombination depends on the development of the meiosis-specific chromosome structure synaptonemal complex (SC). SC is a protein network that pairs homolog chromosomes along their entire length and holds them together. The cohesion complex consists of one filament (lateral elements) on each homologue and central elements linking lateral elements a in ladder like structure. Central elements contain various proteins, including Zip1 (Sym et al., 1993) and SUMO (Cheng et al., 2006). Lateral elements contain meiosis-specific proteins, e.g. Red1, Hop1, Mek1/Mre4, and a cohesion complex that is similar to the mitotic sister chromatid cohesion complex, only that SCC1 is replaced by Rec8 in meiosis (Xu et al., 2005). It has been shown that meiosis-specific kinase Mek1 suppresses meiotic intersister DSB repair by working directly on sister chromatids and that Mek1 acts on Rad51-specific recombination processes (Callender & Hollingsworth, 2010).

4.2.3 Cdc28 in meiotic recombination

Most components of SCs including Zip1, Hop1, Red1, Mre4, and Rec8 are phosphoproteins, although the functional significance of this phosphorylation remains to be characterized

(Zhu et al., 2010). It was shown recently that phosphorylation of Red1 is carried out in Cdc28-dependent and Cdc28-independent manners and that Red1 phosphorylation is independent of meiotic DNA recombination (Lai et al., 2011). Cdc28 is the only CDC (cyclin dependent kinase) in *S.cerevisiae* and plays the main role in cell cycle regulation. From G1 to S phase and in S phase Cdc28 is bound to B-type cyclins Clb5,6-Cdc28 and this complex plays a role in entry into the pre-mitotic and pre-meiotic S-phase. But in meiosis, the Clb5,6-Cdc28 complex also has a role in the recombination process. It regulates DSBs formation by phosphorylation of Mer2, a protein that is bound to Spo11 (Henderson et al., 2006). Mre11-Rad50-Xrs2 complex and Sae2 endonuclease are necessary to remove the covalently attached Spo11 from the DNA ends. It was shown that phosphorylation of Sae2 by Cdc28 is required to initiate meiotic DSB resection by allowing Spo11 removal from DSB ends (Manfrini et al., 2010). Cdc28 is required for the processing of DSBs by providing a mechanism for coordinating DSB resection with progression through the meiotic prophase. But localization of Clb5,6-Cdc28 is independent of DSB formation and is rather dependent on meiosis-specific chromosome components such as Red1, Hop1, and a cohesin subunit Rec8. Recently it was found that compromised Cdc28 activity in the meiotic prophase leads to defective SC formation without affecting DSB formation suggesting that CDK-dependent phosphorylation regulates formation of SC (Zhu et al., 2010). Clb5,6-Cdc28 obviously promotes not only the onset of premeiotic DNA replication but also the formation of meiotic DSBs and SC formation.

4.2.4 Ime2 in meiotic recombination

During meiosis, Ime2, a meiosis-specific protein kinase, assumes some function of the Cdc28 complexes. Ime2 is required for critical events in meiosis, including DNA replication (section 3.1.2.). Transition from G_1 to S phase is prohibited by the Clb5,6-Cdc28 inhibitor Sic1 in both mitosis and meiosis. In mitosis, inactivation of Sic1 by phosphorylation is catalyzed by the Cln1,2-Cdc28 complex (Nash et al., 2001), while in meiosis it is catalyzed by Ime2 (Dirick et al., 1995). Ime2 is obviously required for the initiation of DNA replication in meiosis. On the other hand, Ime2 interacts with RPA, a complex required for stabilization of ssDNA during replication and recombination. In meiosis, Ime2 is required for full RPA phosphorylation (Clifford et al., 2005), thus Ime2 affects meiotic recombination processes as well.

4.2.5 Kinases Mec1 and Tel1 in meiotic recombination

Mec1 (hATR) is an essential protein that mediates two important functions: S-phase checkpoint responses (2.1.) and meiotic recombination. Kinases Mec1 and Tel1 phosphorylate the axial element protein Hop1 and promote meiotic recombination using an intact homologous non-sister chromatid rather than a sister chromatid (Carballo et al., 2008). Without this specific phosphorylation, meiotic DSBs are repaired via a Dmc1-independent intersister repair pathway, resulting in diminished interhomolog crossing-over. Phosphorylation of Hop1 by Mec1/Tel1 is required for activation of Mek1, a meiotic paralogue of the DNA-damage effector kinase, Rad53p.

It was proposed that Mec1 and Tel1 also modulate the switch from the open to closed state of telomeres (Dubrana et al., 2001). Telomeres are not elongated every cell cycle. They can switch to an open state for telomerase recruitment.

4.2.6 Mre11 in meiotic recombination

The Mre11-Rad50-Xrs2 complex is required for the initiation of meiotic recombination - for programmed DSBs catalyzed by Spo11 and for break end resection, which is a key step in homologous recombination. It has been proposed that Mre11 assembles on the DSB sites and ensures a link between DSB formation and the processing of break ends (Borde et al., 2004).

4.2.7 Spo11 and Rec8 in meiosis

The Spo11 protein is the catalytic subunit of the meiotic DSB transesterase and is directly responsible for the initiation of meiotic recombination. Rec8 is a meiosis-specific protein required for meiotic sister chromatid cohesion and meiotic recombination. It has been shown that recombination proteins Spo11 and Rec8 also play distinct roles in meiotic DNA replication (Cha et al., 2000). They modulate the progression of meiotic replication: the mutation of *spo11* decreases the length of the S phase, while mutation of *rec8* increases the length of the S phase. It was proposed that meiotic S-phase progression is linked directly to the development of specific chromosomal features required for meiotic interhomolog interactions. During the process of meiotic replication, the future DSB sites are probably marked. The time delay between replication and DSBs may reflect the time required to assemble the proper protein complexes at the target sites.

5. Common problem: DNA unfolding

Organization of DNA sequences into a chromatin structure represents a barrier to processes acting on DNA, like replication and recombination. During these processes chromatin structure has to be remodeled and reestablished after DNA replication and repair. Replication and recombination need access to the sequence in the interior of the double helix DNA and both require DNA topoisomerase to unwind the DNA helix, DNA helicase to open the DNA helix, and ssDNA-binding protein to protect single stranded DNA.

5.1 DNA topoisomerase and DNA helicase

Topoisomerases are enzymes that are able to unwind and wind DNA. They bind to DNA and cut the phosphate backbone of the DNA, the DNA molecule can then untangle, and the untangled DNA is reconnected. Thus, their function in replication, transcription, and recombination is essential. In *S. cerevisiae*, there are three types of topoisomerases: Top1 and Top2 that relax positively and negatively supercoiled DNA, and Top3 that relaxes single-stranded negatively-supercoiled DNA.

Helicases are able to separate strands of the DNA double helix using energy from ATP hydrolysis and are also required for replication, transcription, and recombination. Helicases Sgs1, Srs2, Rrm3, Dna2, and Rad3 form a complex interacting network with other DNA replication and recombination proteins to preserve genomic integrity. Sgs1 and Srs2 are involved in genome integrity maintenance and meiotic recombination; Rrm3 is involved in telomere and rDNA replication, and Ty1 transposition; nuclease and helicase Dna2 is required for Okazaki fragment processing and DNA repair; Rad3 is involved in nucleotide excision repair and transcription (SGD; http://www.yeastgenome.org/).

Sgs1 is a helicase of the RecQ family, similar to human BLM and WRN proteins that are implicated in Bloom and Werner syndromes. Sgs1 interacts with many proteins and has very complex function, which is a good example of the cooperation between replication and recombination.

- Sgs1 and Srs2 helicases control distinct pathways of HR during DNA replication and the restart of stalled replication forks. Recombination-dependent cruciform structures are formed on damaged chromatids and Sgs1 and Srs2 counteract their formation (Liberi et al., 2005). It was shown that the double mutation *sgs1srs2* leads to a synthetic growth defect and that a mutation in *rad51* fully rescues the *sgs1 srs2* synthetic defect (Gangloff et al., 2000). It was therefore concluded that defects in *sgs1 srs2* mutants are caused by misregulated HR during DNA replication.
  During regulation of HR, Sgs1 functions in a complex with Top3 and Rmi1, a DNA-binding protein with a preference for cruciform structures (Mullen et al., 2005). The Sgs1-Top3-Rmi1 complex is crucial for resolution of recombination intermediates such as Holliday junctions. The complex interacts with recombination protein Rad51. It was shown that Rad51 helps recruit Sgs1-Top3 to sites of replicative damage (Shor et al., 2002).
- During meiosis Sgs1 negatively regulates not all HR mechanisms, but specifically crossovers (Rockmill et al., 2003). The mutation *sgs1* leads to an increase in closely spaced crossovers without an increase in non-crossover products (Oh et al., 2007). The anti-crossover activity of Sgs1 is opposed by the pro-crossover activities of the ZMM proteins. Srs2 play a similar role as Sgs1. Double mutants *sgs1srs2* increase crossovers and overexpression of SRS2 nearly eliminates crossovers (Ira et al., 2003). Sgs1 and Srs2 obviously regulate the processing of recombination intermediates during DNA replication and promote non-crossover products.
  Sgs1 also functions in a Sgs1-Top3-Rmi1 complex during meiosis. Mutants *spo11* that have no recombination between homologous chromosomes, still form viable spores if there is also a *top3* mutation (Gangloff et al., 1999). This result indicates that Top3 is required to complete recombination successfully.
- Sgs1 has a direct role in the DNA damage response during mitotic DNA replication. Sgs1 is one of the components of the S-phase checkpoint response, which senses DNA damage or a blocked fork progression during DNA replication (Frei & Gasser, 2000). Sgs1 associates with signal-transducing kinase Rad53 in S-phase-specific foci.
- Sgs1 interacts with the Top2 topoisomerase, which is the major mitotic post-replication decatenase. In *top2* mutants, chromosomes segregate improperly, leading to chromosome loss and disomy. Because Sgs1 acts along the same pathway as Top2, it has been suggested that Sgs1-Top2 is important for the decatenation of sister chromosomes (Watt et al., 1995). In meiosis, the Sgs1-Top2 complex has the similar role.

5.2 ssDNA-binding protein

Replication protein A (RPA) binds strongly and in long clusters to ssDNA and form a nucleoprotein filament. Because of its protective function on ssDNA ends, RPA has a central role in DNA repair, meiotic recombination, and also in replication checkpoints.

RPA recruits checkpoint kinase Mec1 (hATR) to ssDNA. Such activated Mec1 further phosphorylates its substrates during the DNA damage checkpoint response. It has been proposed that RPA is needed to determine the severity of DNA damage and also to initiate a full checkpoint response (Pellicioli et al., 2001). DNA damage and the extent of ssDNA are probably monitored by the binding of the RPA to ssDNA (Lee et al., 1998).

6. Post-translational modifications

Post-translational modifications, with their key role in controlling protein function, play an important role in the maintenance of genome integrity. Sumoylation, phosphorylation, and ubiquitination are especially important for the operation of replication and recombination proteins in order for them to execute their functions in a rapid and efficient manner. While ubiquitination leads in most cases to proteasomal degradation of the target protein, there are also many non-proteolytic functions of ubiquitin (Ulrich & Walden, 2010). Monoubiquitylation is not directed at proteolysis; it often reveals a new binding domain. Polyubiquitin chains that are linked through distinct Lys residues of ubiquitin also have functions that are independent of proteolysis; they might activate kinases or provide protein interaction changes (Hicke et al., 2005). Non-proteolytic functions of monoubiquitylation and polyubiquitylation are particularly important in the control of the DNA damage response and DNA repair pathways. The small ubiquitin-like modifier (SUMO), which modifies proteins by regulation of their protein-protein interactions, allows the assembly and disassembly of protein complexes to be modulated. Sumoylation and ubiquitination both occur as the result of sequential action of specific enzymes: activating enzyme (E1), conjugating enzyme (E2), and ligase (E3). SUMO and ubiquitin are covalently attached to the target protein; sometimes it is the same lysine residue of a target protein that can be alternatively modified by either SUMO or ubiquitin. Phosphorylation, the addition of a phosphate group (PO4) to a target protein, results in a conformational change in the protein and consequently leads to its altered activity. Reversible phosphorylation is catalysed by kinases (phosphorylation) and phosphatases (dephosphorylation). Beside its central post-translational role, phosphorylation is also a regulator of the SUMO pathway (Hietakangas et al., 2006).

Here are some examples of post-translational modifications of replication and recombination factors:

- RecQ helicase Sgs1 is specifically sumoylated under the stress of DNA double strand breaks (Lu et al., 2010). SUMO together with the Sgs1-Top3 complex counteracts the accumulation of crucial intermediates at replication forks during replication resumption processes (Branzei et al., 2006). Sumoylation of Sgs1 at K621 is uniquely required for its role in telomere–telomere recombination for Type II cells.
- Repair proteins yKu70, Smc5, and Smc6 are modified by SUMO (Zhao & Blobel, 2005). Smc5 is sumoylated by Mms21 SUMO ligase in response to DNA damage and forms a complex with Smc6 that has a role in DNA repair and segregation of repetitive chromosome regions (Cost & Cozzarelli, 2006).
- In the NHEJ pathway the Nej1 protein recruits anti-recombinogenic helicase Srs2 to DSB repressing HR and favoring NHEJ or SSA. Interaction between Nej1 and Srs2 is enhanced by phosphorylation of Nej1 (Carter et al., 2009).
- Phosphorylation of Sae2, a nuclease that regulates DNA end resection in mitotic and meiotic cells, determines whether a DSB is channelled into NHEJ or HR (Huertas et al., 2008).
- Nuclease Exo1 that generates ssDNA is regulated by phosphorylation. Rad53-dependent phosphorylation reduces Exo1 activity (Morin et al., 2008).
- Rad51 has a central role in HR. Human Rad51 is phosphorylated in response to HU. Its phosphorylation has an activating role (Sorensen et al., 2005).
- Rad52 is sumoylated after DNA damage and during meiosis and this sumoylation is essential for activating HR and SSA (Sacher et al., 2006). Rad52 is excluded from the

nucleolus containing rDNA repeats to diminish the negative effect of HR in repetitive sequences. Cells with mutated Rad52, which cannot interact with SUMO, form foci within the nucleolus, resulting in slightly elevated rDNA recombination (Torres-Rosell et al., 2007).

- Several components of the replication fork including Mrc1 are phosphorylated after fork stalling, including Mrc1, which plays roles in both the S phase checkpoint and at the replication fork. Phosphorylation of Mrc1 is required for activation of the Rad53 kinase during the S phase checkpoint but is not required for DNA replication (Lou et al., 2008).
- Phosphorylation of histone H3 has a role in DNA replication. Phosphorylation of H3 Thr45 is mediated by the kinase Cdc7–Dbf4. It has been shown that Thr45 phosphorylation peaks during DNA replication and that the loss of this phosphorylation site causes phenotypes consistent with replicative defects (Baker et al., 2010).
- Topoisomerase Top2 cleavage and re-sealing of the phosphodiester backbone is required for replication and recombination processes. It has been shown that sumoylation is essential for Top2 functioning (Bachant et al., 2002).
- Kinetochore proteins Ndc10, Bir1, Ndc80, Cep3 were also shown to be sumoylated (Montpetit et al., 2006).

Of particular interest are the post-translational modifications of proteins like PCNA that directly connect replication and recombination processes. Sumoylation and different types of ubiquitination on PCNA activate a different set of functions to deal with particular types of replication stresses:

- PCNA is essential in DNA replication and DNA repair. It is loaded on chromatids and functions as a processivity factor for DNA polymerases and other proteins that regulate replication-associated processes. Sumoylation and ubiquitination of PCNA both occur in the S phase: sumoylation during normal S-phase and ubiquitination following DNA damage. Sumoylation of PCNA prevents unwanted recombination repair during DNA replication. PCNA sumoylation favors physical interactions with anti-recombinogenic helicase Srs2 and replication forks (Papouli et al., 2005; Pfander et al., 2005). Helicase Srs2 inhibits recombination by disrupting Rad1 nucleoprotein filaments from ssDNA (Veaute et al., 2003). DNA damage induces mono- or poli-ubiquitination of PCNA. Monoubiquitination of PCNA favors interaction with translesion DNA polymerases and promotes error-prone translesion synthesis, while polyubiquitination on the same residue promotes error-free damage repair, which relies on recombination mechanisms (Hoege et al., 2002). Poliubiquitination with recombination repair is favored over monoubiquitination.

7. Telomere: DNA replication can be replaced by recombination

Telomeres are nucleoprotein structures at the ends of eukaryotic chromosomes. They play a crucial role in maintaining genomic stability by providing chromosome-end protection. Telomeric DNA with repetitive guanine-rich DNA sequences is able to form protective t-loop and G-quartet structures; and together with interacting specific proteins, form a protective 'cap' that distinguish telomeres from DNA double-strand breaks (Simonsson, 2001).

Telomeres are duplicated by special DNA replication using a specific DNA polymerase, telomerase. When this special telomere replication is unavailable, DNA recombination at telomeres can be replaced by recombination mechanisms.

7.1 Telomere DNA replication

Because of single-stranded 3′ overhangs and bound proteins, telomeres are specifically replicated by telomerase. Telomerase is a DNA polymerase that is specifically dedicated to the replication of chromosome ends. It is composed of several components: a reverse transcriptase catalytic subunit - RNA that provides a template for DNA synthesis, an Est2 catalytic subunit, and additional associated proteins, Est1 and Est3. Cdc13 ssDNA telomere binding protein is a key factor in telomerase recruitment. The telomere binding Ku heterodimer (Ku70,80) with its role in the maintenance of telomere DNA structure also plays a positive role in the Cdc13p-dependent recruitment of telomerase. It also stimulates telomerase activity after telomerase is bound to the telomere. The telomere binding protein Rap1 is involved in telomere length regulation and telomeric silencing; Rap1p in complex with Rif1 and Rif2 forms a higher-order structures that is part of a system for telomere length measurement (Ji et al., 2008).

Telomerase activity has been detected throughout the entire cell cycle, but telomere elongation is restricted to late S phase when replication machinery is available. It has been shown that telomere elongation is coincident with normal DNA replication; telomerase action is tightly co-regulated with conventional replication (Diede & Gottschling, 1999).

As regards replication of sub-telomeric regions, there are no converging forks that would complete replication when forks collapse. In sub-telomeric regions, DNA repair mechanisms are absolutely required to restart the collapsed fork.

7.2 Telomere maintenance by recombination

Without telomerase, telomeres shorten with replication and signal cell senescence. The final consequence of telomere erosion is the loss of capping proteins, which leaves telomeres exposed to DNA repair mechanisms, potentially inappropriate recombination events or end-to-end fusion (Blackburn, 2000). However, rare survivors bypass senescence and death. Homologous recombination (HR) could slow senescence and support the growth of the rare survivors. HR is suppressed where telomere sequences are of normal length; however, telomere recombination is allowed when telomeres erode in the absence of telomerase activity or incomplete replication. Most human malignant cells become immortalized by telomere extension due to the activation of telomerase, while about 10% of human cancers activate a recombination-mediated elongation, the so-called alternative lengthening of telomeres (ALT). Recombination mechanisms in budding yeast that enable telomere elongation in the absence of telomerase are analogous to ALT (Lydeard et al., 2007). There are two types of survivors when telomerase is absent and both depend on the Rad52 recombination protein (Chen et al., 2001). Type I cells exhibit the amplification of Y′ sequences and have very short telomere repeats on the chromosome ends. They depend on Rad51, Rad54, Rad55, Rad57 proteins, like DSB repair by HR. Type I cells show accelerated loss of viability. Type II cells exhibit extremely elongated and heterogeneous telomere repeats and only modest Y' amplification. They depend on Rad50, Mre11, and Xrs2 proteins, like DSB repair by SSA. Type II cells show a slower rate of senescence. It was shown that Type II cells with long telomere repeats and dependence on Rad50, resemble human ALT cells (Dunham et al., 2000). Type II cells are as efficient as wild type in maintaining cell survival. Telomere recombination is as efficient as telomerase, but cells using recombination for telomere maintenance instead of replication by telomerase had a shortened replicative life span or accelerated cellular aging (Chen et al., 2009b). In the absence of telomerase and both recombination pathways, cells fail to produce survivors.

It has been shown that short telomere is the preferred substrate of telomerase and is also sufficient to recruit recombination proteins; on the other hand, ssDNA at telomeres does not appear to be sufficient to attract recombination proteins (Pennaneach et al., 2006). The Rad52- Cdc13 focus is found to colocalize with short telomeres in 50% of cells. It has been proposed that a burst of resection at a single telomere marks the transition between recombination-resistant and recombination-prone states at telomeres.

Telomeres bind numerous DNA repair and damage checkpoint proteins as DSBs, but they activate neither DNA repair nor DNA damage checkpoint pathways. Paradoxically DNA repair and checkpoint proteins do still play critical roles in telomere stability (Lydall, 2003).

8. Ecm11, yeast protein with a role in replication and recombination

Ecm11 is a protein of the budding yeast *S.cerevisiae.* The predicted *ECM11* gene product has 302 amino acids and shows no significant similarity to any other protein in the databases. From the microarray hybridization data available in the Stanford Genome Database (SGD; http://www.yeastgenome.org/), it is apparent that the *ECM11* transcript does not oscillate during the cell cycle, but is significantly elevated during meiosis. It was confirmed that the level of protein Ecm11 is in accordance with the mRNA: the level of Ecm11 protein is low in mitosis, but high in meiosis (Zavec et al., 2008). The highest level of Ecm11 is in the early-middle phase of sporulation. The central, unique features of meiosis are homologue pairing, interhomologue recombination, and synaptonemal complex formation. These regulated events are expected to use meiosis-specific regulators and this was the supposed role of Ecm11. In our previous work we have demonstrated that Ecm11 is indeed required in meiosis (Zavec et al., 2004). Mutants *ecm11Δ* exhibit complex defects in meiotic replication and recombination: diminished meiotic DNA synthesis, reduced crossing over, increased gene conversion events and reduced levels of sporulation and spore viability (Fig. 2).

8.1 Ecm11 has important role in meiotic recombination

ECM11 showed an early to middle pattern of induction in meiosis. There are three groups of meiotic genes with the nearly identical expression pattern as *ECM11*: the meiotic recombination genes such as *MND1* and *REC114*, the synaptonemal complex genes such as *RED1* and *MSH4*, and the meiotic specific cohesion gene *REC8* (SGD; http://www.yeastgenome.org/). Such an expression pattern of *ECM11* indicates that Ecm11 could have a role in meiotic recombination process. It has been shown that *ecm11* homozygous diploid strains sporulate more slowly and less efficiently than wild type strains and that the viability of spores was reduced to 50% (Zavec et al., 2004). Using recombination tests, it was shown that *ECM11* is required for crossing over, but not for gene conversion.

8.1.1 The *ecm11* mutation affects sporulation efficiency

In the homozygous *ecm11* mutants, a delay in sporulation was observed and there was about a 30% reduction in the maximal level of asci obtained, compared to the isogenic wild

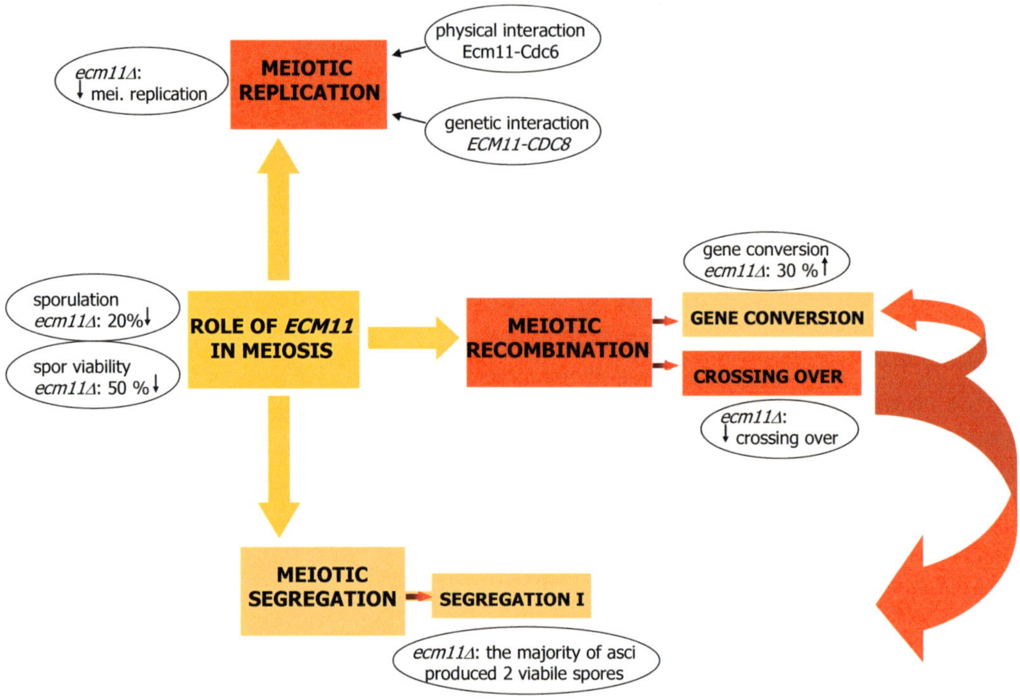

Fig. 2. The role of yeast protein Ecm11: mutants *ecm11Δ* exhibit complex defects in meiotic replication and recombination: diminished meiotic DNA synthesis, reduced crossing over, increased gene conversion events and reduced levels of sporulation and spore viability.

type strain. Heterozygous strains yielded slightly higher sporulation efficiency *ecm11* mutants. Wild type strains carrying additional *ECM11* on the centromeric plasmid also showed reduced sporulation efficiency comparing to wild types. Obviously, sporulation efficiency depends on the copy number of Ecm11 protein in the cell during meiosis. Since more Ecm11 than usual in the cell leads to lower sporulation efficiency, Ecm11 is probably a part of a heterologous protein complex that requires the correct balance among these proteins.

The kinetics of the sporulation process shows that spores appeared about four hours later in *ecm11* mutants than in wild type. Both strains complete sporulation at the same time, but *ecm11* strains produce lowers level of asci. Since deletion of *ECM11* resulted in reduced meiotic process progression with reduced maximal level of asci, Ecm11 was defined as a positive effector of meiosis.

8.1.2 Ecm11 is required for crossing over, but not for gene conversion

Asci of the parental MAS and homozygous *ecm11* mutants were dissected and compared. In the parental strain, 98% of spores germinated after dissection, while only 50% spores of the *ecm11* mutants survived. Beside strongly reduced spore viability in the *ecm11* mutants, a strongly elevated fraction of tetrads exhibiting two viable spores in *ecm11* mutants was observed (Zavec et al., 2004). The majority of *ecm11* asci (56%) produced only two viable spores, while only 1% of such asci were observed in the parental strain. This result shows non-disjunction of homologous chromosomes at the first meiotic division.

Crossing over frequency was measured in two-viable-spores asci in the *ecm11* strain. In 84% of asci both surviving spores had the same URA phenotype, indicating that both functional spores inherited sister chromatids. Obviously, *ECM11* is required for crossing over. Additionally, since in meiosis I homologous chromatids are separated, the effect of Ecm11 in fidelity of chromosome segregation can be confined to meiosis I. Surprisingly, the results of the return-to-growth experiment showed slightly increased gene conversion events in *ecm11* mutants. This result raises the possibility that *ecm11* mutation impairs the crossover process at an early step of recombination, at the differentiation of intermediates into crossovers or non-crossovers.

The *ECM11* gene is required to produce a normal level of crossover, but not noncrossover events, just like genes required for synaptonemal complex formation (*ZIP1, ZIP2, ZIP3*), mutS homologues (*MSH4, MSH5*), some mismatch repair genes (*MLH1, MLH3, EXO1*) and meoisis specific DNA helicase *MER3* (Borner et al., 2004). So, Ecm11 must belong to the specific set of proteins that are required for crossing over. Mutants of some of those genes (*msh5, mer3, zip1, zip2, zip3*) exhibit normal levels of double-strand breaks and noncrossover products but strong coordinate defects in single-end invasions, double Holliday junctions and crossover products, thus implying that those mutants are specifically defective in the formation and functioning of single-end invasions (Borner et al., 2004).

As proper segregation of homologous chromosomes during the reductional division of meiosis does not require gene conversion, but does require crossing over to establish chiasmata, which physically connect homologues after disassembly of the synaptonemal complex, inappropriate segregation of chromosomes in *ecm11* mutants could be due to reduced crossing over in those cells.

8.2 *ECM11* is required for meiotic DNA replication

To determine if deletion of *ECM11* influences meiotic replication, the DNA content of yeast cells was analysed by flow cytometry. FACS analysis show that the fraction of *ecm11* mutants entering S phase is reduced compared to the wild type. The *ecm11* mutants enter S phase at the same time as wild type cells, but it is less efficient in the knockout strain. The replication process was the most intense between the second and the fourth hour of sporulation. In this period, the percentage of 4N cells in the wild type cell population increased by 36%, while in the mutant cells this increase was only 18%. The hindrance of DNA replication caused by the deletion of the *ECM11* gene may be due to many reasons: the lower efficiency of origin firing, the lower progression of DNA replication or as a consequence of modifications in some other meiotic process. Based on our FACS data we cannot exclude any of these possibilities. Since, in all strains tested, deletion of the *ECM11* gene has no impact on generation time during vegetative growth, we assume that the effect of the *ecm11* mutation on S phase is limited to meiosis.

In the two-hybrid screen it was found that Ecm11 strongly interacts with an essential protein Cdc6, which has a pivotal role in the initiation of DNA replication (Zavec et al., 2000). Genetic interactions between Cdc6 and Ecm11 were also observed. Moderate suppression of the *cdc6-1* mutation by overexpression of *ECM11* was detected (Zavec et al., 2000) and deletion of *ECM11* in *cdc6-1* genetic background enhances thermosensitivity of the *cdc6-1* mutation (unpublished result). In addition, *ECM11* shows synthetic lethality with *CDC8*, a gene coding thymidylate kinase, which is required for DNA synthesis (Tong et al., 2004). These data suggest the direct involvment of *ECM11* in DNA replication.

In meiosis, Cdc6 is required for premeiotic DNA replication as in the vegetative cell cycle, but the origin-bound Cdc6 is protected from degradation and occupies origins throughout the meiotic cycle (Ofir et al., 2004). Origin-bound Cdc6 could reflect a change in chromatin structure that occurs in meiosis and Ecm11 bound to Cdc6 could be a part of these changes.

8.3 Ecm11 is modified by SUMO during meiosis

8.3.1 Sumoylation status of Ecm11 during meiosis

In a wide search of protein-protein interactions it was found that Ecm11 interacts with SUMO (Smt3) in the two-hybrid system (Ito et al., 2001; Yu et al., 2008). The Ecm11 protein has two lysine residues, K5 and K101, with a corresponding surrounding sequence IKTE that could accept SUMO. It was confirmed by immunoprecipitation that Ecm11 is sumoylated during meiosis and that Ecm11 interacts with SUMO covalently (Zavec et al., 2008). The majority of Ecm11 protein in the cell is sumoylated during meiosis. The HA antibodies recognized the HA-tagged Ecm11, as well as additional ~10 and ~20 kDa larger species, which correspond to the molecular mass of one or two copies of mature SUMO. Sumoylation of Ecm11 was confirmed by anti-Smt3 reactivity on anti-HA immunoprecipitated samples. Multiple sumoylation was already observed for other sumoylated proteins, e.g. Rpb1, the largest subunit of RNA polymerase II (Pol II) (Chen et al., 2009a).

8.3.2 Sumoylation of Ecm11 is essential for Ecm11 functioning in meiosis

The importance of Ecm11 sumoylation for progression through meiosis was investigated by studying the effect of mutations of predicted SUMO consensus sites in Ecm11 on sporulation efficiency (Zavec et al., 2008). Lysines K5 and K101 in the predicted SUMO consensus sites were mutated to the uncharged amino acid asparagine. Mutation of the predicted sumoylation site K5 affects the biological function of Ecm11 in meiosis. Mutation of K5 led to a reduction of sporulation to the same level as that seen in the mutant with the deleted *ECM11* gene, while mutation of K101 did not affect sporulation level. These results suggest, firstly, that the Lys5 at N-terminus of Ecm11 is modified by SUMO during meiosis and, secondly, that sumoylation is essential for the biological role of Ecm11 in meiosis and directly regulates Ecm11 function in meiosis.

8.3.3 Ecm11 is probably modified by phosphorylation

As described previous (section 5.), beside sumoylation, phosphorylation is the most important modification for replication and recombination proteins. Most components of SCs including Zip1, Hop1, Red1, Mre4, and Rec8 are phosphoproteins, but the functional significance of this phosphorylation and the kinase responsible for the phosphorylation remains to be characterized (Zhu et al., 2010). Ecm11 also contains many predicted phosphorylation sites.

9. Conclusion

In this chapter connections between replication and recombination processes are presented. Studying of proteins that affect both processes will further clarify the relationship between these two processes. One of such proteins is yeast protein Ecm11, which affects meiotic replication and crossing over and is typically modified by sumoylation. Studying such proteins and discussing the relationship between replication and recombination from different points of view may improve understanding of living systems on a higher level.

10. References

Agarwal, S., and G.S. Roeder. (2000). Zip3 provides a link between recombination enzymes and synaptonemal complex proteins. *Cell*, 102, 245-55, 0092-8674 (Print)

Alcasabas, A.A., A.J. Osborn, J. Bachant, F. Hu, P.J. Werler, K. Bousset, K. Furuya, J.F. Diffley, A.M. Carr, and S.J. Elledge. (2001). Mrc1 transduces signals of DNA replication stress to activate Rad53. *Nat Cell Biol*, 3, 958-65, 1465-7392 (Print)

Allers, T., and M. Lichten. (2001). Differential timing and control of noncrossover and crossover recombination during meiosis. *Cell*, 106, 47-57, 0092-8674 (Print)

Bachant, J., A. Alcasabas, Y. Blat, N. Kleckner, and S.J. Elledge. (2002). The SUMO-1 isopeptidase Smt4 is linked to centromeric cohesion through SUMO-1 modification of DNA topoisomerase II. *Mol Cell*, 9, 1169-82, 1097-2765 (Print)

Baker, S.P., J. Phillips, S. Anderson, Q. Qiu, J. Shabanowitz, M.M. Smith, J.R. Yates, 3rd, D.F. Hunt, and P.A. Grant. (2010). Histone H3 Thr 45 phosphorylation is a replication-associated post-translational modification in S. cerevisiae. *Nat Cell Biol*, 12, 294-8, 1476-4679 (Electronic)

Berdichevsky, A., L. Izhar, and Z. Livneh. (2002). Error-free recombinational repair predominates over mutagenic translesion replication in E. coli. *Mol Cell*, 10, 917-24, 1097-2765 (Print)

Blackburn, E.H. (2000). Telomere states and cell fates. *Nature*, 408, 53-6, 0028-0836 (Print)

Boddy, M.N., and P. Russell. (2001). DNA replication checkpoint. *Curr Biol*, 11, R953-6, 0960-9822 (Print)

Borde, V., A.S. Goldman, and M. Lichten. (2000). Direct coupling between meiotic DNA replication and recombination initiation. *Science*, 290, 806-9, 0036-8075 (Print)

Borde, V., W. Lin, E. Novikov, J.H. Petrini, M. Lichten, and A. Nicolas. (2004). Association of Mre11p with double-strand break sites during yeast meiosis. *Mol Cell*, 13, 389-401, 1097-2765 (Print)

Borner, G.V., N. Kleckner, and N. Hunter. (2004). Crossover/noncrossover differentiation, synaptonemal complex formation, and regulatory surveillance at the leptotene/zygotene transition of meiosis. *Cell*, 117, 29-45, 0092-8674 (Print)

Bosco, G., and J.E. Haber. (1998). Chromosome break-induced DNA replication leads to nonreciprocal translocations and telomere capture. *Genetics*, 150, 1037-47, 0016-6731 (Print)

Bousset, K., and J.F. Diffley. (1998). The Cdc7 protein kinase is required for origin firing during S phase. *Genes Dev*, 12, 480-90, 0890-9369 (Print)

Branzei, D., and M. Foiani. (2010). Maintaining genome stability at the replication fork. *Nat Rev Mol Cell Biol*, 11, 208-19, 1471-0080 (Electronic)

Branzei, D., J. Sollier, G. Liberi, X. Zhao, D. Maeda, M. Seki, T. Enomoto, K. Ohta, and M. Foiani. (2006). Ubc9- and mms21-mediated sumoylation counteracts recombinogenic events at damaged replication forks. *Cell*, 127, 509-22, 0092-8674 (Print)

Budd, M.E., K.D. Wittrup, J.E. Bailey, and J.L. Campbell. (1989). DNA polymerase I is required for premeiotic DNA replication and sporulation but not for X-ray repair in Saccharomyces cerevisiae. *Mol Cell Biol*, 9, 365-76, 0270-7306 (Print)

Callender, T.L., and N.M. Hollingsworth. (2010). Mek1 suppression of meiotic double-strand break repair is specific to sister chromatids, chromosome autonomous and independent of Rec8 cohesin complexes. *Genetics*, 185, 771-82, 1943-2631 (Electronic)

Carballo, J.A., A.L. Johnson, S.G. Sedgwick, and R.S. Cha. (2008). Phosphorylation of the axial element protein Hop1 by Mec1/Tel1 ensures meiotic interhomolog recombination. *Cell*, 132, 758-70, 1097-4172 (Electronic)

Carson, D.R., and M.F. Christman. (2001). Evidence that replication fork components catalyze establishment of cohesion between sister chromatids. *Proc Natl Acad Sci U S A*, 98, 8270-5, 0027-8424 (Print)

Carter, S.D., D. Vigasova, J. Chen, M. Chovanec, and S.U. Astrom. (2009). Nej1 recruits the Srs2 helicase to DNA double-strand breaks and supports repair by a single-strand annealing-like mechanism. *Proc Natl Acad Sci U S A*, 106, 12037-42, 1091-6490 (Electronic)

Cha, R.S., B.M. Weiner, S. Keeney, J. Dekker, and N. Kleckner. (2000). Progression of meiotic DNA replication is modulated by interchromosomal interaction proteins, negatively by Spo11p and positively by Rec8p. *Genes Dev*, 14, 493-503, 0890-9369 (Print)

Chen, Q., A. Ijpma, and C.W. Greider. (2001). Two survivor pathways that allow growth in the absence of telomerase are generated by distinct telomere recombination events. *Mol Cell Biol*, 21, 1819-27, 0270-7306 (Print)

Chen, X., B. Ding, D. LeJeune, C. Ruggiero, and S. Li. (2009a). Rpb1 sumoylation in response to UV radiation or transcriptional impairment in yeast. *PLoS One*, 4, e5267, 1932-6203 (Electronic)

Chen, X.F., F.L. Meng, and J.Q. Zhou. (2009b). Telomere recombination accelerates cellular aging in Saccharomyces cerevisiae. *PLoS Genet*, 5, e1000535, 1553-7404 (Electronic)

Cheng, C.H., Y.H. Lo, S.S. Liang, S.C. Ti, F.M. Lin, C.H. Yeh, H.Y. Huang, and T.F. Wang. (2006). SUMO modifications control assembly of synaptonemal complex and polycomplex in meiosis of Saccharomyces cerevisiae. *Genes Dev*, 20, 2067-81, 0890-9369 (Print)

Clifford, D.M., K.E. Stark, K.E. Gardner, S. Hoffmann-Benning, and G.S. Brush. (2005). Mechanistic insight into the Cdc28-related protein kinase Ime2 through analysis of replication protein A phosphorylation. *Cell Cycle*, 4, 1826-33, 1551-4005 (Electronic)

Cost, G.J., and N.R. Cozzarelli. (2006). Smc5p promotes faithful chromosome transmission and DNA repair in Saccharomyces cerevisiae. *Genetics*, 172, 2185-200, 0016-6731 (Print)

Davis, L., M. Barbera, A. McDonnell, K. McIntyre, R. Sternglanz, Q. Jin, J. Loidl, and J. Engebrecht. (2001). The Saccharomyces cerevisiae MUM2 gene interacts with the DNA replication machinery and is required for meiotic levels of double strand breaks. *Genetics*, 157, 1179-89, 0016-6731 (Print)

Diede, S.J., and D.E. Gottschling. (1999). Telomerase-mediated telomere addition in vivo requires DNA primase and DNA polymerases alpha and delta. *Cell*, 99, 723-33, 0092-8674 (Print)

Dirick, L., T. Bohm, and K. Nasmyth. (1995). Roles and regulation of Cln-Cdc28 kinases at the start of the cell cycle of Saccharomyces cerevisiae. *Embo J*, 14, 4803-13, 0261-4189 (Print)

Downs, J.A., N.F. Lowndes, and S.P. Jackson. (2000). A role for Saccharomyces cerevisiae histone H2A in DNA repair. *Nature*, 408, 1001-4, 0028-0836 (Print)

Dubrana, K., S. Perrod, and S.M. Gasser. (2001). Turning telomeres off and on. *Curr Opin Cell Biol*, 13, 281-9, 0955-0674 (Print)

Dunham, M.A., A.A. Neumann, C.L. Fasching, and R.R. Reddel. (2000). Telomere maintenance by recombination in human cells. *Nat Genet*, 26, 447-50, 1061-4036 (Print)

Eggler, A.L., R.B. Inman, and M.M. Cox. (2002). The Rad51-dependent pairing of long DNA substrates is stabilized by replication protein A. *J Biol Chem*, 277, 39280-8, 0021-9258 (Print)

Forsburg, S.L. (2002). Only connect: linking meiotic DNA replication to chromosome dynamics. *Mol Cell*, 9, 703-11, 1097-2765 (Print)

Frei, C., and S.M. Gasser. (2000). The yeast Sgs1p helicase acts upstream of Rad53p in the DNA replication checkpoint and colocalizes with Rad53p in S-phase-specific foci. *Genes Dev*, 14, 81-96, 0890-9369 (Print)

Friedberg, E.C., R. Wagner, and M. Radman. (2002). Specialized DNA polymerases, cellular survival, and the genesis of mutations. *Science*, 296, 1627-30, 1095-9203 (Electronic)

Galhardo, R.S., and S.M. Rosenberg. (2009). Extreme genome repair. *Cell*, 136, 998-1000, 1097-4172 (Electronic)

Gangloff, S., C. Soustelle, and F. Fabre. (2000). Homologous recombination is responsible for cell death in the absence of the Sgs1 and Srs2 helicases. *Nat Genet*, 25, 192-4, 1061-4036 (Print)

Gangloff, S., B. de Massy, L. Arthur, R. Rothstein, and F. Fabre. (1999). The essential role of yeast topoisomerase III in meiosis depends on recombination. *Embo J*, 18, 1701-11, 0261-4189 (Print)

Gurevich, V., and Y. Kassir. (2010). A switch from a gradient to a threshold mode in the regulation of a transcriptional cascade promotes robust execution of meiosis in budding yeast. *PLoS One*, 5, e11005, 1932-6203 (Electronic)

Hayase, A., M. Takagi, T. Miyazaki, H. Oshiumi, M. Shinohara, and A. Shinohara. (2004). A protein complex containing Mei5 and Sae3 promotes the assembly of the meiosis-specific RecA homolog Dmc1. *Cell*, 119, 927-40, 0092-8674 (Print)

Henderson, K.A., K. Kee, S. Maleki, P.A. Santini, and S. Keeney. (2006). Cyclin-dependent kinase directly regulates initiation of meiotic recombination. *Cell*, 125, 1321-32, 0092-8674 (Print)

Heyer, W.D., K.T. Ehmsen, and J. Liu. (2010). Regulation of homologous recombination in eukaryotes. *Annu Rev Genet*, 44, 113-39, 1545-2948 (Electronic)

Hicke, L., H.L. Schubert, and C.P. Hill. (2005). Ubiquitin-binding domains. *Nat Rev Mol Cell Biol*, 6, 610-21, 1471-0072 (Print)

Hietakangas, V., J. Anckar, H.A. Blomster, M. Fujimoto, J.J. Palvimo, A. Nakai, and L. Sistonen. (2006). PDSM, a motif for phosphorylation-dependent SUMO modification. *Proc Natl Acad Sci U S A*, 103, 45-50, 0027-8424 (Print)

Hoege, C., B. Pfander, G.L. Moldovan, G. Pyrowolakis, and S. Jentsch. (2002). RAD6-dependent DNA repair is linked to modification of PCNA by ubiquitin and SUMO. *Nature*, 419, 135-41, 0028-0836 (Print)

Holmes, A.M., and J.E. Haber. (1999). Double-strand break repair in yeast requires both leading and lagging strand DNA polymerases. *Cell*, 96, 415-24, 0092-8674 (Print)

Huertas, P., F. Cortes-Ledesma, A.A. Sartori, A. Aguilera, and S.P. Jackson. (2008). CDK targets Sae2 to control DNA-end resection and homologous recombination. *Nature*, 455, 689-92, 1476-4687 (Electronic)

Ira, G., A. Malkova, G. Liberi, M. Foiani, and J.E. Haber. (2003). Srs2 and Sgs1-Top3 suppress crossovers during double-strand break repair in yeast. *Cell*, 115, 401-11, 0092-8674 (Print)

Ito, T., T. Chiba, R. Ozawa, M. Yoshida, M. Hattori, and Y. Sakaki. (2001). A comprehensive two-hybrid analysis to explore the yeast protein interactome. *Proc Natl Acad Sci U S A*, 98, 4569-74, 0027-8424 (Print)

Ji, H., C.J. Adkins, B.R. Cartwright, and K.L. Friedman. (2008). Yeast Est2p affects telomere length by influencing association of Rap1p with telomeric chromatin. *Mol Cell Biol*, 28, 2380-90, 1098-5549 (Electronic)

Katou, Y., Y. Kanoh, M. Bando, H. Noguchi, H. Tanaka, T. Ashikari, K. Sugimoto, and K. Shirahige. (2003). S-phase checkpoint proteins Tof1 and Mrc1 form a stable replication-pausing complex. *Nature*, 424, 1078-83, 1476-4687 (Electronic)

Kenna, M.A., and R.V. Skibbens. (2003). Mechanical link between cohesion establishment and DNA replication: Ctf7p/Eco1p, a cohesion establishment factor, associates with three different replication factor C complexes. *Mol Cell Biol*, 23, 2999-3007, 0270-7306 (Print)

Kiianitsa, K., J.A. Solinger, and W.D. Heyer. (2006). Terminal association of Rad54 protein with the Rad51-dsDNA filament. *Proc Natl Acad Sci U S A*, 103, 9767-72, 0027-8424 (Print)

Krisko, A., and M. Radman. (2010). Protein damage and death by radiation in Escherichia coli and Deinococcus radiodurans. *Proc Natl Acad Sci U S A*, 107, 14373-7, 1091-6490 (Electronic)

Lai, Y.J., F.M. Lin, M.J. Chuang, H.J. Shen, and T.F. Wang. (2011). Genetic requirements and meiotic function of phosphorylation of the yeast axial element protein Red1. *Mol Cell Biol*, 31, 912-23, 1098-5549 (Electronic)

Lambert, S., A. Watson, D.M. Sheedy, B. Martin, and A.M. Carr. (2005). Gross chromosomal rearrangements and elevated recombination at an inducible site-specific replication fork barrier. *Cell*, 121, 689-702, 0092-8674 (Print)

Lee, S.E., J.K. Moore, A. Holmes, K. Umezu, R.D. Kolodner, and J.E. Haber. (1998). Saccharomyces Ku70, mre11/rad50 and RPA proteins regulate adaptation to G2/M arrest after DNA damage. *Cell*, 94, 399-409, 0092-8674 (Print)

Li, X., C.M. Stith, P.M. Burgers, and W.D. Heyer. (2009). PCNA is required for initiation of recombination-associated DNA synthesis by DNA polymerase delta. *Mol Cell*, 36, 704-13, 1097-4164 (Electronic)

Liberi, G., G. Maffioletti, C. Lucca, I. Chiolo, A. Baryshnikova, C. Cotta-Ramusino, M. Lopes, A. Pellicioli, J.E. Haber, and M. Foiani. (2005). Rad51-dependent DNA structures accumulate at damaged replication forks in sgs1 mutants defective in the yeast ortholog of BLM RecQ helicase. *Genes Dev*, 19, 339-50, 0890-9369 (Print)

Lisby, M., R. Rothstein, and U.H. Mortensen. (2001). Rad52 forms DNA repair and recombination centers during S phase. *Proc Natl Acad Sci U S A*, 98, 8276-82, 0027-8424 (Print)

Lo, H.C., L. Wan, A. Rosebrock, B. Futcher, and N.M. Hollingsworth. (2008). Cdc7-Dbf4 regulates NDT80 transcription as well as reductional segregation during budding yeast meiosis. *Mol Biol Cell*, 19, 4956-67, 1939-4586 (Electronic)

Lopes, M., C. Cotta-Ramusino, A. Pellicioli, G. Liberi, P. Plevani, M. Muzi-Falconi, C.S. Newlon, and M. Foiani. (2001). The DNA replication checkpoint response stabilizes stalled replication forks. *Nature*, 412, 557-61, 0028-0836 (Print)

Lou, H., M. Komata, Y. Katou, Z. Guan, C.C. Reis, M. Budd, K. Shirahige, and J.L. Campbell. (2008). Mrc1 and DNA polymerase epsilon function together in linking DNA replication and the S phase checkpoint. *Mol Cell*, 32, 106-17, 1097-4164 (Electronic)

Lu, C.Y., C.H. Tsai, S.J. Brill, and S.C. Teng. (2010). Sumoylation of the BLM ortholog, Sgs1, promotes telomere-telomere recombination in budding yeast. *Nucleic Acids Res*, 38, 488-98, 1362-4962 (Electronic)

Lucca, C., F. Vanoli, C. Cotta-Ramusino, A. Pellicioli, G. Liberi, J. Haber, and M. Foiani. (2004). Checkpoint-mediated control of replisome-fork association and signalling in response to replication pausing. *Oncogene*, 23, 1206-13, 0950-9232 (Print)

Lydall, D. (2003). Hiding at the ends of yeast chromosomes: telomeres, nucleases and checkpoint pathways. *J Cell Sci*, 116, 4057-65, 0021-9533 (Print)

Lydeard, J.R., S. Jain, M. Yamaguchi, and J.E. Haber. (2007). Break-induced replication and telomerase-independent telomere maintenance require Pol32. *Nature*, 448, 820-3, 1476-4687 (Electronic)

Lydeard, J.R., Z. Lipkin-Moore, Y.J. Sheu, B. Stillman, P.M. Burgers, and J.E. Haber. (2010). Break-induced replication requires all essential DNA replication factors except those specific for pre-RC assembly. *Genes Dev*, 24, 1133-44, 1549-5477 (Electronic)

Maloisel, L., F. Fabre, and S. Gangloff. (2008). DNA polymerase delta is preferentially recruited during homologous recombination to promote heteroduplex DNA extension. *Mol Cell Biol*, 28, 1373-82, 1098-5549 (Electronic)

Manfrini, N., I. Guerini, A. Citterio, G. Lucchini, and M.P. Longhese. (2010). Processing of meiotic DNA double strand breaks requires cyclin-dependent kinase and multiple nucleases. *J Biol Chem*, 285, 11628-37, 1083-351X (Electronic)

Martini, E., R.L. Diaz, N. Hunter, and S. Keeney. (2006). Crossover homeostasis in yeast meiosis. *Cell*, 126, 285-95, 0092-8674 (Print)

Mayer, M.L., I. Pot, M. Chang, H. Xu, V. Aneliunas, T. Kwok, R. Newitt, R. Aebersold, C. Boone, G.W. Brown, and P. Hieter. (2004). Identification of protein complexes required for efficient sister chromatid cohesion. *Mol Biol Cell*, 15, 1736-45, 1059-1524 (Print)

McIlwraith, M.J., A. Vaisman, Y. Liu, E. Fanning, R. Woodgate, and S.C. West. (2005). Human DNA polymerase eta promotes DNA synthesis from strand invasion intermediates of homologous recombination. *Mol Cell*, 20, 783-92, 1097-2765 (Print)

Merrill, B.J., and C. Holm. (1998). The RAD52 recombinational repair pathway is essential in pol30 (PCNA) mutants that accumulate small single-stranded DNA fragments during DNA synthesis. *Genetics*, 148, 611-24, 0016-6731 (Print)

Montpetit, B., T.R. Hazbun, S. Fields, and P. Hieter. (2006). Sumoylation of the budding yeast kinetochore protein Ndc10 is required for Ndc10 spindle localization and regulation of anaphase spindle elongation. *J Cell Biol*, 174, 653-63, 0021-9525 (Print)

Morin, I., H.P. Ngo, A. Greenall, M.K. Zubko, N. Morrice, and D. Lydall. (2008). Checkpoint-dependent phosphorylation of Exo1 modulates the DNA damage response. *Embo J*, 27, 2400-10, 1460-2075 (Electronic)

Mullen, J.R., F.S. Nallaseth, Y.Q. Lan, C.E. Slagle, and S.J. Brill. (2005). Yeast Rmi1/Nce4 controls genome stability as a subunit of the Sgs1-Top3 complex. *Mol Cell Biol*, 25, 4476-87, 0270-7306 (Print)

Nash, P., X. Tang, S. Orlicky, Q. Chen, F.B. Gertler, M.D. Mendenhall, F. Sicheri, T. Pawson, and M. Tyers. (2001). Multisite phosphorylation of a CDK inhibitor sets a threshold for the onset of DNA replication. *Nature*, 414, 514-21, 0028-0836 (Print)

Ofir, Y., S. Sagee, N. Guttmann-Raviv, L. Pnueli, and Y. Kassir. (2004). The role and regulation of the preRC component Cdc6 in the initiation of premeiotic DNA replication. *Mol Biol Cell*, 15, 2230-42, 1059-1524 (Print)

Oh, S.D., J.P. Lao, P.Y. Hwang, A.F. Taylor, G.R. Smith, and N. Hunter. (2007). BLM ortholog, Sgs1, prevents aberrant crossing-over by suppressing formation of multichromatid joint molecules. *Cell*, 130, 259-72, 0092-8674 (Print)

Papouli, E., S. Chen, A.A. Davies, D. Huttner, L. Krejci, P. Sung, and H.D. Ulrich. (2005). Crosstalk between SUMO and ubiquitin on PCNA is mediated by recruitment of the helicase Srs2p. *Mol Cell*, 19, 123-33, 1097-2765 (Print)

Pellicioli, A., S.E. Lee, C. Lucca, M. Foiani, and J.E. Haber. (2001). Regulation of Saccharomyces Rad53 checkpoint kinase during adaptation from DNA damage-induced G2/M arrest. *Mol Cell*, 7, 293-300, 1097-2765 (Print)

Pennaneach, V., C.D. Putnam, and R.D. Kolodner. (2006). Chromosome healing by de novo telomere addition in Saccharomyces cerevisiae. *Mol Microbiol*, 59, 1357-68, 0950-382X (Print)

Petes, T.D. (2001). Meiotic recombination hot spots and cold spots. *Nat Rev Genet*, 2, 360-9, 1471-0056 (Print)

Pfander, B., G.L. Moldovan, M. Sacher, C. Hoege, and S. Jentsch. (2005). SUMO-modified PCNA recruits Srs2 to prevent recombination during S phase. *Nature*, 436, 428-33, 1476-4687 (Electronic)

Rockmill, B., J.C. Fung, S.S. Branda, and G.S. Roeder. (2003). The Sgs1 helicase regulates chromosome synapsis and meiotic crossing over. *Curr Biol*, 13, 1954-62, 0960-9822 (Print)

Sacher, M., B. Pfander, C. Hoege, and S. Jentsch. (2006). Control of Rad52 recombination activity by double-strand break-induced SUMO modification. *Nat Cell Biol*, 8, 1284-90, 1465-7392 (Print)

Sasanuma, H., K. Hirota, T. Fukuda, N. Kakusho, K. Kugou, Y. Kawasaki, T. Shibata, H. Masai, and K. Ohta. (2008). Cdc7-dependent phosphorylation of Mer2 facilitates initiation of yeast meiotic recombination. *Genes Dev*, 22, 398-410, 0890-9369 (Print)

Schwob, E., T. Bohm, M.D. Mendenhall, and K. Nasmyth. (1994). The B-type cyclin kinase inhibitor p40SIC1 controls the G1 to S transition in S. cerevisiae. *Cell*, 79, 233-44, 0092-8674 (Print)

Sclafani, R.A. (2000). Cdc7p-Dbf4p becomes famous in the cell cycle. *J Cell Sci*, 113 (Pt 12), 2111-7, 0021-9533 (Print)

Sherwood, R., T.S. Takahashi, and P.V. Jallepalli. (2010). Sister acts: coordinating DNA replication and cohesion establishment. *Genes Dev*, 24, 2723-31, 1549-5477 (Electronic)

Shimada, K., P. Pasero, and S.M. Gasser. (2002). ORC and the intra-S-phase checkpoint: a threshold regulates Rad53p activation in S phase. *Genes Dev*, 16, 3236-52, 0890-9369 (Print)

Shor, E., S. Gangloff, M. Wagner, J. Weinstein, G. Price, and R. Rothstein. (2002). Mutations in homologous recombination genes rescue top3 slow growth in Saccharomyces cerevisiae. *Genetics*, 162, 647-62, 0016-6731 (Print)

Simonsson, T. (2001). G-quadruplex DNA structures--variations on a theme. *Biol Chem,* 382, 621-8, 1431-6730 (Print)

Skibbens, R.V., L.B. Corson, D. Koshland, and P. Hieter. (1999). Ctf7p is essential for sister chromatid cohesion and links mitotic chromosome structure to the DNA replication machinery. *Genes Dev,* 13, 307-19, 0890-9369 (Print)

Slade, D., A.B. Lindner, G. Paul, and M. Radman. (2009). Recombination and replication in DNA repair of heavily irradiated Deinococcus radiodurans. *Cell,* 136, 1044-55, 1097-4172 (Electronic)

Smith, K.N., A. Penkner, K. Ohta, F. Klein, and A. Nicolas. (2001). B-type cyclins CLB5 and CLB6 control the initiation of recombination and synaptonemal complex formation in yeast meiosis. *Curr Biol,* 11, 88-97, 0960-9822 (Print)

Sorensen, C.S., L.T. Hansen, J. Dziegielewski, R.G. Syljuasen, C. Lundin, J. Bartek, and T. Helleday. (2005). The cell-cycle checkpoint kinase Chk1 is required for mammalian homologous recombination repair. *Nat Cell Biol,* 7, 195-201, 1465-7392 (Print)

Strom, L., C. Karlsson, H.B. Lindroos, S. Wedahl, Y. Katou, K. Shirahige, and C. Sjogren. (2007). Postreplicative formation of cohesion is required for repair and induced by a single DNA break. *Science,* 317, 242-5, 1095-9203 (Electronic)

Stuart, D., and C. Wittenberg. (1998). CLB5 and CLB6 are required for premeiotic DNA replication and activation of the meiotic S/M checkpoint. *Genes Dev,* 12, 2698-710, 0890-9369 (Print)

Sym, M., J.A. Engebrecht, and G.S. Roeder. (1993). ZIP1 is a synaptonemal complex protein required for meiotic chromosome synapsis. *Cell,* 72, 365-78, 0092-8674 (Print)

Tomita, K., A. Matsuura, T. Caspari, A.M. Carr, Y. Akamatsu, H. Iwasaki, K. Mizuno, K. Ohta, M. Uritani, T. Ushimaru, K. Yoshinaga, and M. Ueno. (2003). Competition between the Rad50 complex and the Ku heterodimer reveals a role for Exo1 in processing double-strand breaks but not telomeres. *Mol Cell Biol,* 23, 5186-97, 0270-7306 (Print)

Tong, A.H., G. Lesage, G.D. Bader, H. Ding, H. Xu, X. Xin, J. Young, G.F. Berriz, R.L. Brost, M. Chang, Y. Chen, X. Cheng, G. Chua, H. Friesen, D.S. Goldberg, J. Haynes, C. Humphries, G. He, S. Hussein, L. Ke, N. Krogan, Z. Li, J.N. Levinson, H. Lu, P. Menard, C. Munyana, A.B. Parsons, O. Ryan, R. Tonikian, T. Roberts, A.M. Sdicu, J. Shapiro, B. Sheikh, B. Suter, S.L. Wong, L.V. Zhang, H. Zhu, C.G. Burd, S. Munro, C. Sander, J. Rine, J. Greenblatt, M. Peter, A. Bretscher, G. Bell, F.P. Roth, G.W. Brown, B. Andrews, H. Bussey, and C. Boone. (2004). Global mapping of the yeast genetic interaction network. *Science,* 303, 808-13, 1095-9203 (Electronic)

Torres-Rosell, J., I. Sunjevaric, G. De Piccoli, M. Sacher, N. Eckert-Boulet, R. Reid, S. Jentsch, R. Rothstein, L. Aragon, and M. Lisby. (2007). The Smc5-Smc6 complex and SUMO modification of Rad52 regulates recombinational repair at the ribosomal gene locus. *Nat Cell Biol,* 9, 923-31, 1465-7392 (Print)

Uhlmann, F. (2001). Chromosome cohesion and segregation in mitosis and meiosis. *Curr Opin Cell Biol,* 13, 754-61, 0955-0674 (Print)

Ulrich, H.D., and H. Walden. (2010). Ubiquitin signalling in DNA replication and repair. *Nat Rev Mol Cell Biol,* 11, 479-89, 1471-0080 (Electronic)

Valentin, G., E. Schwob, and F. Della Seta. (2006). Dual role of the Cdc7-regulatory protein Dbf4 during yeast meiosis. *J Biol Chem,* 281, 2828-34, 0021-9258 (Print)

Vanoli, F., M. Fumasoni, B. Szakal, L. Maloisel, and D. Branzei. (2010). Replication and recombination factors contributing to recombination-dependent bypass of DNA lesions by template switch. *PLoS Genet*, 6, e1001205, 1553-7404 (Electronic)

Veaute, X., J. Jeusset, C. Soustelle, S.C. Kowalczykowski, E. Le Cam, and F. Fabre. (2003). The Srs2 helicase prevents recombination by disrupting Rad51 nucleoprotein filaments. *Nature*, 423, 309-12, 0028-0836 (Print)

Wan, L., H. Niu, B. Futcher, C. Zhang, K.M. Shokat, S.J. Boulton, and N.M. Hollingsworth. (2008). Cdc28-Clb5 (CDK-S) and Cdc7-Dbf4 (DDK) collaborate to initiate meiotic recombination in yeast. *Genes Dev*, 22, 386-97, 0890-9369 (Print)

Wang, X., G. Ira, J.A. Tercero, A.M. Holmes, J.F. Diffley, and J.E. Haber. (2004). Role of DNA replication proteins in double-strand break-induced recombination in Saccharomyces cerevisiae. *Mol Cell Biol*, 24, 6891-9, 0270-7306 (Print)

Wang, Z., I.B. Castano, A. De Las Penas, C. Adams, and M.F. Christman. (2000). Pol kappa: A DNA polymerase required for sister chromatid cohesion. *Science*, 289, 774-9, 0036-8075 (Print)

Watt, P.M., E.J. Louis, R.H. Borts, and I.D. Hickson. (1995). Sgs1: a eukaryotic homolog of E. coli RecQ that interacts with topoisomerase II in vivo and is required for faithful chromosome segregation. *Cell*, 81, 253-60, 0092-8674 (Print)

Xu, H., C. Boone, and H.L. Klein. (2004). Mrc1 is required for sister chromatid cohesion to aid in recombination repair of spontaneous damage. *Mol Cell Biol*, 24, 7082-90, 0270-7306 (Print)

Xu, H., M.D. Beasley, W.D. Warren, G.T. van der Horst, and M.J. McKay. (2005). Absence of mouse REC8 cohesin promotes synapsis of sister chromatids in meiosis. *Dev Cell*, 8, 949-61, 1534-5807 (Print)

Yu, H., P. Braun, M.A. Yildirim, I. Lemmens, K. Venkatesan, J. Sahalie, T. Hirozane-Kishikawa, F. Gebreab, N. Li, N. Simonis, T. Hao, J.F. Rual, A. Dricot, A. Vazquez, R.R. Murray, C. Simon, L. Tardivo, S. Tam, N. Svrzikapa, C. Fan, A.S. de Smet, A. Motyl, M.E. Hudson, J. Park, X. Xin, M.E. Cusick, T. Moore, C. Boone, M. Snyder, F.P. Roth, A.L. Barabasi, J. Tavernier, D.E. Hill, and M. Vidal. (2008). High-quality binary protein interaction map of the yeast interactome network. *Science*, 322, 104-10, 1095-9203 (Electronic)

Zavec, A.B., U. Lesnik, R. Komel, and A. Comino. (2004). The Saccharomyces cerevisiae gene ECM11 is a positive effector of meiosis. *FEMS Microbiol Lett*, 241, 193-9, 0378-1097 (Print)

Zavec, A.B., A. Comino, M. Lenassi, and R. Komel. (2008). Ecm11 protein of yeast Saccharomyces cerevisiae is regulated by sumoylation during meiosis. *FEMS Yeast Res*, 8, 64-70, 1567-1356 (Print)

Zavec, P.B., A. Comino, P. Watt, and R. Komel. (2000). Interaction trap experiment with CDC6. *Pflugers Arch*, 439, R94-6, 0031-6768 (Print)

Zhao, X., and G. Blobel. (2005). A SUMO ligase is part of a nuclear multiprotein complex that affects DNA repair and chromosomal organization. *Proc Natl Acad Sci U S A*, 102, 4777-82, 0027-8424 (Print)

Zhou, B.B., and S.J. Elledge. (2000). The DNA damage response: putting checkpoints in perspective. *Nature*, 408, 433-9, 0028-0836 (Print)

Zhu, Z., S. Mori, H. Oshiumi, K. Matsuzaki, M. Shinohara, and A. Shinohara. (2010). Cyclin-dependent kinase promotes formation of the synaptonemal complex in yeast meiosis. *Genes Cells*, 15, 1036-50, 1365-2443 (Electronic)

4

DNA Replication in Repair

Kevin M. McCabe
University of Colorado at Boulder
United States of America

1. Introduction

All living organisms face a constant barrage of DNA damage from anthropogenic and naturally occurring external and endogenous sources, yet DNA provides the blueprint for all other cellular structures. Unlike these other structural and functional molecules, DNA is not turned over in a cycle of breakdown and rebuild; DNA, by the nature of its function as an informational macromolecule and its double stranded structure, is faithfully repaired and copied to maintain the encoded information. In the case of multicellular organisms, the focus of this review, fidelity of information prevents disease, both heritable (e.g. genetic disorders), and within an individual (e.g. cancer). However, errors in DNA replication and repair serve as the grist of evolution; in some sense, these errors are essential to life as we know it.

With few exceptions, the repair of DNA damage requires the action of one or more DNA polymerases. In many cases, these are specialized polymerases, recruited to the site of damage for their specific biochemical properties. In this literature review, I will present different types of DNA damage, the biochemical systems utilized in the repair of this damage, the role of various enzymes in this repair - emphasizing the role of specific DNA polymerases - and the outcome of repair - including the resulting mutation spectrum - where relevant.

2. DNA polymerases

DNA polymerases are responsible for the replication of DNA. They perform this function by adding free deoxynucleotides to the 3′ end of a DNA strand or RNA primer and extending the strand in the 5′ direction; they are not able to synthesize DNA *de novo* without this 3′ hydroxyl (Baker & Bell 1998; Hubscher *et al.* 2002). They are typically composed of several subunits, but an in depth discussion of polymerase components is beyond the scope of this chapter; please see Kawasaki and Sugino for a more in depth discussion of polymerase subunits (Kawasaki & Sugino 2001). The mechanism of nucleotide insertion by a polymerase is a process consisting of 6 steps binding of the DNA template, binding of the incoming dNTP, undergoing a change in conformation to become more catalytically effective, formation of the phosphodiester bond, release of the pyrophosphate group, and translocation to the next template base or dissociation from DNA (Kuchta *et al.* 1988; Kuchta *et al.* 1987; Patel *et al.* 1991; Washington *et al.* 2000; Washington *et al.* 2001; Wong *et al.* 1991). The structure of a polymerase is similar to that of a right human hand grasping a DNA strand, and is thus described as having finger, palm and thumb subdomains (Steitz 1998). Synthesis is carried out using the opposite strand as a template—the semi-conservative model of DNA synthesis (Meselson & Stahl 1958).

2.1 DNA polymerase families

Polymerases are organized into 7 families by their sequence, structure, and function. These polymerase families are: A, B, C, D, X, Y and RT. Each family has different properties and roles. For example, A Family polymerases are responsible for the bulk of S-phase DNA synthesis, and Y Family polymerases are responsible for Translesion Synthesis (TLS) and the bypass of some DNA lesions. A brief discussion of bacterial polymerase families follows, as does a more detailed discussion of multicellular eukaryotic polymerase families, representative members, and roles (summarized in Table 1).

A Family polymerases are replicative and repair polymerases that include the *E. coli* replicative polymerase polI, *T. aquaticus* polI, and the human mitochondrial polymerase, polϒ. This family also includes the E. coli T7 polymerase, one of the most studied polymerases. Orthologues of this family include members of the B Family of eukaryotic polymerases (Hubscher *et al.* 2002). The tight active site and 3′ primer interactions prevent base pair mismatches, and thus these polymerases have a low error rate. polθ is a low fidelity A Family member with roles in repair, possibly including Base Excision Repair (BER) and Interstrand Crosslink Repair (ICLR) (Chan *et al.* 2010; Prasad *et al.* 2009).

The B Family of polymerases is closely related to the A Family in structure and function. They are DNA directed DNA polymerases and this family includes the eukaryotic replicative and repair polymerases polα, polδ, and polε. polα with its accompanying primase is responsible for initiation of DNA synthesis (Harrington & Perrino 1995). polδ and polε cooperate to accomplish leading and lagging strand DNA synthesis (Chilkova *et al.* 2007). polδ and polε are also involved in Homologous Recombination Repair (HRR) of DNA (Asturias *et al.* 2006; Kelman 1997; Maloisel *et al.* 2008). Another B Family member, polζ, is involved in TLS (Haracska *et al.* 2003).

C Family polymerases represent the main bacterial chromosomal synthetic polymerases (Lamers *et al.* 2006). They are fast moving, have proofreading capability, and are structurally and possibly evolutionarily distinct from the other polymerase families (Bloom *et al.* 1997; Lamers *et al.* 2006). Another distinct family are the D Family polymerases. They are archaeal polymerases that are assumed to function as replicative polymerases (Ishino *et al.* 1998; Yamasaki *et al.* 2010).

X Family polymerases are extensively involved in a variety of DNA repair mechanisms. This family includes polβ, polσ, polλ, and polμ, as well as terminal deoxynucleotidyl transferase (TdT). Some of the X Family members, including polβ and polλ, can cleave a 5′ abasic deoxyribose sugar, a critical function in BER and possibly required for Non-Homologous End Joining (NHEJ) (Fan & Wu 2004; Garcia-Diaz *et al.* 2001). TdT expression is limited to developing leukocyte lineages where where it plays a critical role in V(D)J Recombination, a specific type of NHEJ (Mahajan *et al.* 1999). polλ and polμ are required for NHEJ (Fan & Wu 2004; Mahajan *et al.* 2002). polσ works in concert with polε in sister chromatid cohesion and HRR (Edwards *et al.* 2003).

The Y Family of polymerases, including polη, polι, polκ, and REV-1 are involved in TLS. Each polymerase in this family has a different bypass preference. For example, polη will bypass cyclothymine dimers (CTD), inserting two adenines opposite the lesion in an error free manner. Loss of polη because of its involvement in CTD bypass gives a Xeroderma pigmentosum variant phenotype as with many Nucleotide Excision Repair (NER) enzymes (Johnson *et al.* 1999b; Washington *et al.* 2000). polι is not able to replicate past a CTD, however, it is involved in the nucleotide incorporation opposite an abasic site and the 3′ thymine of a (6-4) photoproduct (Johnson *et al.* 2000). Although it can insert bases opposite the lesion, this polymerase cannot extend the nascent DNA strand. While polκ cannot insert bases opposite damage as polηand polι can, it does extend opposite the 3′ end of the lesion (Washington *et al.* 2002). REV-1 is thought to play a supporting role as well, triggering synthesis of the other Y family members at these lesions (Guo *et al.* 2003; Ohashi *et al.* 2004; Tissier *et al.* 2004). The roles of polymerases in TLS are discussed in more detail below.

Polymerase Family	Polymerase	Role in DNA Replication	DNA Repair Pathway Participation
A	polθ	N/A	BER?, ICLR?
B	polα	Initiation of Replication	N/A
	polδ	Processive Synthesis	HRR
	polε	Processive Synthesis	Long Range HRR DNA Synthesis, SSA
	polζ	N/A	TLS, HRR?
X	polβ	N/A	BER
	polλ	N/A	NHEJ
	polμ	N/A	NHEJ
	polσ	N/A	Stimulates polε
	TdT	N/A	V(D)J Recombination
Y	polη	N/A	TLS past CTD
	polι	N/A	TLS past abasic and 6-4 photoproduct
	polκ	N/A	Extension from 3′ of bypass by polη and polι
	REV-1	N/A	Triggering Synthesis by the Other Y Family Members

Table 1. DNA Polymerases Involved in DNA Repair and Their Roles

The RT Family of polymerases includes RNA-directed DNA polymerases that use RNA primers or are involved in viral reverse transcription, like the eukaryotic polymerases responsible for telomere maintenance, telomerase (Gotte *et al.* 1999; Greider & Blackburn 1989). RT stands for Reverse Transcriptase, the primary function of members of this polymerase family.

3. DNA repair

The goal of all DNA repair is to maintain the integrity of the genome with minimal, and ideally no changes to the original DNA sequence. In the case of single strand damage, such as spontaneous depurination, oxidation, alkylation, and ultraviolet (UV) light photoproducts, this is readily achieved by Direct Reversal Repair (DRR), in which an enzyme directly returns the lesion to its former, undamaged state, or utilizing the

antiparallel DNA strand as template, as in TLS, or following excision of the damage as in BER and NER. However, when both strands are damaged, repair mechanisms including Double Strand Break Repair (DSBR) and Interstrand Crosslink Repair (ICLR) are utilized, and repair becomes increasingly complicated and in many cases mutagenic.
The type of DNA damage incurred dictates the mechanism(s) of DNA repair. Initial recognition of the lesion directly recruits, or signals for the recruitment of repair factors. The exact repair mechanism implemented for a specific type of lesion may vary, depending upon available factors or cell cycle status.

3.1 Direct reversal repair

DRR represents a set of enzymes that catalyze direct repair of the damaged base/s, returning the DNA to its previous, undamaged configuration and sequence. Examples of DNA damage and their repair proteins would include O^6-alkylguanine being repaired by O^6-alkylguanine DNA alkyltransferase (AGT), 1-alkyladenine being repaired by AlkB dioxygenase human homologues AHB2 and AHB3, cyclopyrimidine dimers (CPD) being repaired by DNA photolyase and 6-4 photoproducts being repaired by 6-4 photolyase (Duncan *et al.* 2002; Kim *et al.* 1993; Wibley *et al.* 2000; Zhao, X. *et al.* 1997). As these specific enzyme mechanisms execute a direct catalytic repair of DNA damage, they do not require DNA synthesis in repair. However, some of these same forms of DNA damage, for example CPD, can be repaired through alternate, DNA polymerase requiring mechanisms, such as NER.

3.2 Base excision repair

BER is utilized in the repair of DNA damage incurred on a single strand, where there is little structural alteration of the DNA backbone. This damage includes apurinic sites resulting from spontaneous depurination, oxidized or alkylated bases, or base mismatches resulting from 5-methylcytosine deamination (T/G mismatch) or polymerase errors. Because there is little backbone distortion, these lesions tend not to block replicative polymerases, and as a result, this damage can be highly mutagenic if not detected and repaired. For example, an unrepaired 8-oxoguanine at DNA synthesis will lead to G:C to T:A transversions common to many solid tumors (Bruner *et al.* 2000).

3.2.1 Steps of BER

In BER, specific glycosylases recognize and bind specific lesions (Banerjee *et al.* 2006; Bruner *et al.* 2000; Engelward *et al.* 1997; Klungland *et al.* 1999; Parsons 2003) with the assistance of accessory proteins such as MutM (Banerjee *et al.* 2006) (Figure 1). Examples include 8-oxoguanine DNA glycosylase recognizing and binding 8-oxoguanine (Bruner *et al.* 2000) or alkyladenine DNA glycosylase recognizing and binding alkyladenine (Engelward *et al.* 1997). The damaged base is flipped out and cleaved by the glycosylase (Banerjee *et al.* 2006) generating an abasic site. Apurinic-apyrimidinic endonuclease (APE1) will then nick or break the DNA backbone (Mol *et al.* 2000; Srivastava *et al.* 1998) (Figure 1).
At this point, two possible pathways, Short Patch Repair (SPR) and Long Patch Repair (LPR), diverge (Kubota *et al.* 1996). In SPR, polβ will cleave the 5′ abasic sugar and replace the missing nucleotide (Garcia-Diaz *et al.* 2001). X-ray Repair Cross Complementing Protein 1 (XRCC1), along with its binding partner, DNA Ligase III will seal the backbone nick. In LPR, Replication Factor C (RFC) loads Proliferating Cell Nuclear Antigen (PCNA) at the

incision (Kelman 1997). PCNA will facilitate polβ binding (a common step in the recruitment of many polymerases to damaged sites) and polβ will synthesize a stretch of DNA, creating a 5′ flap (Srivastava *et al.* 1998). This flap is trimmed by Flap Endonuclease 1 (FEN1), and DNA Ligase I seals the remaining nick or break in the DNA backbone (Prasad *et al.* 2000; Srivastava *et al.* 1998) (Figure 1). In both cases, the DNA is repaired in an error-free manner, if the damage is recognized before S-phase and DNA synthesis.

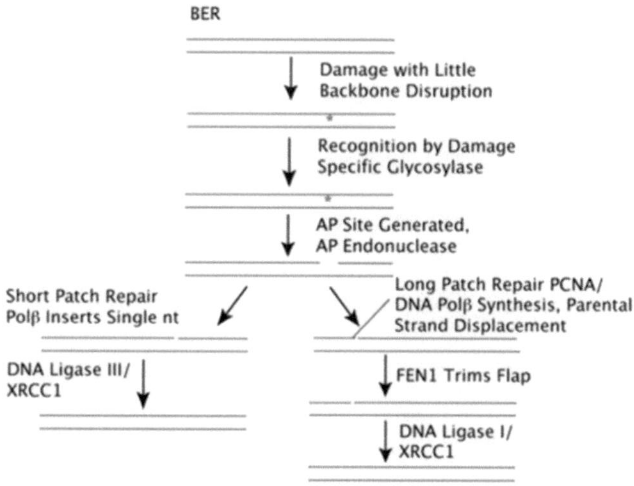

Fig. 1. The generalized steps of BER

3.3 Nucleotide excision repair

Whereas the damage to which BER responds does not significantly distort the DNA backbone, NER explicitly recognizes this backbone distortion utilizing two different systems—Transcription Coupled Repair (TCR, (Bohr *et al.* 1985; Mellon *et al.* 1987)) and Global Genome Repair (GGR, (Aboussekhra *et al.* 1995; Araujo *et al.* 2000)). The types of damage recognized by these systems primarily consist of bulky adducts, including UV photoproducts (cyclopyrimidine dimmers and 6-4 photoproducts (Mellon *et al.* 1987; Ng *et al.* 2003)) or N-acetoxy-2acetyl-aminofluorene induced adducts (Ng *et al.* 2003). These bulky adducts will stall DNA polymerases as well as transcription machinery, and are therefore less mutagenic than the types of damage repaired by BER, but they can be cytotoxic (Mitchell *et al.* 2003).

3.3.1 Steps of NER

TCR is activated by the stalling of RNA polymerase II upon encountering a bulky adduct. This recruits Cockayne Syndrome Proteins A and B (CSA and CSB, (Henning *et al.* 1995)), Xeroderma Pigmentosum Protein A (XPA), Binding Protein 2 (XAB2, (Nakatsu *et al.* 2000)), and High Mobility Group Nucleosome Binding Protein 1 (HMGN1, (Birger *et al.* 2003)) to the site of damage. This system for sensing DNA damage can only function on actively transcribed genes. With GGR, the bulky adducts are recognized by the Xeroderma Pigmentosum Protein C (XPC)-Homologue of RAD23 B (HR23B) complex (Figure 2), with help from Xeroderma Pigmentosum Protein E (XPE, also known as Damaged DNA Binding Protein 2 (DDB2)) in the case of photodimers (Kulaksiz *et al.* 2005; Yokoi *et al.* 2000).

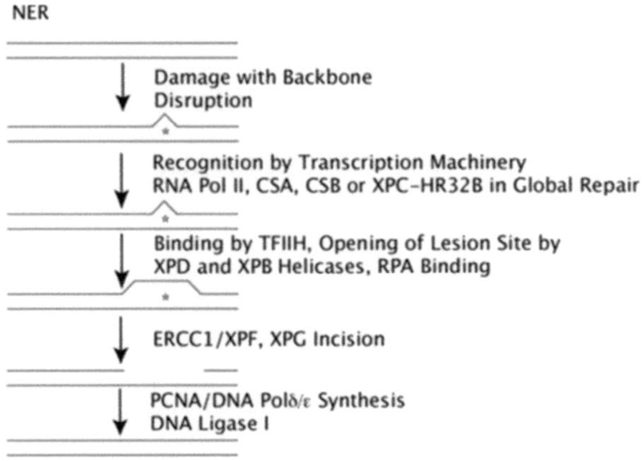

Fig. 2. Generalized Steps of NER

Following damage recognition, these two repair systems utilize the same enzymes to catalyze repair. These include the basal transcription factor (TFIIH), with the helicases Xeroderma Pigmentosum Protein B (XPB, 3′ to 5′ helicase) and Xeroderma Pigmentosum Protein D (XPD, 5′ to 3′ helicase), as well as Xeroderma Pigmentosum Protein A (XPA) and Xeroderma Pigmentosum Group G (XPG)(Tantin 1998; Tantin *et al.* 1997). Once bound, the TFIIH complex opens the lesion. XPA recruits Replication Protein A (RPA), which stabilizes the single stranded DNA (ssDNA) (Li *et al.* 1995a; Li *et al.* 1995b). The Excision Repair Cross Complementation Group 1–Xeroderma Pigmentosum Group F (ERCC1-XPF) heterodimer then incises the DNA backbone 5′ of the damage, while XPG incises the backbone on the 3′ side of the adduct (O'Donovan *et al.* 1994; Sijbers *et al.* 1996).

With 25-30nt surrounding the lesion removed, RFC loads PCNA, as in BER (Kelman 1997). At this stage, variations in the final steps may be observed with dividing and non-dividing cells (Fousteri & Mullenders 2008). In the case of dividing cells, DNA polδ and polε will syntheize DNA across the gap, and DNA Ligase I will seal the resulting nick (Aboussekhra *et al.* 1995; Araujo *et al.* 2000; Araujo & Wood 1999). In the DNA of non-dividing cells (out of S-phase), polκ might instead be utilized to bridge the gap, with XRCC1-DNA Ligase III sealing the nick (Moser *et al.* 2007; Ogi & Lehmann 2006). Again, as with BER, the utilization of the undamaged strand results in error-free repair.

3.4 Translesion synthesis

The DNA lesions produced in cells by a variety of chemical or physical agents can sometimes escape the repair mechanisms of the cells, including NER. Because these lesions distort the structure of the DNA, the high-fidelity polymerases are no longer able to bind and replicate past the lesions. Other polymerases, the low-fidelity, TLS polymerases, are recruited at the replication fork and are involved in replication past the DNA damage (Burgers *et al.* 2001; Ohmori *et al.* 2001). As noted above, the most significant classes of TLS enzymes encountered in eukaryotes are the members of the Y-family of DNA polymerases (polη, ι, κ and Rev1) also known as UmuC/DinB/Rev1/Rad30 superfamily, in addition to a member of the B-family of polymerases, polζ (Ohmori *et al.* 2001; Zhao, B. *et al.* 2004).

3.4.1 Steps of TLS

The first step in DNA repair is the recruitment of TLS polymerases at the stalled replication fork by a monoubiquitnated, sumoulated, or otherwise modified PCNA (Haracska *et al.* 2001a; Haracska *et al.* 2001b; Waters *et al.* 2009). Rev-1 is suspected to act as a trigger in mobilizing the other polymerases, polη, polι, and polκ, to insert a base or bases opposite the damaged nucleotide/s (Guo *et al.* 2003; Ohashi *et al.* 2004; Tissier *et al.* 2004). After bringing the polymerases to the lesion site during the repair process, the same Rev-1 will bind polζ. polζ is a member of the B-family of polymerases that is not very efficient in inserting the nucleotides opposite lesions, but can extend the primer termini (Haracska *et al.* 2003). Once this polymerase binds, it will begin to synthesize a stretch of DNA opposite the damage site, completing the bypass of the lesion. Two generalized models for TLS include polymerase switching, in which a replicative polymerase stalls, PCNA is modified, and a TLS polymerase extends from the lesion, and once bypassed, replication resumes. The other model is gap filling, in which a gap is left following replication fork stalling at a damaged site, and TLS fills this gap. These models are reviewed in Waters *et al.* (Waters *et al.* 2009).

3.5 Double strand break repair

Unlike the damage repaired by DRR, BER, and NER, DSB involve both strands of DNA. This eliminates the ability of DSBR to utilize DNA's built in backup, the opposing DNA strand, as it too is damaged. This damage is typically caused by ionizing radiation, neighboring single strand breaks, natural processes such as V(D)J recombination, meiotic and mitotic crossing over, yeast mating type switching, and the collapse or stalling of replication forks (Khanna & Jackson 2001; Sugawara *et al.* 2000).

There are three main pathways for the repair of DSB:— Single Strand Annealing (SSA), NHEJ, and HRR. Local differences in DNA sequence, the availability of repair factors, the availability of a homologous sequence, and cell cycle status affect which mechanism of DSBR is utilized. NHEJ, of which there are two alternate biochemical pathways, the primary, Ligase IV dependent NHEJ (D-NHEJ) and the backup, Ligase III dependent NHEJ (B-NHEJ), is utilized for most DSB in mammalian cells (Mladenov & Iliakis 2011). SSA can occur where there are direct repeats in DNA sequence, and there are lower levels of NHEJ components (Fishman-Lobell *et al.* 1992). HRR functions predominantly in S and G2 phases of the cell cycle, when homologous substrates are readily available (Aylon *et al.* 2004).

3.5.1 Steps of NHEJ

DSBR by NHEJ can follow a main D-NHEJ (named for the requirement of DNA-PKcs) pathway responsible for the bulk of DSBR in mammalian cells, or a Backup B-NHEJ. Both pathways repair DSB in similar manners, but utilize different proteins at each step (Mladenov & Iliakis 2011). For simplicity, Figure 3 will only list D-NHEJ, but B-NHEJ follows similar catalytic steps, as discussed below.

In mammalian D-NHEJ, the DSB is recognized and bound by Ku70/Ku80 heterodimer. This leads to binding of the DNA Dependent Protein Kinase catalytic subunit (DNA-PKcs) yielding a functional DNA-PK holoenzyme (Cary et al. 1997). The ends are modified by polynucleotide kinase (PNK) and terminal deoxynucleotide transferase (TDT), also, an as yet unidentified endonuclease (possibly Artemis, a substrate of DNA-PK) will then resect the 5′ ends leaving 3′ ssDNA. These ends will be filled by DNA polλ and μ, and joined by the DNA Ligase IV-XRCC4 complex, enhanced by XRCC4 Like Factor (XLF) (Bryans et al. 1999; Fan & Wu 2004; Mahajan et al. 2002; Yano et al. 2008) (Figure 3).

Less is known about B-NHEJ then D-NHEJ, but B-NHEJ seems to act more slowly than D-NHEJ, though it can ultimately achieve the same ends, the repair of DSB (Iliakis 2009; Wang, H. et al. 2003; Wang, M. et al. 2006; Wu et al. 2008). This alternate pathway was identified in cell lines deficient in many of the D-NHEJ proteins (Nevaldine et al. 1997; Wang, H. et al. 2001a; Wang, H. et al. 2001b). In B-NHEJ, Poly [ADP-ribose] polymerase 1 (PARP-1), usually associated with single strand break repair, is responsible for end recognition and binding (McKinnon & Caldecott 2007; Wang, M. et al. 2006). A role for the MRN complex in processing of the break has been suggested based upon reduced end joining in D-NHEJ deficient cells when Mre11 is inhibited (Rass et al. 2009). DNA Ligase III and XRCC1 are regulated by PARP-1, and a role for Ligase III has been demonstrated in NHEJ (McKinnon & Caldecott 2007; Windhofer et al. 2007). Enhancement of Ligase III activity by Histone H1, suggests a role in B-NHEJ as well (Rosidi et al. 2008). No direct evidence for the role of a specific polymerase has been identified in B-NHEJ, however, it in known that PARP-1 interacts with DNA polα, suggesting possible involvement in this pathway (Dantzer et al. 1998).

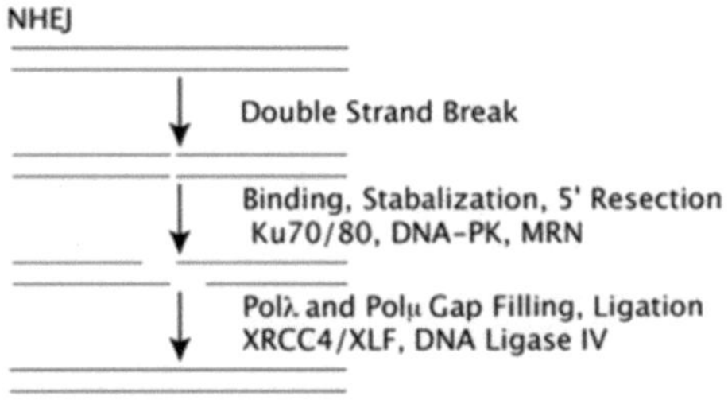

Fig. 3. Generalized steps of NHEJ

If the two ends that are joined by NHEJ are from a single double strand break, the outcome can be conservative or lead to deletions of varying sizes, depending upon the extent of processing of the ends. If, however, the two ends that are rejoined were from separate DSBs, the result will be a translocation. While NHEJ is quite proficient at rejoining DSB ends and eliminating this highly cytotoxic DNA damage, it does not involve a mechanism to choose which ends to rejoin, and is, thus, considered to be a non-conservative mechanism for DNA repair.

3.5.2 Steps of SSA

SSA requires a more specific set of conditions than NHEJ, specifically neighboring repeats either side of the DSB, and will predominantly occur in S-phase (Frankenberg-Schwager *et al.* 2009; Sugawara *et al.* 2000). At the site of the DSB, there is a 5′ to 3′ resection, likely by the MRN complex, that leaves 3′ tails. RAD52 binds the 3′ ends, and these tails are stabilized by the ssDNA binding protein, RPA (Stasiak *et al.* 2000; Van Dyck *et al.* 1999; Wold 1997). These factors are sufficient for annealing of the repeat sequences. FEN1 or ERCC1/XPF then trim the 3′ overhangs (Al-Minawi *et al.* 2008; Gottlich *et al.* 1998). The remaining gaps are filled and ligated by DNA polε and DNA Ligase III (Gottlich *et al.* 1998) (Figure 4).
As neighboring repeats are annealed, sometimes at distances of 40bp to 1-2kb apart, SSA results in deletions of varying sizes (Gottlich *et al.* 1998; Richardson & Jasin 2000). With multiple genomic DSB, SSA has also been demonstrated to yield translocations (Richardson & Jasin 2000). Presumably, these result from homologous sequences on non-homologous chromosomes annealing and being joined by the SSA machinery.

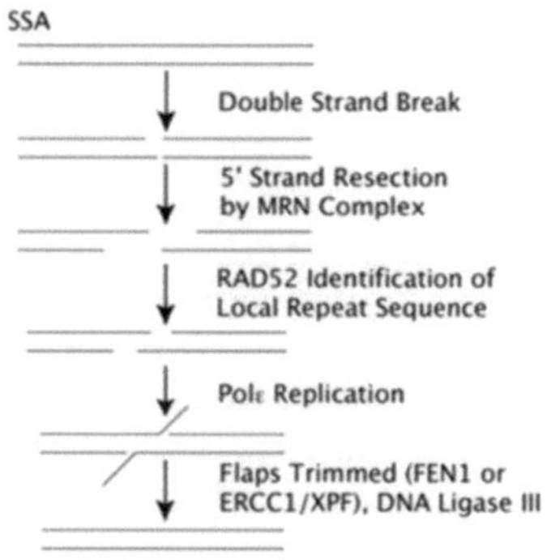

Fig. 4. Generalized Steps of SSA

3.5.3 Steps of HRR

Like SSA, HRR requires a homologous sequence, typically a sister chromatid; thus most HRR occurs in late S or G2 phases of the cell cycle. Following DSB formation, there is a 5′ resection leaving 3′ tails. Rad51 recombinase (made up of Rad51B and Rad51C) binds these single stranded regions, a homologous region is identified, and a D-loop is formed (Sung & Robberson 1995). This complicated process utilizes a number of other proteins, including the MRN complex which, along with BRCA1 and CtIP, again serves a role in resection; BRCA2, which facilitates Rad51 loading and facilitates recombination; RPA, which acts to stabilize the ssDNA and promote strand exchange with Rad51; Rad54, which aids in chromatin remodeling; and Hop2-Mnd1, which help promote D-loop capture and processing (Chen *et al.* 2008; Pellegrini *et al.* 2002; Solinger *et al.* 2001; Stauffer & Chazin 2004; Sung & Robberson 1995; Vignard *et al.* 2007). (Other protein systems are responsible for meiotic recombination and are not discussed in detail here, but are reviewed in (Smith & Nicolas 1998)).

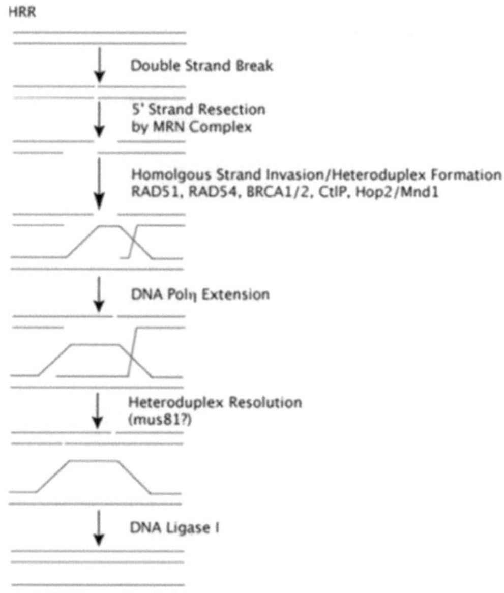

Fig. 5. Generalized Steps of HRR

DNA polη will then extend from the 3′ end of the invading strand, elongating the D-loop (McIlwraith *et al.* 2005). The invading strand is then displaced and anneals with the second DSB end, being ligated by DNA Ligase I (Goetz *et al.* 2005) (Figure 5). This mechanism of repair avoids the formation of a Holiday junction and the risk of crossover (referred to as Synthesis Dependent Strand Annealing or SDSA) (Ferguson & Holloman 1996). However, where the goal is crossover, as in meiotic recombination, the extended D-loop will bind the second DSB end creating a Holiday junction, leading to crossover and non-crossover products (referred to as the DSBR pathway) (Szostak *et al.* 1983).

A specialized version of HRR, called Break Induced Replication (BIR), acts to preserve single DSB ends such as those at chromosomal termini, or, as we will discuss in ICLR, at stalled replication forks. In BIR similar factors are utilized to process the ends, invade a homologous or repeat sequence, extend, and resolve the lesion. Of note, the polα primase is required for initiation of replication by polδ (Maloisel *et al.* 2008). polε is required for long-range synthesis, and, unique to BIR, Pol32 is required but does not function in other HRR pathways (Asturias *et al.* 2006; Lydeard *et al.* 2007).

HRR is the only truly conservative repair mechanism for double strand breaks, with both SDSA and DSBR, when a hololologous chromosome provides the template for repair. Unlike NHEJ and SSA, it does not typically lead to translocations or deletions, but DSBR can lead to crossing over of chromatids. In BIR, if the substrate for recombination is a homologous chromatid, repair is conservative; however, if a repeat from a non-homologous sequence is utilized, a translocation may result.

3.6 Interstrand crosslink repair

There are certain chemicals, endogenous and exogenous, that covalently link both strands of a DNA molecule together; these agents include malondialdehyde, mitomycin C, or psorlen (Scharer 2005). With an ICL, much like a DSB, the anti-parallel strands can no longer be used as template for one another. ICLs covalently link both strands of DNA together preventing strand separation required for transcription and replication, making ICL inducing agents particularly potent killers of cycling cells (Dronkert & Kanaar 2001). For this reason, many ICL inducing agents are used as chemotherapeutic agents in the treatment of cancer (Lawley & Phillips 1996; Lord *et al.* 2002; Ryu *et al.* 2004). Stalled replication forks will also utilize ICLR under certain circumstances (McCabe *et al.* 2008).

The genetic disorder Fanconi Anemia (FA) is intimately associated with ICLR, much the way Xeroderma Pigmentosum is associated with NER. There are currently 15 FA groups, representing defects in 15 proteins involved in ICL repair. These genes are, FANCA, B (Fanconi Anemia Associated Protein of 95kDa, FAAP95), C, D1 (BRCA2), D2, E, F, G, I, J (BRCA1 Interacting Protein C-terminal Helicase 1, BRIP1), L, M (Fanconi Anemia Associated Protein of 250KD, FAAP250), N (Partner and Localizer of BRCA2, PALB2), O (Rad51C), and P (SLX4) (Kitao & Takata 2011). The numerous proteins involved in ICLR reflect the complexity of repairing this type of damage. The model presented here (Figure 6) is speculative; it is based upon published biochemical functions of the proteins involved and the formation of recombination intermediates in FA cells between non-homologous chromosomes (Newell *et al.* 2004). The ICLR pathway likely represents a last ditch mechanism of repair for this extremely cytotoxic damage where there are no homologous substrates for HRR of these lesions (McCabe *et al.* 2009). TLS is one other option for damage bypass, but does not constitute repair.

3.6.1 TLS in response to ICL

If there are incisions on both sides of an ICL on one strand, TLS has been proposed to replicate past the lesion, reducing its cytotoxicity and permitting continuation of the cell cycle. TLS utilizing error prone polζ or polη might replicate past the ICL following DSB formation (reviewed in (Dronkert & Kanaar 2001)). However, polη mutants show normal sensitivity to ICL, suggesting no role for this polymerase in repair (Grossmann *et al.* 2001). Little is known about this pathway compared to NER and HR repair; however, it is thought that this pathway helps the cells to bypass an ICL to reduce cytotoxicity as opposed to actually repairing the lesion (Dronkert & Kanaar 2001). Further, the severity of the FA phenotype with respect to ICL damage suggests TLS is, at most, a minor mechanism of ICL repair.

3.6.2 Steps of ICLR

It has been suggested that the distortion created by the ICL or the ensuing chromatin change could be one of the initial signals for repair (Dronkert & Kanaar 2001). DSB signaling, including ATM kinase activity, also plays a clear role in ICLR, as DSB are an important intermediate in repair, though data suggests that DSB do not activate the FA pathway (Rogakou *et al.* 1999; Sobeck *et al.* 2007). The collapsed replication fork at the site of ICL damage, or in response to hydroxyurea treatment, collapses and regresses with the help of RECA (Robu *et al.* 2001). This leads to loading of the FA core complex via the DNA translocase activity of FANCM/MHF complex (Singh *et al.* 2010; Yan *et al.* 2010). The FA core complex is comprised of FANCA, B, C, E, F, G, L and M, and is required for monoubiquitination of FANCD2 by the E3 ligase FANCL, in concert with the E2 subunit UBE2T (Machida *et al.* 2006) (Figure 6).

Central to the FA pathway are FANCD2 and its paralog FANCI (Smogorzewska *et al.* 2007). FANCD2 monoubiqitination is traditionally looked upon as the marker of activation of the FA pathway. Monoubiquitination is required for FANCD2 and FANCI localization to chromatin (Garcia-Higuera *et al.* 2001; Smogorzewska *et al.* 2007). Monoubiquitinated FANCD2/FANCI colocalizes with BRCA1 in response to DNA damage and at synaptonemal complexes (Garcia-Higuera *et al.* 2001). Additionally, FANCD2 has been shown to interact in a constitutive manner with FANCD1/BRCA2 and co-localizes with RAD51 in nuclear foci (Hussain *et al.* 2004). FANCD2 also interacts with the MRN complex, which may serve a role in processing a recombination intermediate (Nakanishi *et al.* 2002).

FANCA, a core complex component, has been shown to interact with several other proteins. Independently of the other FA proteins, FANCA interacts directly with BRCA1 without the requirement for DNA damage, suggesting a constitutive interaction (Folias *et al.* 2002). Additionally, FANCA has been suggested to aid in the recruitment of the SWI/SNF complex subunit, brahma-related gene 1 (BRG1), and may be involved in chromatin remodeling at the site of action of the FA pathway (Otsuki *et al.* 2001).

Biochemical studies have identified several proteins forming large complexes with the FA proteins. Included in the BRAFT complex are five FA proteins (FANCA, C, E, F, and G), the Bloom syndrome helicase (BLM), replication protein A (RPA) and topoisomerase IIIa (Topo3a). This complex has a DNA duplex unwinding capability that requires BLM, but not FANCA. However, BLM is not required for FANCD2 monoubiqitination, suggesting BLM functions in this pathway downstream of core complex signaling for activation of the FA pathway (Meetei *et al.* 2003). FANCJ is a BRCA1 interacting protein that functions as an ATP- dependent 5′-3′ helicase (Cantor *et al.* 2001; Cantor *et al.* 2004). Combined with the interaction of FA proteins with BLM, a 3′-5′ helicase, these data suggest the ability of FA complexes to open stretches of DNA in both directions (Ellis *et al.* 1995).

The discovery of FANCD1 as BRCA2 directly linked the FA pathway and HRR pathway (Hirsch *et al.* 2004). BRCA2 is known to regulate RAD51 controlling the formation of the RAD51/ssDNA nucleoprotein filament required for strand pairing during HRR in DSBR (Davies *et al.* 2001; Sharan *et al.* 1997). In addition, BRCA2 binds FANCD2 and G placing the core complex and FANCD2 at sites of homologous recombination repair (Hussain *et al.* 2004). Another recombination and FA was uncovered with the identification of FANCN as the partner and localizer of BRCA2 (PALB2) (Reid *et al.* 2007; Tischkowitz *et al.* 2007; Xia *et al.* 2006). As its name suggests, PALB2 interacts with BRCA2 and is responsible for its localization to chromatin; thus, PALB2 is required for BRCA2's function in homologous recombination repair and cell cycle checkpoints (Xia *et al.* 2007; Xia *et al.* 2006). FANCM, in addition to its early binding role, also serves a catalytic function in the processing or resolution of the recombination intermediate, as cells from a FANCM patient form radials in response to ICL inducing agents, but the FANCM defect does not impact FANCD2 monoubiquitination (Singh *et al.* 2009).

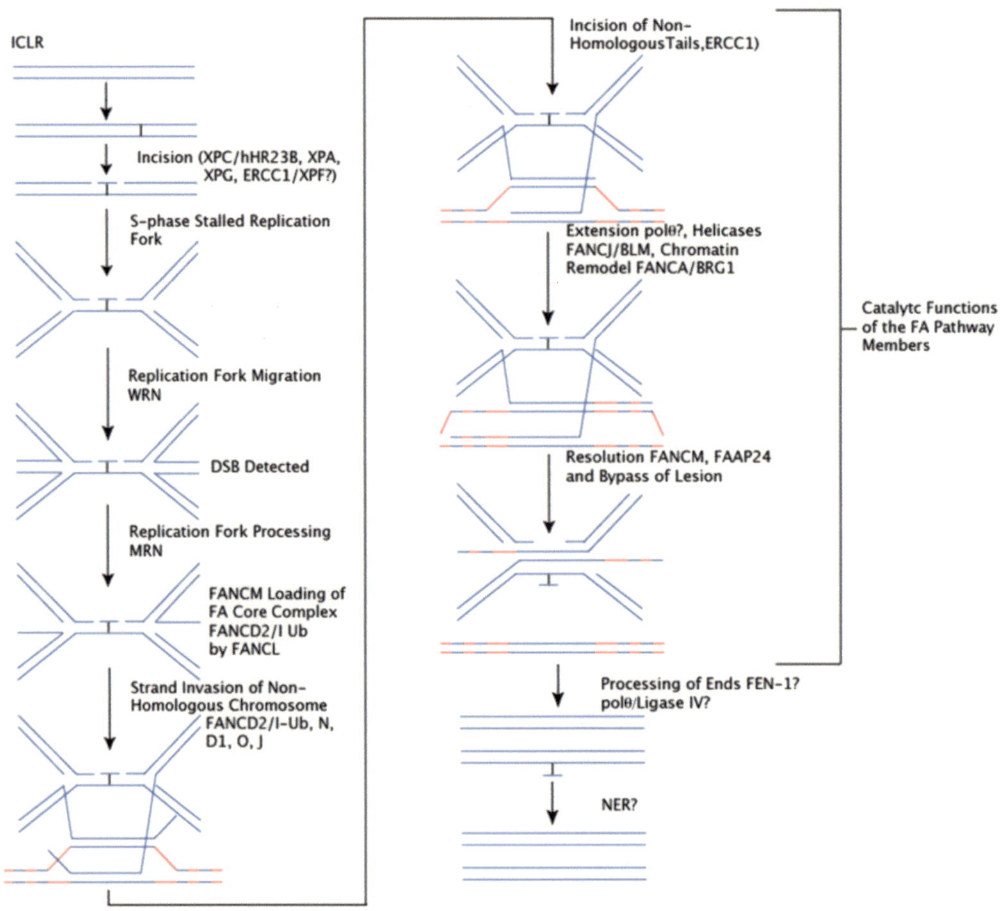

Fig. 6. Hypothetical Steps of ICLR

All of this suggests the next step in repair involves a HRR or HRR like repair mechanism, likely similar to BIR with a non-homologous substrate, as failure to complete repair yields a radial formation (Figure 7), and these radials are between non-homologous chromosomes (Newell *et al.* 2004). It would seem the variety of functions pulled together for ICLR serve to stabilize the stalled replication fork, initiate recombination in the absence of an available direct homologue by identifying repeats or microhomology suitable for recombination on non-homologous chromosomes, synthesis along this sequence past the region affected by the ICL (possibly involving polθ/Ligase IV, (Chan *et al.* 2010)), and subsequent resolution of the recombination intermediate (Figure 6).

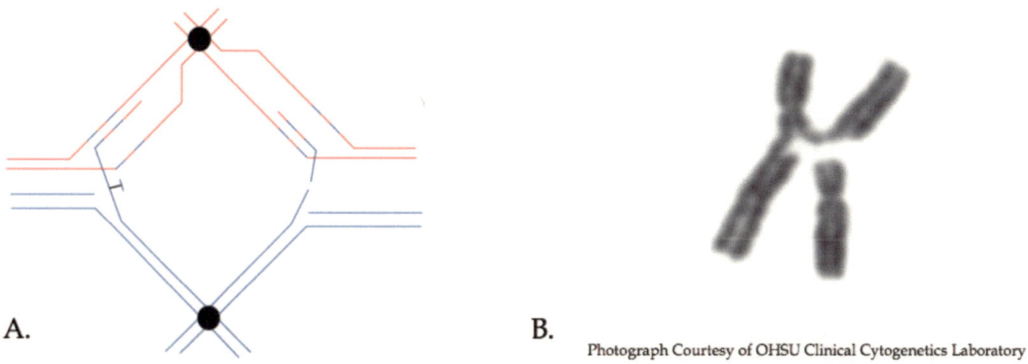

A. B.

Photograph Courtesy of OHSU Clinical Cytogenetics Laboratory

Fig. 7. A. Reorganization of non-homologous chromosome recombination intermediates from the model in Figure 6 into a chromosomal context (large circles represent centromeres) demonstrates the possibility for intermediates from this mechanism to yield radials. B. Portion of a metaphase spread of ICL treated FA mutant cells and a radial formation.

4. Discussion

With the exception of DRR and possibly a small subset of NHEJ, DNA damage repair requires DNA replication. BrdU incorporation, a general marker of DNA synthesis, has been successfully used as a surrogate marker for DNA damage repair (Kalle *et al.* 1993; Kao *et al.* 2001). The requirement of replication for repair relates to the double stranded structure of DNA, and the idea of having a built in backup copy of information on the opposing strand. To a certain extent, this holds true even in the case of double stranded damage, though the backup may be a repeat sequence on the same stretch of DNA or on a non-homologous chromosome, in the case of SSA and ICLR respectively.

Different types of DNA damage will utilize any of a variety of DNA polymerases, based upon the structure/function of this polymerase. The evolution of various DNA polymerase families with specific roles supports the importance of replication as an indispensible tool in the repair of DNA damage. TLS utilizes polymerases with open active sites to permit synthesis past an adduct (Trincao *et al.* 2001). Long-range synthesis in HRR requires polε, because of its processivity (Asturias *et al.* 2006). BIR requires the normally dispensable polδ subunit, pol32, to facilitate replication restart in response to this specific recombination based repair mechanism (Lydeard *et al.* 2007). The importance of polη in NER, is demonstrated by the similarity of disease spectrum present in XP variant and the XP group genes constituting catalytic functions in the repair of bulky adducts (Johnson *et al.* 1999a).

The evolutionary persistence of many of these polymerases demonstrates that this intimate involvement of DNA replication in repair is an indispensible facet of life, as we know it.

5. Acknowledgements

I would like to thank Alina M. Handorean, PhD for her contributions to the sections on Translesion Synthesis and Y Family Polymerases. The photo of the metaphase chromosomes in a radial formation was generously provided by Susan Olson, PhD and Amy Hanlon-Newell, PhD of the Oregon Health and Science University Clinical Cytogenetics Laboratories.

6. References

Aboussekhra, A., Biggerstaff, M., Shivji, M. K., Vilpo, J. A., Moncollin, V., Podust, V. N., Protic, M., Hubscher, U., Egly, J. M. and Wood, R. D. (1995). Mammalian DNA nucleotide excision repair reconstituted with purified protein components. *Cell* 80, (6):859-68.

Al-Minawi, A. Z., Saleh-Gohari, N. and Helleday, T. (2008). The ERCC1/XPF endonuclease is required for efficient single-strand annealing and gene conversion in mammalian cells. *Nucleic Acids Res* 36, (1):1-9.

Araujo, S. J., Tirode, F., Coin, F., Pospiech, H., Syvaoja, J. E., Stucki, M., Hubscher, U., Egly, J. M. and Wood, R. D. (2000). Nucleotide excision repair of DNA with recombinant human proteins: definition of the minimal set of factors, active forms of TFIIH, and modulation by CAK. *Genes Dev* 14, (3):349-59.

Araujo, S. J. and Wood, R. D. (1999). Protein complexes in nucleotide excision repair. *Mutat Res* 435, (1):23-33.

Asturias, F. J., Cheung, I. K., Sabouri, N., Chilkova, O., Wepplo, D. and Johansson, E. (2006). Structure of Saccharomyces cerevisiae DNA polymerase epsilon by cryo-electron microscopy. *Nat Struct Mol Biol* 13, (1):35-43.

Aylon, Y., Liefshitz, B. and Kupiec, M. (2004). The CDK regulates repair of double-strand breaks by homologous recombination during the cell cycle. *EMBO J* 23, (24):4868-75.

Baker, T. A. and Bell, S. P. (1998). Polymerases and the replisome: machines within machines. *Cell* 92, (3):295-305.

Banerjee, A., Santos, W. L. and Verdine, G. L. (2006). Structure of a DNA glycosylase searching for lesions. *Science* 311, (5764):1153-7.

Birger, Y., West, K. L., Postnikov, Y. V., Lim, J. H., Furusawa, T., Wagner, J. P., Laufer, C. S., Kraemer, K. H. and Bustin, M. (2003). Chromosomal protein HMGN1 enhances the rate of DNA repair in chromatin. *EMBO J* 22, (7):1665-75.

Bloom, L. B., Chen, X., Fygenson, D. K., Turner, J., O'Donnell, M. and Goodman, M. F. (1997). Fidelity of Escherichia coli DNA polymerase III holoenzyme. The effects of beta, gamma complex processivity proteins and epsilon proofreading exonuclease on nucleotide misincorporation efficiencies. *J Biol Chem* 272, (44):27919-30.

Bohr, V. A., Smith, C. A., Okumoto, D. S. and Hanawalt, P. C. (1985). DNA repair in an active gene: removal of pyrimidine dimers from the DHFR gene of CHO cells is much more efficient than in the genome overall. *Cell* 40, (2):359-69.

Bruner, S. D., Norman, D. P. and Verdine, G. L. (2000). Structural basis for recognition and repair of the endogenous mutagen 8-oxoguanine in DNA. *Nature* 403, (6772):859-66.
Bryans, M., Valenzano, M. C. and Stamato, T. D. (1999). Absence of DNA ligase IV protein in XR-1 cells: evidence for stabilization by XRCC4. *Mutat Res* 433, (1):53-8.
Burgers, P. M., Koonin, E. V., Bruford, E., Blanco, L., Burtis, K. C., Christman, M. F., Copeland, W. C., Friedberg, E. C., Hanaoka, F., Hinkle, D. C., Lawrence, C. W., Nakanishi, M., Ohmori, H., Prakash, L., Prakash, S., Reynaud, C. A., Sugino, A., Todo, T., Wang, Z., Weill, J. C. and Woodgate, R. (2001). Eukaryotic DNA polymerases: proposal for a revised nomenclature. *J Biol Chem* 276, (47):43487-90.
Cantor, S., Bell, D. W., Ganesan, S., Kass, E. M., Drapkin, R., Grossman, S., Wahrer, D. C., Sgroi, D. C., Lane, W. S., Haber, D. A. and Livingston, D. M. (2001). BACH1, a novel helicase-like protein, interacts directly with BRCA1 and contributes to its DNA repair function. *Cell* 105, (1):149-60.
Cantor, S., Drapkin, R., Zhang, F., Lin, Y., Han, J., Pamidi, S. and Livingston, D. M. (2004). The BRCA1-associated protein BACH1 is a DNA helicase targeted by clinically relevant inactivating mutations. *Proc Natl Acad Sci U S A* 101, (8):2357-62.
Cary, R. B., Peterson, S. R., Wang, J., Bear, D. G., Bradbury, E. M. and Chen, D. J. (1997). DNA looping by Ku and the DNA-dependent protein kinase. *Proc Natl Acad Sci U S A* 94, (9):4267-72.
Chan, S. H., Yu, A. M. and McVey, M. (2010). Dual roles for DNA polymerase theta in alternative end-joining repair of double-strand breaks in Drosophila. *PLoS Genet* 6, (7):e1001005.
Chen, L., Nievera, C. J., Lee, A. Y. and Wu, X. (2008). Cell cycle-dependent complex formation of BRCA1.CtIP.MRN is important for DNA double-strand break repair. *J Biol Chem* 283, (12):7713-20.
Chilkova, O., Stenlund, P., Isoz, I., Stith, C. M., Grabowski, P., Lundstrom, E. B., Burgers, P. M. and Johansson, E. (2007). The eukaryotic leading and lagging strand DNA polymerases are loaded onto primer-ends via separate mechanisms but have comparable processivity in the presence of PCNA. *Nucleic Acids Res* 35, (19):6588-97.
Dantzer, F., Nasheuer, H. P., Vonesch, J. L., de Murcia, G. and Menissier-de Murcia, J. (1998). Functional association of poly(ADP-ribose) polymerase with DNA polymerase alpha-primase complex: a link between DNA strand break detection and DNA replication. *Nucleic Acids Res* 26, (8):1891-8.
Davies, A. A., Masson, J. Y., McIlwraith, M. J., Stasiak, A. Z., Stasiak, A., Venkitaraman, A. R. and West, S. C. (2001). Role of BRCA2 in control of the RAD51 recombination and DNA repair protein. *Mol Cell* 7, (2):273-82.
Dronkert, M. L. and Kanaar, R. (2001). Repair of DNA interstrand cross-links. *Mutat Res* 486, (4):217-47.
Duncan, T., Trewick, S. C., Koivisto, P., Bates, P. A., Lindahl, T. and Sedgwick, B. (2002). Reversal of DNA alkylation damage by two human dioxygenases. *Proc Natl Acad Sci U S A* 99, (26):16660-5.
Edwards, S., Li, C. M., Levy, D. L., Brown, J., Snow, P. M. and Campbell, J. L. (2003). Saccharomyces cerevisiae DNA polymerase epsilon and polymerase sigma interact physically and functionally, suggesting a role for polymerase epsilon in sister chromatid cohesion. *Mol Cell Biol* 23, (8):2733-48.

Ellis, N. A., Groden, J., Ye, T. Z., Straughen, J., Lennon, D. J., Ciocci, S., Proytcheva, M. and German, J. (1995). The Bloom's syndrome gene product is homologous to RecQ helicases. *Cell* 83, (4):655-66.

Engelward, B. P., Weeda, G., Wyatt, M. D., Broekhof, J. L., de Wit, J., Donker, I., Allan, J. M., Gold, B., Hoeijmakers, J. H. and Samson, L. D. (1997). Base excision repair deficient mice lacking the Aag alkyladenine DNA glycosylase. *Proc Natl Acad Sci U S A* 94, (24):13087-92.

Fan, W. and Wu, X. (2004). DNA polymerase lambda can elongate on DNA substrates mimicking non-homologous end joining and interact with XRCC4-ligase IV complex. *Biochem Biophys Res Commun* 323, (4):1328-33.

Ferguson, D. O. and Holloman, W. K. (1996). Recombinational repair of gaps in DNA is asymmetric in Ustilago maydis and can be explained by a migrating D-loop model. *Proc Natl Acad Sci U S A* 93, (11):5419-24.

Fishman-Lobell, J., Rudin, N. and Haber, J. E. (1992). Two alternative pathways of double-strand break repair that are kinetically separable and independently modulated. *Mol Cell Biol* 12, (3):1292-303.

Folias, A., Matkovic, M., Bruun, D., Reid, S., Hejna, J., Grompe, M., D'Andrea, A. and Moses, R. (2002). BRCA1 interacts directly with the Fanconi anemia protein FANCA. *Hum Mol Genet* 11, (21):2591-7.

Fousteri, M. and Mullenders, L. H. (2008). Transcription-coupled nucleotide excision repair in mammalian cells: molecular mechanisms and biological effects. *Cell Res* 18, (1):73-84.

Frankenberg-Schwager, M., Gebauer, A., Koppe, C., Wolf, H., Pralle, E. and Frankenberg, D. (2009). Single-strand annealing, conservative homologous recombination, nonhomologous DNA end joining, and the cell cycle-dependent repair of DNA double-strand breaks induced by sparsely or densely ionizing radiation. *Radiat Res* 171, (3):265-73.

Garcia-Diaz, M., Bebenek, K., Kunkel, T. A. and Blanco, L. (2001). Identification of an intrinsic 5'-deoxyribose-5-phosphate lyase activity in human DNA polymerase lambda: a possible role in base excision repair. *J Biol Chem* 276, (37):34659-63.

Garcia-Higuera, I., Taniguchi, T., Ganesan, S., Meyn, M. S., Timmers, C., Hejna, J., Grompe, M. and D'Andrea, A. D. (2001). Interaction of the Fanconi anemia proteins and BRCA1 in a common pathway. *Mol Cell* 7, (2):249-62.

Goetz, J. D., Motycka, T. A., Han, M., Jasin, M. and Tomkinson, A. E. (2005). Reduced repair of DNA double-strand breaks by homologous recombination in a DNA ligase I-deficient human cell line. *DNA Repair (Amst)* 4, (6):649-54.

Gotte, M., Li, X. and Wainberg, M. A. (1999). HIV-1 reverse transcription: a brief overview focused on structure-function relationships among molecules involved in initiation of the reaction. *Arch Biochem Biophys* 365, (2):199-210.

Gottlich, B., Reichenberger, S., Feldmann, E. and Pfeiffer, P. (1998). Rejoining of DNA double-strand breaks in vitro by single-strand annealing. *Eur J Biochem* 258, (2):387-95.

Greider, C. W. and Blackburn, E. H. (1989). A telomeric sequence in the RNA of Tetrahymena telomerase required for telomere repeat synthesis. *Nature* 337, (6205):331-7.

Grossmann, K. F., Ward, A. M., Matkovic, M. E., Folias, A. E. and Moses, R. E. (2001). S. cerevisiae has three pathways for DNA interstrand crosslink repair. *Mutat Res* 487, (3-4):73-83.

Guo, C., Fischhaber, P. L., Luk-Paszyc, M. J., Masuda, Y., Zhou, J., Kamiya, K., Kisker, C. and Friedberg, E. C. (2003). Mouse Rev1 protein interacts with multiple DNA polymerases involved in translesion DNA synthesis. *EMBO J* 22, (24):6621-30.

Haracska, L., Johnson, R. E., Unk, I., Phillips, B., Hurwitz, J., Prakash, L. and Prakash, S. (2001a). Physical and functional interactions of human DNA polymerase eta with PCNA. *Mol Cell Biol* 21, (21):7199-206.

Haracska, L., Kondratick, C. M., Unk, I., Prakash, S. and Prakash, L. (2001b). Interaction with PCNA is essential for yeast DNA polymerase eta function. *Mol Cell* 8, (2):407-15.

Haracska, L., Prakash, S. and Prakash, L. (2003). Yeast DNA polymerase zeta is an efficient extender of primer ends opposite from 7,8-dihydro-8-Oxoguanine and O6-methylguanine. *Mol Cell Biol* 23, (4):1453-9.

Harrington, C. and Perrino, F. W. (1995). Initiation of RNA-primed DNA synthesis in vitro by DNA polymerase alpha-primase. *Nucleic Acids Res* 23, (6):1003-9.

Henning, K. A., Li, L., Iyer, N., McDaniel, L. D., Reagan, M. S., Legerski, R., Schultz, R. A., Stefanini, M., Lehmann, A. R., Mayne, L. V. and Friedberg, E. C. (1995). The Cockayne syndrome group A gene encodes a WD repeat protein that interacts with CSB protein and a subunit of RNA polymerase II TFIIH. *Cell* 82, (4):555-64.

Hirsch, B., Shimamura, A., Moreau, L., Baldinger, S., Hag-alshiekh, M., Bostrom, B., Sencer, S. and D'Andrea, A. D. (2004). Association of biallelic BRCA2/FANCD1 mutations with spontaneous chromosomal instability and solid tumors of childhood. *Blood* 103, (7):2554-9.

Hubscher, U., Maga, G. and Spadari, S. (2002). Eukaryotic DNA polymerases. *Annu Rev Biochem* 71, 133-63.

Hussain, S., Wilson, J. B., Medhurst, A. L., Hejna, J., Witt, E., Ananth, S., Davies, A., Masson, J. Y., Moses, R., West, S. C., de Winter, J. P., Ashworth, A., Jones, N. J. and Mathew, C. G. (2004). Direct interaction of FANCD2 with BRCA2 in DNA damage response pathways. *Hum Mol Genet* 13, (12):1241-8.

Iliakis, G. (2009). Backup pathways of NHEJ in cells of higher eukaryotes: cell cycle dependence. *Radiother Oncol* 92, (3):310-5.

Ishino, Y., Komori, K., Cann, I. K. and Koga, Y. (1998). A novel DNA polymerase family found in Archaea. *J Bacteriol* 180, (8):2232-6.

Johnson, R. E., Kondratick, C. M., Prakash, S. and Prakash, L. (1999a). hRAD30 mutations in the variant form of xeroderma pigmentosum. *Science* 285, (5425):263-5.

Johnson, R. E., Prakash, S. and Prakash, L. (1999b). Efficient bypass of a thymine-thymine dimer by yeast DNA polymerase, Poleta. *Science* 283, (5404):1001-4.

Johnson, R. E., Washington, M. T., Haracska, L., Prakash, S. and Prakash, L. (2000). Eukaryotic polymerases iota and zeta act sequentially to bypass DNA lesions. *Nature* 406, (6799):1015-9.

Kalle, W. H., Hazekamp-van Dokkum, A. M., Lohman, P. H., Natarajan, A. T., van Zeeland, A. A. and Mullenders, L. H. (1993). The use of streptavidin-coated magnetic beads and biotinylated antibodies to investigate induction and repair of DNA damage: analysis of repair patches in specific sequences of uv-irradiated human fibroblasts. *Anal Biochem* 208, (2):228-36.

Kao, G. D., McKenna, W. G. and Yen, T. J. (2001). Detection of repair activity during the DNA damage-induced G2 delay in human cancer cells. *Oncogene* 20, (27):3486-96.

Kawasaki, Y. and Sugino, A. (2001). Yeast replicative DNA polymerases and their role at the replication fork. *Mol Cells* 12, (3):277-85.

Kelman, Z. (1997). PCNA: structure, functions and interactions. *Oncogene* 14, (6):629-40.

Khanna, K. K. and Jackson, S. P. (2001). DNA double-strand breaks: signaling, repair and the cancer connection. *Nat Genet* 27, (3):247-54.

Kim, S. T., Malhotra, K., Smith, C. A., Taylor, J. S. and Sancar, A. (1993). DNA photolyase repairs the trans-syn cyclobutane thymine dimer. *Biochemistry* 32, (28):7065-8.

Kitao, H. and Takata, M. (2011). Fanconi anemia: a disorder defective in the DNA damage response. *Int J Hematol* 73(4):417-24.

Klungland, A., Rosewell, I., Hollenbach, S., Larsen, E., Daly, G., Epe, B., Seeberg, E., Lindahl, T. and Barnes, D. E. (1999). Accumulation of premutagenic DNA lesions in mice defective in removal of oxidative base damage. *Proc Natl Acad Sci U S A* 96, (23):13300-5.

Kubota, Y., Nash, R. A., Klungland, A., Schar, P., Barnes, D. E. and Lindahl, T. (1996). Reconstitution of DNA base excision-repair with purified human proteins: interaction between DNA polymerase beta and the XRCC1 protein. *EMBO J* 15, (23):6662-70.

Kuchta, R. D., Benkovic, P. and Benkovic, S. J. (1988). Kinetic mechanism whereby DNA polymerase I (Klenow) replicates DNA with high fidelity. *Biochemistry* 27, (18):6716-25.

Kuchta, R. D., Mizrahi, V., Benkovic, P. A., Johnson, K. A. and Benkovic, S. J. (1987). Kinetic mechanism of DNA polymerase I (Klenow). *Biochemistry* 26, (25):8410-7.

Kulaksiz, G., Reardon, J. T. and Sancar, A. (2005). Xeroderma pigmentosum complementation group E protein (XPE/DDB2): purification of various complexes of XPE and analyses of their damaged DNA binding and putative DNA repair properties. *Mol Cell Biol* 25, (22):9784-92.

Lamers, M. H., Georgescu, R. E., Lee, S. G., O'Donnell, M. and Kuriyan, J. (2006). Crystal structure of the catalytic alpha subunit of E. coli replicative DNA polymerase III. *Cell* 126, (5):881-92.

Lawley, P. D. and Phillips, D. H. (1996). DNA adducts from chemotherapeutic agents. *Mutat Res* 355, (1-2):13-40.

Li, L., Lu, X., Peterson, C. A. and Legerski, R. J. (1995a). An interaction between the DNA repair factor XPA and replication protein A appears essential for nucleotide excision repair. *Mol Cell Biol* 15, (10):5396-402.

Li, L., Peterson, C. A., Lu, X. and Legerski, R. J. (1995b). Mutations in XPA that prevent association with ERCC1 are defective in nucleotide excision repair. *Mol Cell Biol* 15, (4):1993-8.

Lord, R. V., Brabender, J., Gandara, D., Alberola, V., Camps, C., Domine, M., Cardenal, F., Sanchez, J. M., Gumerlock, P. H., Taron, M., Sanchez, J. J., Danenberg, K. D., Danenberg, P. V. and Rosell, R. (2002). Low ERCC1 expression correlates with prolonged survival after cisplatin plus gemcitabine chemotherapy in non-small cell lung cancer. *Clin Cancer Res* 8, (7):2286-91.

Lydeard, J. R., Jain, S., Yamaguchi, M. and Haber, J. E. (2007). Break-induced replication and telomerase-independent telomere maintenance require Pol32. *Nature* 448, (7155):820-3.

Machida, Y. J., Machida, Y., Chen, Y., Gurtan, A. M., Kupfer, G. M., D'Andrea, A. D. and Dutta, A. (2006). UBE2T is the E2 in the Fanconi anemia pathway and undergoes negative autoregulation. *Mol Cell* 23, (4):589-96.

Mahajan, K. N., Gangi-Peterson, L., Sorscher, D. H., Wang, J., Gathy, K. N., Mahajan, N. P., Reeves, W. H. and Mitchell, B. S. (1999). Association of terminal deoxynucleotidyl transferase with Ku. *Proc Natl Acad Sci U S A* 96, (24):13926-31.

Mahajan, K. N., Nick McElhinny, S. A., Mitchell, B. S. and Ramsden, D. A. (2002). Association of DNA polymerase mu (pol mu) with Ku and ligase IV: role for pol mu in end-joining double-strand break repair. *Mol Cell Biol* 22, (14):5194-202.

Maloisel, L., Fabre, F. and Gangloff, S. (2008). DNA polymerase delta is preferentially recruited during homologous recombination to promote heteroduplex DNA extension. *Mol Cell Biol* 28, (4):1373-82.

McCabe, K. M., Hemphill, A., Akkari, Y., Jakobs, P. M., Pauw, D., Olson, S. B., Moses, R. E. and Grompe, M. (2008). ERCC1 is required for FANCD2 focus formation. *Mol Genet Metab* 95, (1-2):66-73.

McCabe, K. M., Olson, S. B. and Moses, R. E. (2009). DNA interstrand crosslink repair in mammalian cells. *J Cell Physiol* 220, (3):569-73.

McIlwraith, M. J., Vaisman, A., Liu, Y., Fanning, E., Woodgate, R. and West, S. C. (2005). Human DNA polymerase eta promotes DNA synthesis from strand invasion intermediates of homologous recombination. *Mol Cell* 20, (5):783-92.

McKinnon, P. J. and Caldecott, K. W. (2007). DNA strand break repair and human genetic disease. *Annu Rev Genomics Hum Genet* 8, 37-55.

Meetei, A. R., Sechi, S., Wallisch, M., Yang, D., Young, M. K., Joenje, H., Hoatlin, M. E. and Wang, W. (2003). A multiprotein nuclear complex connects Fanconi anemia and Bloom syndrome. *Mol Cell Biol* 23, (10):3417-26.

Mellon, I., Spivak, G. and Hanawalt, P. C. (1987). Selective removal of transcription-blocking DNA damage from the transcribed strand of the mammalian DHFR gene. *Cell* 51, (2):241-9.

Meselson, M. and Stahl, F. W. (1958). The Replication of DNA in Escherichia Coli. *Proc Natl Acad Sci U S A* 44, (7):671-82.

Mitchell, J. R., Hoeijmakers, J. H. and Niedernhofer, L. J. (2003). Divide and conquer: nucleotide excision repair battles cancer and ageing. *Curr Opin Cell Biol* 15, (2):232-40.

Mladenov, E. and Iliakis, G. (2011). Induction and repair of DNA double strand breaks: The increasing spectrum of non-homologous end joining pathways. *Mutat Res* 711(1-2):61-72.

Mol, C. D., Hosfield, D. J. and Tainer, J. A. (2000). Abasic site recognition by two apurinic/apyrimidinic endonuclease families in DNA base excision repair: the 3' ends justify the means. *Mutat Res* 460, (3-4):211-29.

Moser, J., Kool, H., Giakzidis, I., Caldecott, K., Mullenders, L. H. and Fousteri, M. I. (2007). Sealing of chromosomal DNA nicks during nucleotide excision repair requires XRCC1 and DNA ligase III alpha in a cell-cycle-specific manner. *Mol Cell* 27, (2):311-23.

Nakanishi, K., Taniguchi, T., Ranganathan, V., New, H. V., Moreau, L. A., Stotsky, M., Mathew, C. G., Kastan, M. B., Weaver, D. T. and D'Andrea, A. D. (2002). Interaction of FANCD2 and NBS1 in the DNA damage response. *Nat Cell Biol* 4, (12):913-20.

Nakatsu, Y., Asahina, H., Citterio, E., Rademakers, S., Vermeulen, W., Kamiuchi, S., Yeo, J. P., Khaw, M. C., Saijo, M., Kodo, N., Matsuda, T., Hoeijmakers, J. H. and Tanaka, K. (2000). XAB2, a novel tetratricopeptide repeat protein involved in transcription-coupled DNA repair and transcription. *J Biol Chem* 275, (45):34931-7.

Nevaldine, B., Longo, J. A. and Hahn, P. J. (1997). The scid defect results in much slower repair of DNA double-strand breaks but not high levels of residual breaks. *Radiat Res* 147, (5):535-40.

Newell, A. E., Akkari, Y. M., Torimaru, Y., Rosenthal, A., Reifsteck, C. A., Cox, B., Grompe, M. and Olson, S. B. (2004). Interstrand crosslink-induced radials form between non-homologous chromosomes, but are absent in sex chromosomes. *DNA Repair (Amst)* 3, (5):535-42.

Ng, J. M., Vermeulen, W., van der Horst, G. T., Bergink, S., Sugasawa, K., Vrieling, H. and Hoeijmakers, J. H. (2003). A novel regulation mechanism of DNA repair by damage-induced and RAD23-dependent stabilization of xeroderma pigmentosum group C protein. *Genes Dev* 17, (13):1630-45.

O'Donovan, A., Davies, A. A., Moggs, J. G., West, S. C. and Wood, R. D. (1994). XPG endonuclease makes the 3' incision in human DNA nucleotide excision repair. *Nature* 371, (6496):432-5.

Ogi, T. and Lehmann, A. R. (2006). The Y-family DNA polymerase kappa (pol kappa) functions in mammalian nucleotide-excision repair. *Nat Cell Biol* 8, (6):640-2.

Ohashi, E., Murakumo, Y., Kanjo, N., Akagi, J., Masutani, C., Hanaoka, F. and Ohmori, H. (2004). Interaction of hREV1 with three human Y-family DNA polymerases. *Genes Cells* 9, (6):523-31.

Ohmori, H., Friedberg, E. C., Fuchs, R. P., Goodman, M. F., Hanaoka, F., Hinkle, D., Kunkel, T. A., Lawrence, C. W., Livneh, Z., Nohmi, T., Prakash, L., Prakash, S., Todo, T., Walker, G. C., Wang, Z. and Woodgate, R. (2001). The Y-family of DNA polymerases. *Mol Cell* 8, (1):7-8.

Otsuki, T., Furukawa, Y., Ikeda, K., Endo, H., Yamashita, T., Shinohara, A., Iwamatsu, A., Ozawa, K. and Liu, J. M. (2001). Fanconi anemia protein, FANCA, associates with BRG1, a component of the human SWI/SNF complex. *Hum Mol Genet* 10, (23):2651-60.

Parsons, B. L. (2003). MED1: a central molecule for maintenance of genome integrity and response to DNA damage. *Proc Natl Acad Sci U S A* 100, (25):14601-2.

Patel, S. S., Wong, I. and Johnson, K. A. (1991). Pre-steady-state kinetic analysis of processive DNA replication including complete characterization of an exonuclease-deficient mutant. *Biochemistry* 30, (2):511-25.

Pellegrini, L., Yu, D. S., Lo, T., Anand, S., Lee, M., Blundell, T. L. and Venkitaraman, A. R. (2002). Insights into DNA recombination from the structure of a RAD51-BRCA2 complex. *Nature* 420, (6913):287-93.

Prasad, R., Dianov, G. L., Bohr, V. A. and Wilson, S. H. (2000). FEN1 stimulation of DNA polymerase beta mediates an excision step in mammalian long patch base excision repair. *J Biol Chem* 275, (6):4460-6.

Prasad, R., Longley, M. J., Sharief, F. S., Hou, E. W., Copeland, W. C. and Wilson, S. H. (2009). Human DNA polymerase theta possesses 5'-dRP lyase activity and functions in single-nucleotide base excision repair in vitro. *Nucleic Acids Res* 37, (6):1868-77.

Rass, E., Grabarz, A., Plo, I., Gautier, J., Bertrand, P. and Lopez, B. S. (2009). Role of Mre11 in chromosomal nonhomologous end joining in mammalian cells. *Nat Struct Mol Biol* 16, (8):819-24.

Reid, S., Schindler, D., Hanenberg, H., Barker, K., Hanks, S., Kalb, R., Neveling, K., Kelly, P., Seal, S., Freund, M., Wurm, M., Batish, S. D., Lach, F. P., Yetgin, S., Neitzel, H., Ariffin, H., Tischkowitz, M., Mathew, C. G., Auerbach, A. D. and Rahman, N. (2007). Biallelic mutations in PALB2 cause Fanconi anemia subtype FA-N and predispose to childhood cancer. *Nat Genet* 39, (2):162-4.

Richardson, C. and Jasin, M. (2000). Frequent chromosomal translocations induced by DNA double-strand breaks. *Nature* 405, (6787):697-700.

Robu, M. E., Inman, R. B. and Cox, M. M. (2001). RecA protein promotes the regression of stalled replication forks in vitro. *Proc Natl Acad Sci U S A* 98, (15):8211-8.

Rogakou, E. P., Boon, C., Redon, C. and Bonner, W. M. (1999). Megabase chromatin domains involved in DNA double-strand breaks in vivo. *J Cell Biol* 146, (5):905-16.

Rosidi, B., Wang, M., Wu, W., Sharma, A., Wang, H. and Iliakis, G. (2008). Histone H1 functions as a stimulatory factor in backup pathways of NHEJ. *Nucleic Acids Res* 36, (5):1610-23.

Ryu, J. S., Hong, Y. C., Han, H. S., Lee, J. E., Kim, S., Park, Y. M., Kim, Y. C. and Hwang, T. S. (2004). Association between polymorphisms of ERCC1 and XPD and survival in non-small-cell lung cancer patients treated with cisplatin combination chemotherapy. *Lung Cancer* 44, (3):311-6.

Scharer, O. D. (2005). DNA interstrand crosslinks: natural and drug-induced DNA adducts that induce unique cellular responses. *Chembiochem* 6, (1):27-32.

Sharan, S. K., Morimatsu, M., Albrecht, U., Lim, D. S., Regel, E., Dinh, C., Sands, A., Eichele, G., Hasty, P. and Bradley, A. (1997). Embryonic lethality and radiation hypersensitivity mediated by Rad51 in mice lacking Brca2. *Nature* 386, (6627):804-10.

Sijbers, A. M., de Laat, W. L., Ariza, R. R., Biggerstaff, M., Wei, Y. F., Moggs, J. G., Carter, K. C., Shell, B. K., Evans, E., de Jong, M. C., Rademakers, S., de Rooij, J., Jaspers, N. G., Hoeijmakers, J. H. and Wood, R. D. (1996). Xeroderma pigmentosum group F caused by a defect in a structure-specific DNA repair endonuclease. *Cell* 86, (5):811-22.

Singh, T. R., Bakker, S. T., Agarwal, S., Jansen, M., Grassman, E., Godthelp, B. C., Ali, A. M., Du, C. H., Rooimans, M. A., Fan, Q., Wahengbam, K., Steltenpool, J., Andreassen, P. R., Williams, D. A., Joenje, H., de Winter, J. P. and Meetei, A. R. (2009). Impaired FANCD2 monoubiquitination and hypersensitivity to camptothecin uniquely characterize Fanconi anemia complementation group M. *Blood* 114, (1):174-80.

Singh, T. R., Saro, D., Ali, A. M., Zheng, X. F., Du, C. H., Killen, M. W., Sachpatzidis, A., Wahengbam, K., Pierce, A. J., Xiong, Y., Sung, P. and Meetei, A. R. (2010). MHF1-MHF2, a histone-fold-containing protein complex, participates in the Fanconi anemia pathway via FANCM. *Mol Cell* 37, (6):879-86.

Smith, K. N. and Nicolas, A. (1998). Recombination at work for meiosis. *Current Opinion in Genetics & Development* 8, (2):200-211.

Smogorzewska, A., Matsuoka, S., Vinciguerra, P., McDonald, E. R., 3rd, Hurov, K. E., Luo, J., Ballif, B. A., Gygi, S. P., Hofmann, K., D'Andrea, A. D. and Elledge, S. J. (2007). Identification of the FANCI protein, a monoubiquitinated FANCD2 paralog required for DNA repair. *Cell* 129, (2):289-301.

Sobeck, A., Stone, S. and Hoatlin, M. E. (2007). DNA structure-induced recruitment and activation of the Fanconi anemia pathway protein FANCD2. *Mol Cell Biol* 27, (12):4283-92.

Solinger, J. A., Lutz, G., Sugiyama, T., Kowalczykowski, S. C. and Heyer, W. D. (2001). Rad54 protein stimulates heteroduplex DNA formation in the synaptic phase of DNA strand exchange via specific interactions with the presynaptic Rad51 nucleoprotein filament. *J Mol Biol* 307, (5):1207-21.

Srivastava, D. K., Berg, B. J., Prasad, R., Molina, J. T., Beard, W. A., Tomkinson, A. E. and Wilson, S. H. (1998). Mammalian abasic site base excision repair. Identification of the reaction sequence and rate-determining steps. *J Biol Chem* 273, (33):21203-9.

Stasiak, A. Z., Larquet, E., Stasiak, A., Muller, S., Engel, A., Van Dyck, E., West, S. C. and Egelman, E. H. (2000). The human Rad52 protein exists as a heptameric ring. *Curr Biol* 10, (6):337-40.

Stauffer, M. E. and Chazin, W. J. (2004). Physical interaction between replication protein A and Rad51 promotes exchange on single-stranded DNA. *J Biol Chem* 279, (24):25638-45.

Steitz, T. A. (1998). A mechanism for all polymerases. *Nature* 391, (6664):231-2.

Sugawara, N., Ira, G. and Haber, J. E. (2000). DNA length dependence of the single-strand annealing pathway and the role of Saccharomyces cerevisiae RAD59 in double-strand break repair. *Mol Cell Biol* 20, (14):5300-9.

Sung, P. and Robberson, D. L. (1995). DNA strand exchange mediated by a RAD51-ssDNA nucleoprotein filament with polarity opposite to that of RecA. *Cell* 82, (3):453-61.

Szostak, J. W., Orr-Weaver, T. L., Rothstein, R. J. and Stahl, F. W. (1983). The double-strand-break repair model for recombination. *Cell* 33, (1):25-35.

Tantin, D. (1998). RNA polymerase II elongation complexes containing the Cockayne syndrome group B protein interact with a molecular complex containing the transcription factor IIH components xeroderma pigmentosum B and p62. *J Biol Chem* 273, (43):27794-9.

Tantin, D., Kansal, A. and Carey, M. (1997). Recruitment of the putative transcription-repair coupling factor CSB/ERCC6 to RNA polymerase II elongation complexes. *Mol Cell Biol* 17, (12):6803-14.

Tischkowitz, M., Xia, B., Sabbaghian, N., Reis-Filho, J. S., Hamel, N., Li, G., van Beers, E. H., Li, L., Khalil, T., Quenneville, L. A., Omeroglu, A., Poll, A., Lepage, P., Wong, N., Nederlof, P. M., Ashworth, A., Tonin, P. N., Narod, S. A., Livingston, D. M. and Foulkes, W. D. (2007). Analysis of PALB2/FANCN-associated breast cancer families. *Proc Natl Acad Sci U S A* 104, (16):6788-93.

Tissier, A., Kannouche, P., Reck, M. P., Lehmann, A. R., Fuchs, R. P. and Cordonnier, A. (2004). Co-localization in replication foci and interaction of human Y-family members, DNA polymerase pol eta and REVl protein. *DNA Repair (Amst)* 3, (11):1503-14.

Trincao, J., Johnson, R. E., Escalante, C. R., Prakash, S., Prakash, L. and Aggarwal, A. K. (2001). Structure of the catalytic core of S. cerevisiae DNA polymerase eta: implications for translesion DNA synthesis. *Mol Cell* 8, (2):417-26.

Van Dyck, E., Stasiak, A. Z., Stasiak, A. and West, S. C. (1999). Binding of double-strand breaks in DNA by human Rad52 protein. *Nature* 398, (6729):728-31.

Vignard, J., Siwiec, T., Chelysheva, L., Vrielynck, N., Gonord, F., Armstrong, S. J., Schlogelhofer, P. and Mercier, R. (2007). The interplay of RecA-related proteins and the MND1-HOP2 complex during meiosis in Arabidopsis thaliana. *PLoS Genet* 3, (10):1894-906.

Wang, H., Perrault, A. R., Takeda, Y., Qin, W. and Iliakis, G. (2003). Biochemical evidence for Ku-independent backup pathways of NHEJ. *Nucleic Acids Res* 31, (18):5377-88.

Wang, H., Zeng, Z. C., Bui, T. A., Sonoda, E., Takata, M., Takeda, S. and Iliakis, G. (2001a). Efficient rejoining of radiation-induced DNA double-strand breaks in vertebrate cells deficient in genes of the RAD52 epistasis group. *Oncogene* 20, (18):2212-24.

Wang, H., Zeng, Z. C., Perrault, A. R., Cheng, X., Qin, W. and Iliakis, G. (2001b). Genetic evidence for the involvement of DNA ligase IV in the DNA-PK-dependent pathway of non-homologous end joining in mammalian cells. *Nucleic Acids Res* 29, (8):1653-60.

Wang, M., Wu, W., Rosidi, B., Zhang, L., Wang, H. and Iliakis, G. (2006). PARP-1 and Ku compete for repair of DNA double strand breaks by distinct NHEJ pathways. *Nucleic Acids Res* 34, (21):6170-82.

Washington, M. T., Johnson, R. E., Prakash, L. and Prakash, S. (2002). Human DINB1-encoded DNA polymerase kappa is a promiscuous extender of mispaired primer termini. *Proc Natl Acad Sci U S A* 99, (4):1910-4.

Washington, M. T., Johnson, R. E., Prakash, S. and Prakash, L. (2000). Accuracy of thymine-thymine dimer bypass by Saccharomyces cerevisiae DNA polymerase eta. *Proc Natl Acad Sci U S A* 97, (7):3094-9.

Washington, M. T., Prakash, L. and Prakash, S. (2001). Yeast DNA polymerase eta utilizes an induced-fit mechanism of nucleotide incorporation. *Cell* 107, (7):917-27.

Waters, L. S., Minesinger, B. K., Wiltrout, M. E., D'Souza, S., Woodruff, R. V. and Walker, G. C. (2009). Eukaryotic translesion polymerases and their roles and regulation in DNA damage tolerance. *Microbiol Mol Biol Rev* 73, (1):134-54.

Wibley, J. E., Pegg, A. E. and Moody, P. C. (2000). Crystal structure of the human O(6)-alkylguanine-DNA alkyltransferase. *Nucleic Acids Res* 28, (2):393-401.

Windhofer, F., Wu, W. and Iliakis, G. (2007). Low levels of DNA ligases III and IV sufficient for effective NHEJ. *J Cell Physiol* 213, (2):475-83.

Wold, M. S. (1997). Replication protein A: a heterotrimeric, single-stranded DNA-binding protein required for eukaryotic DNA metabolism. *Annu Rev Biochem* 66, 61-92.

Wong, I., Patel, S. S. and Johnson, K. A. (1991). An induced-fit kinetic mechanism for DNA replication fidelity: direct measurement by single-turnover kinetics. *Biochemistry* 30, (2):526-37.

Wu, W., Wang, M., Mussfeldt, T. and Iliakis, G. (2008). Enhanced use of backup pathways of NHEJ in G2 in Chinese hamster mutant cells with defects in the classical pathway of NHEJ. *Radiat Res* 170, (4):512-20.

Xia, B., Dorsman, J. C., Ameziane, N., de Vries, Y., Rooimans, M. A., Sheng, Q., Pals, G., Errami, A., Gluckman, E., Llera, J., Wang, W., Livingston, D. M., Joenje, H. and de

Winter, J. P. (2007). Fanconi anemia is associated with a defect in the BRCA2 partner PALB2. *Nat Genet* 39, (2):159-61.

Xia, B., Sheng, Q., Nakanishi, K., Ohashi, A., Wu, J., Christ, N., Liu, X., Jasin, M., Couch, F. J. and Livingston, D. M. (2006). Control of BRCA2 cellular and clinical functions by a nuclear partner, PALB2. *Mol Cell* 22, (6):719-29.

Yamasaki, K., Urushibata, Y., Yamasaki, T., Arisaka, F. and Matsui, I. (2010). Solution structure of the N-terminal domain of the archaeal D-family DNA polymerase small subunit reveals evolutionary relationship to eukaryotic B-family polymerases. *FEBS Lett* 584, (15):3370-5.

Yan, Z., Delannoy, M., Ling, C., Daee, D., Osman, F., Muniandy, P. A., Shen, X., Oostra, A. B., Du, H., Steltenpool, J., Lin, T., Schuster, B., Decaillet, C., Stasiak, A., Stasiak, A. Z., Stone, S., Hoatlin, M. E., Schindler, D., Woodcock, C. L., Joenje, H., Sen, R., de Winter, J. P., Li, L., Seidman, M. M., Whitby, M. C., Myung, K., Constantinou, A. and Wang, W. (2010). A histone-fold complex and FANCM form a conserved DNA-remodeling complex to maintain genome stability. *Mol Cell* 37, (6):865-78.

Yano, K., Morotomi-Yano, K., Wang, S. Y., Uematsu, N., Lee, K. J., Asaithamby, A., Weterings, E. and Chen, D. J. (2008). Ku recruits XLF to DNA double-strand breaks. *EMBO Rep* 9, (1):91-6.

Yokoi, M., Masutani, C., Maekawa, T., Sugasawa, K., Ohkuma, Y. and Hanaoka, F. (2000). The xeroderma pigmentosum group C protein complex XPC-HR23B plays an important role in the recruitment of transcription factor IIH to damaged DNA. *J Biol Chem* 275, (13):9870-5.

Zhao, B., Xie, Z., Shen, H. and Wang, Z. (2004). Role of DNA polymerase eta in the bypass of abasic sites in yeast cells. *Nucleic Acids Res* 32, (13):3984-94.

Zhao, X., Liu, J., Hsu, D. S., Zhao, S., Taylor, J. S. and Sancar, A. (1997). Reaction mechanism of (6-4) photolyase. *J Biol Chem* 272, (51):32580-90.

5

The Role of MutS Homologues MSH4 and MSH5 in DNA Metabolism and Damage Response

Xiling Wu[1], Keqian Xu[2] and Chengtao Her[1]
[1]*School of Molecular Biosciences, College of Veterinary Medicine, Washington State University, Pullman,*
[2]*Department of Medical Laboratory, Xiangya Medical School, Central South University, Changsha, Hunan*
[1]*USA*
[2]*P.R. China*

1. Introduction

The DNA mismatch repair (MMR) pathway is one of the most important genome surveillance systems involved in governing faithful transmission of genetic information during DNA replication and homologous recombination (Jiricny 2006). MMR deficiency attributes to a phenotype known as microsatellite instability (MSI), a condition that predisposes individuals to a heightened risk of cancer development (Harfe & Jinks-Robertson 2000; Iyer *et al.* 2006; Jiricny 2006; Kunkel & Erie 2005). Notably, hereditary nonpolyposis colorectal cancer (HNPCC) or Lynch syndrome is the most common malignancy identified in individuals with MMR gene mutations. The MMR pathway relies on the coordinated functions of a family of proteins that recognize mismatched nucleotides and initiate subsequent repair actions ranging from excision of a fragment of DNA containing the mismatched nucleotide to DNA repair synthesis. The MMR system is well conserved evolutionarily from bacteria to humans, of which the eukaryotic MMR pathway is evolved to possess multiple homologous genes that carry out conserved and diverse functions corresponding to their bacterial counterparts (Modrich 1991). Genes encoding homologues of the bacterial MMR proteins such as MutS and MutL have been identified in a variety of eukaryotes including yeast, plants, nematodes, and mammals. However, the bacterial MutH appears to be an exception—this methylation-sensitive endonuclease, exclusively functioning in gram-negative bacteria, directs the action of MMR to hemimethylated newly synthesized bacterial DNA (Iyer *et al.* 2006).

All eukaryotic organisms possess multiple MutS homologues—collectively known as MSH proteins—which may number as high as seven (MSH1 to MSH7), although the mitochondrial-localizing MSH1 of *Saccharomyces cerevisiae* (Reenan & Kolodner 1992) and the *Arabadopsis thalia* MSH7 (Culligan & Hays 1997) do not appear to be fully conserved (Fishel & Wilson 1997). The functionality of these proteins is similar to that of their counterparts in bacteria such as *Eschericia coli*. Prokaryotic MutS exists as a homodimer, while eukaryotic MSH proteins form heterodimers in the forms of MSH2-MSH3, MSH2-MSH6 and MSH4-MSH5. Two of these eukaryotic heterodimers (MSH2-MSH3 and MSH2-

MSH6) play fundamental roles in mitotic post-replicative MMR (Fishel & Wilson 1997; Kolodner 1996), in which incorrectly matched bases are replaced with proper partners.

In spite of the high levels of sequence homology to the other MSH proteins, what role, if any, of the MutS homologues MSH4 and MSH5 in the process of MMR has yet to be experimentally determined, and the biochemical function(s) of the heterocomplex formed by MSH4 and MSH5 also awaits to be further delineated (Her *et al.* 2007). Nevertheless, high levels of expression of both genes in the testes and ovaries implicate a direct role for hMSH4 and hMSH5 in development and meiosis (Bocker *et al.* 1999; Her & Doggett 1998; Moens *et al.* 2002). Genetic studies in *S. cerevisiae*, *Caenorhabditis elegans*, and *Mus musculus* highlight an important role for MSH4 and MSH5 in meiotic development of viable gametes, but provide no evidence to substantiate their potential role in the repair of mismatched bases like the other MutS homologues (de Vries *et al.* 1999; Edelmann *et al.* 1999; Hollingsworth *et al.* 1995; Kelly *et al.* 2000; Kneitz *et al.* 2000; Ross-Macdonald & Roeder 1994; Zalevsky *et al.* 1999). The observation that purified recombinant hMSH4-hMSH5 heterocomplex can specifically bind to recombination intermediate structures such as the Holliday junction (Snowden *et al.* 2004) has implicated a direct role for hMSH4-hMSH5 in the process of meiotic and mitotic recombinational double-strand break (DSB) repair. Gene knockout of *Msh4* and/or *Msh5* in mice results in defective chromosome synapsis in meiotic prophase I, and therefore sterility—likely attributed to defective homologous recombination (de Vries *et al.* 1999; Edelmann *et al.* 1999; Kneitz *et al.* 2000). Although the expression patterns of MSH4 and MSH5 mRNA in testis support their functional role in meiosis, low levels of MSH4 and MSH5 expression have been identified in many other, non-meiotic organs, and these two genes are not necessarily expressed in concert (de Vries *et al.* 1999; Edelmann *et al.* 1999; Her *et al.* 2001; Her *et al.* 2003; Her *et al.* 1999; Kneitz *et al.* 2000; Paquis-Flucklinger *et al.* 1997; Winand *et al.* 1998), implicating MSH4 and/or MSH5 can function in other pathways beyond the scope of meiosis and may function separately as well (Her *et al.* 2007). In fact, recent evidence supports the notion that MSH4 and MSH5 are involved in the process of mitotic DNA DSB repair, and may be also involved in other aspects of DNA damage repair and response (Tompkins et al. 2009; Sekine et al. 2007).

2. Structural and functional features of MSH4 and MSH5

2.1 Gene structure and expression of MSH4 and MSH5

2.1.1 *S. cerevisiae* MSH4 and MSH5

The identification of *MSH4* and *MSH5* was first performed in the budding yeast *S. cerevisiae*, and that led to the classification of these proteins as meiosis-specific members of the MutS homologue family. *MSH4* was isolated by a transposon insertion screen resulting in the generation of *lacZ* fusion genes expressed specifically in meiotic cells (Burns *et al.* 1994). Following electrophoretic separation of yeast chromosomes, the *MSH4* gene was mapped to chromosome VI by Southern blot analysis, located 2 cM from *SEC4*. Sequence analysis of an *MSH4*-complementing subclone identified an open reading frame (ORF) of 2634 bp encoding the 878-amino acid MSH4 protein. As a member of the MutS family, MSH4 shows 35% identity to *E. coli* MutS and 31-36% identity to the other yeast MutS homologues. The similarity is most pronounced in the C-terminal region, which contains the putative ATP-binding domain and helix-turn-helix DNA-binding motif. Despite its extensive homology to bacterial MutS, which functions in the initiation of MMR through direct binding of mispaired bases, MSH4 is meiosis specific. Expression of mutant MSH4 results in defective reciprocal recombination and nondisjunction of homologous chromosomes at meiosis I and consequently spore inviability. The MSH4 protein is specifically expressed in meiotic cells where it localizes to discrete chromosomal locations with no apparent involvement in MMR (Ross-Macdonald & Roeder 1994).

The *MSH5* gene is mapped to chromosome IV, located 1.9 cM from *CDC36*. The *MSH5* ORF is composed of 2703 nucleotides and encodes a protein of 901 amino acids with a predicted molecular mass of 102 kDa (Hollingsworth *et al.* 1995). Although MSH5 exhibits strong homology to the MutS family of proteins, like MSH4, it is not involved in MMR. Diploids lacking *MSH5* display decreased spore viability, increased chromosomal nondisjunction during meiosis I, with a concomitant decrease in reciprocal exchange between—but not within—homologous chromosomes. However, lack of *MSH5* expression does not correlate to a decrease in gene conversion. Mutants lacking *MSH4* or *MSH5* are phenotypically comparable, indicating that these two yeast genes are in the same epistasis group and are likely to serve similar functions (Hollingsworth *et al.* 1995).

2.1.2 Mouse MSH4 and MSH5

Sequence analysis revealed that the mouse *Msh4* ORF is 2874 bp in length with a 196 bp 3'-UTR followed by a poly(A) tract. A polyadenylation signal (AATAAA) is located 24 nucleotides 5' upstream from the poly(A) tract. The 958-amino acid protein encoded by this ORF contains the highly conserved sequence motifs present in all MutS homologues. The cDNA shares 84.1% and 89.3% sequence identities with its human orthologue in nucleotide and amino acid sequences, respectively. The amino terminus of Msh4, on the other hand, is the most divergent and shares no sequence homology with that of the human hMSH4 (Her *et al.* 2001; Kneitz *et al.* 2000). Northern blot analysis has indicated that *Msh4* is predominantly expressed in the testis, but low levels of expression are also present in the heart, brain, and liver, whereas dot-blot analysis, besides confirming the Northern results, has also revealed low levels of Msh4 expression in several other non-meiotic tissues (Her *et al.* 2001).

The mouse *Msh5* gene is located on chromosome 17 in a region that is syntenic to the locus on human chromosome 6 harboring the human gene. The gene for Msh5 contains 24 exons and spans approximately 18 kb with exon length varying from 36 bp for exon 7 to 392 bp for exon 24; intron lengths range from 79 bp for intron 17 to 4687 bp for intron 11. The first 248 nucleotides of exon 1 and the last 133 nucleotides of exon 24 are noncoding. Comparison between the human and mouse homologues reveals that the mouse *Msh5* gene shares a high degree of structural homology with that of the human *hMSH5* gene. The locations of most exon-intron splicing junctions as well as the lengths of all internal coding exons of *Msh5* are identical to that of *hMSH5*. The mouse Msh5 ORF is 2502 bp in length and encodes an 833-amino acid polypeptide with a predicted molecular weight of 92.6 kDa and an isoelectric point of 6.33. Msh5 contains the same set of highly conserved sequence motifs that present in all other MutS proteins (de Vries *et al.* 1999; Edelmann *et al.* 1999; Her *et al.* 1999). Like Msh4, high levels of Msh5 expression are largely confined to the testis while relatively low levels of Msh5 expression are detectable from heart, spleen, liver, and lung (Her *et al.* 1999).

Both male and female mice lacking *Msh4* or *Msh5* are infertile as a result of meiotic arrest (de Vries *et al.* 1999; Edelmann *et al.* 1999; Kneitz *et al.* 2000). Spermatocyte chromosomes of *Msh4* or *Msh5* deficient mice do not synapse properly in late zygonema and early pachynema despite DSB formation. Chromosome pairing, normally triggered by meiotic

DSB, involves mainly nonhomologous chromosomes in *Msh4* or *Msh5* deficient mice, of which only a fraction of nuclei in *Msh5*-null males show partial pairing; while in *Msh4*-null spermatocyte pairing is typically higher at 70% of all nuclei. As a consequence, germ cells in *Msh4* or *Msh5* deficient mice fail to enter pachynema and die by apoptosis, leading to testes devoid of post-leptotene spermatocytes. In comparison, female mice deficient in *Msh4* or *Msh5* suffer similar consequences as in males experiencing pre-pachytene meiotic catastrophe, particularly oocytes become apoptototic prior to birth. In female mice lacking both *Msh4* and *Msh5*, the oocyte pool is completely lost and is accompanied by ovarian degeneration during the first eight to ten weeks of postnatal period (Kneitz *et al.* 2000).

2.1.3 Human hMSH4 and hMSH5

The human *hMSH4* gene is composed of 20 exons and spans 116 Kb on chromosome 1p31. With a 2808 bp ORF, the *hMSH4* gene encodes a protein of 936 amino acids with a predicted molecular mass of 104.8 kDa (Paquis-Flucklinger *et al.* 1997). In contrast, the *hMSH5* gene contains 26 exons and spans approximately 25 Kb within the MHC class III region on human chromosome 6p21.3. The *hMSH5* gene harbors a 2501 bp ORF encoding an 834-amino acid protein with a predicted molecular mass of 92.9 kDa (Her & Doggett 1998; Winand *et al.* 1998). Moderate levels of hMSH4 transcripts are present in the testis and low levels of hMSH4 transcripts are also detectable in several non-meiotic tissues including the thymus, ovary, colon, pancreas, brain, heart, liver, and placenta (Her *et al.* 2003; Paquis-Flucklinger *et al.* 1997). In contrast, the full-length hMSH5 transcripts are detectable in virtually all tissues examined with the most abundant expression in the testis. Northern blot analysis shows the presence of distinct hMSH5 hybridization signals in a variety of tissues such as the thymus, skeletal muscle, bone marrow, spinal cord, brain, trachea, ovary, and lymph node (Bocker *et al.* 1999; Her and Doggett 1998; Winand *et al.* 1998). This wide hMSH5 tissue distribution pattern has been also recapitulated in RT-PCR analysis of various human tissues and is well reflected in the human EST database. The difference in the expression patterns of these two genes raises the possibility that hMSH4 and hMSH5 may function independently of one another in certain tissue types beyond the meiotic arena (Her *et al.* 2007).

2.1.4 Splicing variants and nonsynonymous polymorphisms of hMSH4 and hMSH5 in humans

Recent evidence substantiates the existence of multiple alternatively spliced transcripts for *hMSH4* and *hMSH5* in human cells (Table 1). Although the functional significance of these alternatively spliced transcripts is presently unknown, the expression profiles and some properties of the proteins encoded by the splicing variants are being characterized. For instance, one hMSH4 splicing variant, hMSH4sv, resulting from exon 19-skipping, has been analyzed. hMSH4sv harbors a frameshift of 7 amino acids followed by a stop codon in exon 20, thus producing an 850-amino acid polypeptide. Truncated at the carboxyl terminal, the hMSH4sv contains most of the conserved sequence motifs presented in all MutS homologues except for the carboxyl terminal helix-turn-helix motif (Her *et al.* 2003). The tissue distribution profile of hMSH4sv is similar but not identical to that of hMSH4, suggesting that hMSH4sv might be subjected to differential regulation in some tissue types including the heart, liver, placenta, and ovary (Her *et al.* 2003). Intriguingly, the protein encoded by *hMSH4sv* is incapable of interacting with hMSH5, but it does interact with von

Hippel-Lindau tumor suppressor-binding protein 1(VBP1) (Her *et al.* 2003). Also of note is another hMSH4 exon-skipping variant (ΔhMSH4) that lacks the entire exon 6 leading to an in-frame deletion of hMSH4 amino acid residues 273 to 330 (Her *et al.* 2003; Santucci-Darmanin *et al.* 1999). The hMSH4 homodimerization domain, residing in between amino acid residues 148 and 387 (Her *et al.* 2003), significantly overlaps with the region encoded by *hMSH4* exon 6, thus ΔhMSH4 is expected to be defective in homotypic interaction.

The *hMSH5* gene produces multiple alternative transcripts, of which four hMSH5 variants that maintain the reading frame have been identified (hMSH5a, hMSH5b, hMSH5c, and hMSH5d; UniGene database) and hMSH5c appears to be identical to that of the originally described human hMSH5. Referenced by the deduced amino acid sequence of hMSH5, it is evident that hMSH5a (hMSH5sv) encodes an 851-amino acid protein containing a 17-amino acid insertion between codons 179 and 180, owing to the retention of the last 51-bp of hMSH5 intron 6 (Yi *et al.* 2005), whereas hMSH5b harbors one extra amino acid residue between codons 654 and 655—due to the retention of the last 3 nucleotides of *hMSH5* intron 20 (Her & Doggett 1998). hMSH5d represents the shortest hMSH5 variant. Although it contains the 17-amino acid insertion and the one extra amino acid residue described above, hMSH5d lacks 30 amino acid residues corresponding to codons 744 to 773. The existence of different hMSH5 variant transcripts keenly supports the possibility that *hMSH5* may encode multiple products; a thorough understanding of the functional aspects of these potential protein isoforms requires detailed experimental examination of these variants. In particular, it is necessary to determine whether these hMSH5 variants are resulted from sequence variations within the corresponding introns, or they are created by a yet-to-be-defined mechanism. Presently, besides hMSH5, only one splicing variant, hMSH5sv, has been experimentally analyzed (Yi *et al.* 2005). The expression profile of hMSH5sv appears to be distinguishable from that of hMSH5; for example, the expression of hMSH5sv, but not hMSH5, is absent or below the detection limit in the brain, heart, and skeletal muscle. In addition, the expression of hMSH5sv displays a large variation in tumor cell lines with breast and lung carcinomas showing the most abundant expression. In contrast to hMSH4sv, displaying impaired interaction with hMSH5, hMSH5sv has maintained its capacity to interact with hMSH4 (Yi *et al.* 2005).

In addition to the existence of multiple alternatively spliced transcripts, potential diverse functions involved with the *hMSH4* and *hMSH5* genes are also being reflected by the fact that both genes are associated with many coding region single nucleotide polymorphisms (SNPs), of which many are non-synonymous. There are at least seven non-synonymous SNPs that have been identified for each of the genes (Table 1). For hMSH4 and hMSH5, the corresponding single amino acid changes caused by these SNPs are hMSH4 A60V, A90T, A97T, E162K, I365V, Y589C, S914N, and hMSH5 P29S, L85F, Y202C, V206F, R351G, L377F, P786S. However, the allele frequencies, haplotypes, and functional implications of most, if not all, SNPs are largely undetermined; in fact only one non-synonymous SNP (rs2075789), hMSH5 C85T ($hMSH5^{P29S}$), has been characterized experimentally as a common genetic polymorphism with an allele frequency of 11.6% in an American Caucasian population of 99 individuals and 17% in a Chinese population of 279 individuals (Her *et al.* 2007; Yi *et al.* 2005). Located within the hMSH5 amino terminal proline-rich interacting domain for hMSH4 and c-Abl, the Pro^{29} to Ser alteration causes a moderate reduction of protein interaction with hMSH4, whereas this alteration promotes the activation of c-Abl kinase activity and therefore enhances ionizing radiation (IR) induced p73-dependent apoptosis

	Variants and nonsynonymous polymorphisms	Changes in amino acid (aa) residues
	hMSH4sv	Exon 19 skipping leading to the production of a 850 aa polypeptide, of which the last 7 aa are frame-shifted
hMSH4	ΔhMSH4	Exon 6 skipping leading to the deletion of aa 273 to 330
	A60V	Ala^{60} to Val
	A90T	Ala^{90} to Thr
	A97T	Ala^{97} to Thr
	E162K	Glu^{162} to Lys
	I365V	Ile^{365} to Val
	Y589C	Tyr^{589} to Cys
	S914N	Ser^{914} to Asn
	hMSH5a (hMSH5sv)	17 aa insertion between aa position 179 and 180
	hMSH5b	1 aa insertion between aa position 654 and 655
hMSH5	hMSH5d	17 aa insertion between aa position 179 and 180 1 aa inertion between aa position 654 and 655 and deletion of aa 744 to 773
	P29S	Pro^{29} to Ser
	L85F	Leu^{85} to Phe
	Y202C	Tyr^{202} to Cys
	V206F	Val^{206} to Phe
	R351G	Arg^{351} to Gly
	L377F	Leu^{377} to Phe
	P786S	Pro^{786} to Ser

Table 1. hMSH4 and hMSH5 splicing variants and nonsynonymous polymorphisms.

(Tompkins *et al.* 2009; Yi *et al.* 2006; Yi *et al.* 2005). Given the essential role of Msh5 in ovarian and testicular development in mice (de Vries *et al.* 1999; Edelmann *et al.* 1999), it is interesting to note that the hMSH5 C85T SNP is relatively enriched in ovarian cancer patients and is associated with a higher risk for azoospermia or severe oligozoospermia in humans (Xu *et al.* 2010; Yi *et al.* 2005). Another noteworthy hMSH5 variant is hMSH5$^{L85F/P786S}$—encoded by an *hMSH5* allele harboring two co-segregating SNPs (C253T and C2356T)—that displays compromised ability to interact with hMSH4. Intriguingly, the allele for hMSH5$^{L85F/P786S}$ has been associated with the occurrence of human immunoglobulin deficiency syndromes, *i.e.* IgA deficiency (IgAD) and common variable immune deficiency (CVID) (Sekine *et al.* 2007).

It is also important to note that two hMSH5 noncoding SNPs have been linked to conditions in humans as well. A recent genome-wide association study (GWAS) of 511,919 SNPs in populations with Caucasian origin has identified a high risk factor for lung cancer development within the *hMSH5* gene locus at 6p21.33 (Wang *et al.* 2008). Specifically, a significant increase in lung cancer susceptibility is associated with rs3131379, a SNP located within intron 10 of the *hMSH5* gene. Another study, designed to identify genetic markers for the adverse reaction associated with the use of Allopurinol—a common medication for gout and hyperuricemia, has revealed a tight link with the *hMSH5* locus (Hung *et al.* 2005). The evidence from this study demonstrates a significant association of a separate hMSH5 SNP (rs1150793) with the risk of developing severe cutaneous adverse reactions (SCAR) in Han Chinese patients treated with Allopurinol.

Although the existence of multiple hMSH4 and hMSH5 splicing variants and various SNPs poses a daunting task for a thorough appreciation of their functions, close analysis of their properties at molecular and cellular levels, especially for those with clinical significance, would be necessary for delineating the mechanistic basis underlying their potential link to disease conditions in humans. It is highly plausible that functional effects similar to those observed for hMSH5 P29S could also be conferred by other hMSH5 and/or hMSH4 non-synonymous SNPs. It should not be a surprise that different combinations of these SNPs might associate with an array of subtle functional alterations; that, to a certain extent, could also affect the dynamic interplay among hMSH4-hMSH5 associated proteins and subsequent downstream events.

2.2 Structural properties of MSH4 and MSH5 proteins

2.2.1 General molecular structure of MutS homologues

A common characteristic of MutS homologous proteins is their essential role in binding and recognizing mismatched base pairs—a function facilitated by their ability to act as DNA-binding ATPases. Whilst structures of eukaryotic MSH proteins remains undetermined, insights towards the mechanistic aspects of mismatch recognition may be inferred from the crystal structure of bacterial MutS protein. Crystallographic studies of homologues in *T. aquaticus* and *E. coli* suggest that the MutS homodimer binds to heteroduplex DNA during mismatch recognition as a "structural heterodimer" (Junop *et al.* 2001; Lamers *et al.* 2000; Obmolova *et al.* 2000). The homodimerization of MutS protein is mediated through the region harboring MutS ATPase activity. The dimerization domain is far apart from the DNA binding domain, but these regions coordinate through conformational changes triggered by MutS binding to heteroduplex DNA or ATP (Lamers *et al.* 2004; Lamers *et al.* 2003). In essence, these studies indicate that MutS is a modular protein with separate domains which, when dimerized at their carboxyl termini, act to encircle mismatch-containing DNA during the initiation stages of repair process. Deletion analysis of MutS protein confirms that the carboxyl terminus, which also includes a P-loop motif for nucleoside triphosphate binding, is involved in homodimerization. The amino terminal end is necessary for binding to mismatch-containing DNA, and through the binding and hydrolysis of ATP in the carboxyl terminal, MutS may dissociate from mismatched DNA once repair is underway. Although no crystallographic analysis of eukaryotic MSH proteins is presently available, noting the high degree of homology between MutS homologues and their bacterial counterparts, it is not difficult to conjecture that the MSH proteins found in yeast, mouse, and humans may contain similar structural features to those of prokaryotic MutS proteins.

2.2.2 Eukaryotic MSH4-MSH5 complex

Whereas functional bacterial MutS protein exists as homodimers, the eukaryotic MSH family is far more complex and contains multiple heterodimers composed of different MSH proteins. MSH heterodimers carry out diverse cellular functions including MMR and DNA damage response. However, MSH4 and MSH5 are unique in their intracellular roles. Although they contain the conserved sequence motifs found in all MutS homologues—such as the ATP binding domain and a helix-turn-helix structural motif located at the carboxyl terminal half of the protein (Burns *et al.* 1994; Her & Doggett 1998; Her *et al.* 2001; Her *et al.* 1999; Hollingsworth *et al.* 1995; Paquis-Flucklinger *et al.* 1997)—neither MSH4 nor MSH5 interact with the other MSH proteins known to function in MMR. MSH4 and MSH5 interact with each other exclusively, forming a distinctive heterocomplex (Bocker *et al.* 1999; Her *et al.* 2001; Her *et al.* 1999; Winand *et al.* 1998; Yi *et al.* 2005). Unlike other MSH proteins, which contain specific amino acid residues for recognition and binding of mismatched base pairs, MSH4 and MSH5, either individually or as a heterocomplex, are unable to detect or respond to mismatches as they lack structural motifs for binding of mismatched base pairs (Obmolova *et al.* 2000). It is postulated that the MSH4-MSH5 heterocomplex may configure in a way that can accommodate large recombination intermediate DNA structures such as Holliday junction intermediates (Obmolova *et al.* 2000). Evidence obtained with the purified recombinant hMSH4-hMSH5 heterocomplex points to their role in the recognition and binding of artificial DNA structures resembling four-way junctions (Snowden *et al.* 2004), suggesting that the hMSH4-hMSH5 heterocomplex is uniquely equipped for processing recombinational intermediates.

The human hMSH4 and hMSH5 interact with one another via the carboxyl terminal region of hMSH4 and both the amino and carboxyl terminal regions of hMSH5. The first 109 and the last 103 amino acid residues of hMSH5 are necessary for the formation of a composite hMSH4-interacting domain; however, only the carboxyl terminal 93 amino acid residues of hMSH4 are required to interact with hMSH5 (Yi *et al.* 2005), suggesting an asymmetric structural partition of hMSH4 and hMSH5 in the heterocomplex. The hMSH4-hMSH5 heterocomplex is suggested to form a sliding clamp structure that stabilizes and preserves Holliday junctions during prophase of meiosis I or in the repair of DSBs. A model for hMSH4-hMSH5 in meiotic recombination has been proposed (Snowden *et al.* 2004), implicating their role in linking DSB repair to the regulation of crossover (CO) formation. It is known that the amino terminal region of hMSH4, composed of amino acid residues 148-387, is involved in mediating homotypic interaction (Her *et al.* 1999; Lee *et al.* 2006). Due to the physical separation of the hetero- and homo-interacting domains on hMSH4, it has been suggested that hMSH4 and hMSH5 may form a multimeric protein complex such as a tetramer. In addition, it has been demonstrated that the interface of hMSH4-hMSH5 heterocomplex forms a composite interaction domain for GPS2; the latter is a protein factor involved in intracellular signaling and DNA damage response (Jin *et al.* 1997; Lee *et al.* 2006; Peng *et al.* 2001; Spain *et al.* 1996). The interplay of GPS2 with the hMSH4-hMSH5 heterocomplex may provide a link to downstream molecular events required for Holliday junction processing and subsequent resolution.

2.2.3 Protein interacting partners of MSH4 and MSH5

The MSH4-MSH5 heterocomplex is thought to participate in a limited array of functions, leaving the individual proteins to coordinate specific cellular processes independent of one another throughout various mammalian tissues. It has been shown that hMSH4 physically interacts with hMLH1 as well as its binding partner hMLH3, in which the amino terminal region of hMSH4 interacts with hMLH1 proteolytic degradation products, rather than the full-length hMLH1 (Lipkin *et al.* 2000; Santucci-Darmanin *et al.* 2002; Santucci-Darmanin *et al.* 2000). Furthermore, hMSH4 interacts with VBP1, Rad51, and DMC1 (Her *et al.* 2003; Her *et al.* 2007; Neyton *et al.* 2004). In addition to its interacting partner hMSH4, hMSH5 has been shown to interact with the non-receptor tyrosine kinase c-Abl, hMRE11, and histone demethylase SMCY (Akimoto *et al.* 2008; Kato *et al.* 2007; Yi *et al.* 2006), of which the interaction with c-Abl mediates hMSH5 tyrosine phosphorylation in response to IR-induced DSBs (Yi *et al.* 2006). Coherent with this observation, the ubiquitous DNA damage repair protein hRad51 coexists in the protein complex containing both hMSH5 and c-Abl (Her *et al.* 2007).

Interaction with different protein partners may provide a foundation for hMSH4 and hMSH5 to act independently in specific cellular processes, during which protein interactions can also modulate the functions of hMSH4 and hMSH5. For example, the interaction of VBP1 with hMSH4 negatively regulates the formation of hMSH4-hMSH5 heterocomplex (Her *et al.* 2003). The biological relevance of this observation in mitotic cells is presently not known. It is reported that, during early stages of mouse testis development, the up-regulation of GPS2 coincides with the down-regulation of VBP1 immediately prior to, or at the onset of, the first meiotic wave, presumably facilitating the formation of Msh4-Msh5 heterocomplex (Lee *et al.* 2006). The hMSH4-hMSH5 interaction is also subjected to regulation by c-Abl-mediated hMSH5 tyrosine phosphorylation. In particular, hMSH5 is shown to undergo IR-induced c-Abl-dependent tyrosine phosphorylation, and consequently this posttranslational modification leads to the dissociation of hMSH4-hMSH5 heterocomplex (Tompkins *et al.* 2009; Yi *et al.* 2006). Since the formation of hMSH4-hMSH5 heterocomplex is required for the interaction with GPS2 (likely in a complex with HDAC3), it is expected that hMSH5 tyrosine phosphorylation will result in a dynamic transformation of the hMSH4-hMSH5 associated protein complex, which might be functionally required during recombinational DSB repair.

Recent evidence suggests that factors influence the hMSH4-hMSH5 interaction will also affect their subcellular localization. It appears that hMSH4-hMSH5 dimerization enhances their nuclear localization—possibly facilitated by a nuclear localization signal (NLS) located in the middle of hMSH5 protein, or by masking of a CRM1-dependent nuclear export signal (NES) on the carboxyl terminal region of hMSH5 within the hMSH4-interacting domain (Lahaye *et al.* 2010; Neyton *et al.* 2007).

2.3 Functions of MSH4 and MSH5

2.3.1 Role in meiotic recombination

Meiotic recombination occurs in meiotic prophase starting with the formation of programmed DSBs induced by the expression of SPO11, a protein highly conserved and enriched in germ cells at recombination hotspots (Baudat & de Massy 2007; Keeney *et al.* 1997). After 5′ end resection at the break, the emerging 3′ single-stranded overhang invades undamaged homologous chromosome or sister chromatid, leading to the formation of meiotic recombination intermediate structures including the Holliday junction and thus facilitating DSB repair (Szostak *et al.* 1983). The completion of meiotic homologous recombination is achieved through the resolution of Holliday junction structures by cleavage and rejoining to re-form two separate DNA molecules. The two major outcomes of meiotic homologous recombinational DSB repair are chromosomal reciprocal exchange or CO and gene conversion or non-crossover (Mahadevaiah *et al.* 2001). While non-crossover is important for conserving genetic identities, chromosomal CO is crucial for creating genetic diversity and therefore promoting survival along the way of evolution. Furthermore, COs are critical for successful meiosis, of which both the frequency and the distribution of COs are well controlled in a way that governs the fidelity of chromosome segregation (Youds & Boulton 2011).

Studies carried out in budding yeast have provided evidence to indicate that both MSH4 and MSH5 are involved in meiotic recombination but not in MMR (Hollingsworth *et al.* 1995; Ross-Macdonald & Roeder 1994). *MSH4*-null mutation in *S. cerevisiae* is not associated with elevated rate in mismatches of reporter genes Can^R (Reenan & Kolodner 1992) and Thr+ (Kramer *et al.* 1989) or defective gene conversion, instead the *MSH4*-null strain displays 2 to 3-fold reduction in CO and an increase in homologous chromosome nondisjunction, leading to reduced spore viability (Ross-Macdonald & Roeder 1994). Similar effects are evident in *S. cerevisiae* with mutant *MSH5*, in which MMR is proficient in the processes of both meiosis and mitosis, and meiotic gene conversion frequency is not significantly different from the wild type. However, CO is reduced 2 to 3-fold and homologous chromosome nondisjunction is elevated in meiosis I. As a consequence, spore viability is reduced to 37% from 72% observed in the wild type (Hollingsworth *et al.* 1995). *S. cerevisiae* strain lacking both *MSH4* and *MSH5* does not show a synergistic effect on CO frequency in meiosis I, and the spore viability is compatible with either mutants, indicating *MSH4* and *MSH5* act in the same pathway that facilitate meiotic crossing over recombination (Hollingsworth *et al.* 1995). Decreased crossover interference and delayed or incomplete chromosome synapsis are also observed in *MSH4* mutant yeast, suggesting a role for MSH4 in the regulation of crossover distribution (Novak *et al.* 2001).

Like budding yeast, *C. elegans MSH4* and *MSH5* are functionally conserved with respect to their role in promoting meiotic CO. With a null mutation in *him-14*, the *C. elegans* ortholog of *MSH4*, CO is abolished during meiosis I in both oocytes and spermatocytes. As a result, formation of chiasmata is absent and chromosome segregation is severely defective. Most of the *him-14* embryos, although produced in normal amounts, fail to hatch; and and among the hatched that reached to adulthood, 45% are males (Zalevsky *et al.* 1999; Zetka & Rose 1995). This is consistent with an increase in non-disjunction, because males are normally arisen through spontaneous non-disjunction with a frequency of about 0.1% in the hermaphrodite germ line. The *him-14* mutants, however, do not show any abnormality in meiotic chromosome pairing and synapsis (Zalevsky *et al.* 1999). Similar to their budding yeast counterparts, the mutant worms do not display increased "mutator" phenotype, assayed by the means of levamisole resistance, indicating that Him-14 is not required for MMR in *C. elegans* (Zalevsky *et al.* 1999). In spite of high degree of conservation, *C. elegans* and *S. cerevisiae MSH4* mutants differ significantly in their effects on CO. Without *MSH4*, CO is completely abrogated in *C. elegans* (Zalevsky *et al.* 1999), yet about 30-50% is retained in the budding yeast (Ross-Macdonald & Roeder 1994). This difference has helped to fashion the current view that *C. elegans* has a single or a dominant pathway to create meiotic CO for which *MSH4* is indispensible, and budding yeast has alternative *MSH4*-independent pathway(s) for CO generation. While MSH4 is crucial for proper chromosome segregation, in contrast to yeast, *C. elegans* Him-14 does not appear to act on chromosome pairing and synapsis.

Likewise germ cells from *C. elegans msh-5* mutants are able to progress through meiosis with normal chromosome pairing and synapsis. *Msh-5* mutants lay eggs at a same rate as the wild type, and they produce a normal number of embryos, however, more than 97% of the embryos fail to hatch and 42% of those survived to adulthood are males, owing to defective segregation of homologous chromosomes (Kelly *et al.* 2000). Similar to the *him-14* mutants, CO frequency in *Msh-5* mutants is reduced to about 1% of the wild type, and these mutants lack chiasmata formation (Kelly *et al.* 2000). On the basis of their nearly identical effect on meiotic recombination, it is conceivable that both MSH4 and MSH5 are indispensible for *C. elegans* meiotic CO, and these two MutS homologues act in the same process through apparently the only pathway in this species.

In mice, meiotic recombination is also initiated by Spo11-dependent DSBs (Mahadevaiah *et al.* 2001). *Msh5* knockout mice are generally healthy and undergo normal development, however their reproductive organs do not develop properly. For example, testes in *Msh5*-null animals are significantly smaller in size and ovaries quickly become rudimentary after birth (de Vries *et al.* 1999; Edelmann *et al.* 1999). Although their mating behavior appears normal, *Msh5*-null mice are sterile. Histological analysis demonstrates that the testes of *Msh5*-null mice are completely devoid of epididymal spermatozoa, presumably due to apoptosis before pachytene—the stage of meiosis when crossover structures between homologous chromosomes become experimentally visible (de Vries *et al.* 1999; Edelmann *et al.* 1999). Closer examination of *Msh5*-null spermatocytes and oocytes reveals disrupted chromosome pairing and impaired synaptonemal complex formation, indicating *Msh5* is essential for homologous chromosome pairing and synapsis during meiosis I in mice (de Vries *et al.* 1999; Edelmann *et al.* 1999). Since the single strand DNA binding protein Rad51 typically represents a marker for recombination initiation (Bishop 1994; Moens *et al.* 2002), the observed Rad51 foci formation on unsynapsed chromosomes in *Msh5*-null mice tends to suggest that Msh5 is not involved in the initiation of meiotic recombination (Edelmann *et al.* 1999).

Similarly, *Msh4*-null mice develop normally but are infertile. These mutant mice display severe abnormality in chromosome pairing in early prophase I (Kneitz *et al.* 2000), indicating Msh4 is also required for meiotic homologous chromosome pairing. However, *Msh4* deficiency appears to cause less severe defect in chromosome pairing in comparison to *Msh5*-null animals. Approximately 69% of nuclei in *Msh4*-null spermatocytes have some degree of chromosome pairing, but less than 10% of the nuclei contain very few paired chromosomes in *Msh5*-null mice (Kneitz *et al.* 2000). Meiotic phenotypes of *Msh4* and *Msh5* double-knockout mice are similar to the *Msh5*-null mice, suggesting that Msh4 and Msh5 act together in promoting meiotic chromosome pairing and synapsis in the early phase of meiotic recombination, possibly with Msh5 upstream of Msh4 (Kneitz *et al.* 2000).

In human oocytes, both hMSH4 and hMSH5 proteins are localized on meiotic chromosomes throughout meiotic prophase I and become co-localized at zygonema with SYCP3, a key component of synaptonemal complex, thus supporting the idea that human hMSH4 and hMSH5 may possess meiotic properties similar to their mouse counterparts (Lenzi *et al.* 2005). This view is further supported by the physical interaction observed between hMSH4 and hRad51 as well as the co-localization of their counterparts in mouse spermatocytes (Neyton *et al.* 2004)—indicative of an early role for MSH4, presumably for MSH5 as well, in meiotic recombination. The presence of hMSH4 and hMSH5 foci on meiotic chromosomes after synaptonemal complex formation is highly suggestive of an additional role for these proteins in the late stages of meiotic recombination (Lenzi *et al.* 2005). Consistent with this speculation is the observed *in vitro* physical interaction between hMSH4 and hMLH1, the later is commonly regarded as a marker for crossing over recombination (Lynn *et al.* 2004). Together with the co-localization of these two proteins in mouse spermatocytes (Santucci-Darmanin *et al.* 2000), it is suggested that MSH4 and MSH5 play at least two separate roles in meiosis I—an early role in homology searching that leads to proper chromosome pairing and a late role in the processing of recombination intermediate structures. Binding of purified hMSH4-hMSH5 heterocomplex to the core of the Holliday junction intermediate structures has provided *in vitro* evidence to support the late role of these two proteins. It is hypothesized that the binding of progenitor Holliday junction DNA provokes ATP binding to both hMSH4 and hMSH5 in the heterocomplex, and the loading of hMSH4-hMSH5 is projected to stabilize and preserve meiotic recombination intermediates prior to proper resolution (Snowden *et al.* 2004).

In short, both MSH4 and MSH5 play important roles in meiotic recombination. The similarity in phenotypes among *MSH4*-null, *MSH5*-null, and *MSH4*-null/*MSH5*-null organisms suggests that these two MutS proteins act in the same pathways and likely function as a heterocomplex at least during certain phases of the recombination process. Although *MSH4* and *MSH5* homologues in lower eukaryotes and mammals appear to share conserved properties supporting their common function in meiosis, their precise effects diverge in different species. For instance, the major action of MSH4 and MSH5 in lower eukaryotes is on the generation and control of COs, whereas in mammals these two MutS homologues have evolved to exert an early role in governing homologous chromosome pairing and synapsis.

2.3.2 Role in mitotic recombination and DNA damage response

The most described function of MMR proteins is the repair of base-pairing errors arising from DNA replication or recombination. Defects in MMR proteins lead to mutations and MSI. Mutations in MMR genes are known to cause Lynch syndrome (or HNPCC) and to increase the risk and progression of a wide-variety of sporadic cancers. During MMR, replication errors are recognized either by MutSα, a heterodimer of MSH2 and MSH6 that binds to single base-base mismatches or small insertion-deletion loops, or by MutSβ, a heterodimer of MSH2 and MSH3 that binds to larger insertion-deletion loops (Jiricny 2006). The repair process then proceeds with the recruitment of a MutL activity (*i.e.* one of these three complexes: MLH1-PMS2, MLH1-PMS1 or MLH1-MLH3) and exonucleases to facilitate subsequent excision followed by DNA repair synthesis.

The MMR proteins are frequently recognized as major players in mediating cellular responses to DNA damage. As components of the BRCA-1-associated genome surveillance complex (Wang *et al.* 2000), MMR proteins are thought to mediate DNA damage response through either direct sensing of various DNA distortions or functioning as transducers to couple damage detection and the control of cell cycle progression (Jiricny 2006). For instance, MMR proteins are involved in provoking a G2/M phase cell cycle arrest that is vital for both DNA repair and cell death by apoptosis, especially for cells carrying excessive DNA lesions. To this end, it is important to note that MMR deficiency has been linked to DNA damage tolerance, and MMR deficient cells are found to be frequently resistant to killing by various chemotherapeutics including alkylating agents and antimetabolites. Given that resistance to chemotherapeutic agents is of a great concern in cancer treatment, a thorough understanding of the molecular mechanisms involved with MMR in cellular DNA damage response will undoubtedly pave a way for devising more effective therapeutic strategies.

Although MSH4 and MSH5 have not been indicated experimentally to function in the process of MMR, cumulating evidence has pointed to their potential involvement in mitotic DNA repair and damage response in addition to their role in meiosis. The discrepant expression patterns of MSH4 and MSH5 in mammalian tissues have suggested that these two proteins may function independently of one another and may operate beyond meiosis

(Her *et al.* 2007; Yi *et al.* 2005). Studies in yeast have raised the possibility that MSH5 may be involved in cellular response to DNA damage induced by alkylating agents. Specifically, a mutant *MSH5* allele (*i.e. msh5-14*, encoding $MSH5^{Y823H}$) but not *MSH5*-null mutant in the yeast strain XS-14 (lacking O^6-methylguanine methyltransferase) confers cellular tolerance to alkylating compound N-methyl-N'-nitro-N-nitrosoguanidine (MNNG) (Bawa and Xiao 1997; 2003). Although the exact mechanism of action remains to be explored, these studies do indicate that this gain-of-function MSH5 mutant is involved in mediating mitotic cellular response to DNA damage.

It is evident that many of the proteins involved in meiotic recombination are also important players in mitotic recombinational DSB repair. Thus, the involvement of MSH5 in meiotic recombination is suggestive of a potential role for MSH5 in mitotic recombinational DSB repair. DSBs are considered to be the most lethal form of DNA lesion that may arise from replication fork collapse, exposure to DNA damaging agents, or programmed cellular processes including the initiation of meiotic recombination in germ cells, class-switch recombination (CSR), and V(D)J recombination in lymphocytes (Ataian & Krebs 2006). In response to DSB formation, dividing cells usually undergo G2/M phase arrest, then either repair the lesion and resume cell cycle or enter the path of apoptosis depending on the extent of damage. Cells lacking proper G2/M cell cycle arrest, apoptosis, or damage repair are often at a higher risk for malignant transformation. The repair of DSBs requires either the non-homologous end joining (NHEJ) or the homologous recombination pathways. While NHEJ is a rapid means utilized by somatic cells to repair DSBs, it is error-prone and can result in alteration of DNA sequences for non-compatible breaks (Dery & Masson 2007; Helleday *et al.* 2007). On the other hand, homologous recombination is a more accurate repair pathway during S/G2 phases as it utilizes the homologous template usually provided by a sister chromatid or homologous chromosome (Saleh-Gohari & Helleday 2004). Similar to meiotic homologous recombination, this homology-directed DSB repair will also produce two alternative outcomes, CO or non-crossover/gene conversion. Loss of essential homologous recombination gene products often results in chromosome instability, by which cells exhibit increased sensitivities to a variety of DNA damage agents such as IR, cisplatin, and gemcitabine. In addition, homologous recombination deficient cells may also display DNA damage tolerance and resistance to killing by DNA damaging agents as well (Crul *et al.* 2003; Khanna & Jackson 2001; Takata *et al.* 2001; van Waardenburg *et al.* 2004; Zdraveski *et al.* 2000).

As supported by the observed interactions with hRad51, c-Abl, and hMRE11 as well as structures resembling Holliday junctions (Her *et al.* 2007; Kato *et al.* 2007; Neyton *et al.* 2004; Snowden *et al.* 2004; Yi *et al.* 2006), hMSH4 and hMSH5 are expected to play functional roles in mitotic DNA damage response. In *C. elegans* oocytes, silencing of *RAD51* on a *MSH5* deficient background results in chromosome fragmentation, while a comparable defect is also noted when *MSH4* and *BRCA1* homologues are concomitantly silenced, indicating the existence of functional interplay of these proteins in the maintenance of chromosome integrity (Adamo *et al.* 2008; Rinaldo *et al.* 2002). The interaction between hMSH5 and c-Abl can provoke two different cellular actions depending on the severity of DNA damage (Tompkins *et al.* 2009). Endogenous hMSH5 protein undergoes IR dose and time dependent induction, and it appears that increased levels of hMSH5 can promote IR-triggered apoptosis. However, this effect is more prominent in cells treated with a relatively high dose of IR (> 2 Gy). This is reminiscent of a previous observation that the linear correlation between DSB repair and the number of γH2Ax foci only exists in cells irradiated with IR at doses below 2 Gy (Bouquet *et al.* 2006), suggesting the existence of a dynamic regulatory mechanism controlling DSB repair and apoptosis. Present evidence is compatible with the view that the expression of hMSH5 is normally maintained at a low level in unperturbed cells, and DNA damage-triggered hMSH5 induction promotes c-Abl activation and subsequent initiation of a p73-mediated caspase 3-dependent apoptotic response (Tompkins *et al.* 2009). Coherently, the peculiar interaction between $hMSH5^{P29S}$ and c-Abl is capable of over-activating c-Abl, leading to increased cellular radiosensitivity. In contrast, moderate hMSH5 induction is expected to facilitate recombinational DSB repair. Recent experimental results have demonstrated a functional requirement for c-Abl-mediated hMSH5 phosphorylation in DSB repair (Her *et al.* 2007; Tompkins *et al.* 2009). It is demonstrated, by the use of a chromosomally integrated recombination reporter, that hMSH5 tyrosine phosphorylation is an essential early event for non-crossover DSB repair. In fact, cells harboring a phosphorylation deficient hMSH5 mutant are more sensitive to DSB-inducing anticancer drug cisplatin. Collectively, these studies tend to suggest a dual role for the induction of hMSH5 protein in recombinational DSB repair and DNA damage-triggered apoptotic response.

2.3.3 Role in immunoglobulin diversification

Genomic rearrangement that occurs during B-cell development in the form of V(D)J recombination is essential for the generation of antibody repertoire, and additional diversity is achieved by elevated mutation rate and gene sequence shuffling in corresponding processes known as somatic hypermutation (SHM) and CSR (Li *et al.* 2004b; Schroeder & Cavacini 2010). While SHM targets the "hot spots" in variable (V) region of immunoglobulin (Ig) to enhance antigen recognition, CSR is responsible for Ig isotype switching by way of recombining the switch (S) regions upstream of each functional genes (C_H) in the constant (C) region of Ig heavy (H) chain, *i.e.* switching from IgM or IgD to other isotypes that mediate diverse effector functions in the daughter cells (Li *et al.* 2004b; Schroeder & Cavacini 2010). Both SHM and CSR start from deamination of dC to dU by activation-induced cytidine deaminase, a centroblast B-cell specific protein (Muramatsu *et al.* 2000; Muramatsu *et al.* 1999). Deamination of dCs leads to G-U mismatches and may subsequently generate C to T or G to A mutations. In addition, uracil N-glycosylase, apurinic/apyrimidinic endonucleases, and MMR proteins are required to generate extended single base mutations and single-stranded DNA nicks (Di Noia & Neuberger 2002; Ehrenstein & Neuberger 1999; Ehrenstein *et al.* 2001; Guikema *et al.* 2007; Imai *et al.* 2003; Martin & Scharff 2002; Rada *et al.* 2002; Schrader *et al.* 1999). During CSR, DSBs have to be generated in the S regions, possibly by way of single-strand breaks, to allow intrachromosomal deletion via recombination between the two S regions (Wuerffel *et al.* 1997), in which DSBs are primarily repaired by NHEJ. The tandem repeats of short consensus sequences in the S regions are too short for homologous recombination, however they are enough for microhomology-mediated end joining (MMEJ), a specified type of NHEJ using small homologous regions to anneal the two overhangs at the break site. It is generally accepted that MMEJ represents a prominent process of NHEJ in CSR (Kenter 1999), and the length of microhomology at S-S junctions may change due to impaired MMEJ (Stavnezer 2000).

It is well documented that proteins involved in MMR and DSB repair are also involved in the process of CSR. In fact, *Msh2*, *Msh6*, *Mlh1*, and *Pms2* knockout mice all exhibit impaired CSR and SHM (Ehrenstein & Neuberger 1999; Martin & Scharff 2002; Schrader *et al.* 1999). Mice deficient for early DSB response factors ATM or H2AX, and NHEJ proteins Ku70, Ku80, or DNA-PKcs, show reduced CSR activities but with normal SHM (Bemark *et al.* 2000; Casellas *et al.* 1998; Manis *et al.* 2002; Manis *et al.* 1998; Reina-San-Martin *et al.* 2004; Reina-San-Martin *et al.* 2003). MutS and MutL homologues are not only required to assist MMEJ, but they also play overlapping and distinct roles in the process of switch recombination (Ehrenstein *et al.* 2001; Li *et al.* 2004a; Schrader *et al.* 1999; Schrader *et al.* 2002). This assessment is mainly obtained through analyzing microhomology at the S-S junctions as well as the distribution of breakpoints in the absence of each protein (Ehrenstein *et al.* 2001; Li *et al.* 2004a; Schrader *et al.* 1999; Wu *et al.* 2006). Collectively, deficiency of MutS and MutL homologues has been associated with three different phenotypes at the S-S junctions—*Msh2* or *Mlh3* deficiency leads to a decrease in the length of microhomology (Schrader *et al.* 2002; Wu *et al.* 2006), *Msh6*-null B cells show no change of microhomology (Li *et al.* 2004a), and an increase in the length of microhomology is evident in *Mlh1*- or *Pms2*-null B cells (Ehrenstein *et al.* 2001; Schrader *et al.* 2002). MLH1-PMS2 acts downstream of MSH2-MSH6 during MMR, similar effect would be anticipated if the process of MMR played a predominant role. The presence of different microhomology phenotypes indicates that these MMR proteins are involved, at least in part, in different sub-pathways during MMEJ. Indeed, PMS2 has been speculated to interact and stabilize MMEJ intermediates, whereas MSH2 might participate in DNA end processing (Ehrenstein *et al.* 2001; Schrader *et al.* 1999; Schrader *et al.* 2002).

Present evidence suggests that MSH4 and MSH5 are additional players in CSR. These two MutS homologues are known to function in the early and late steps of meiotic recombination as well as in mitotic DNA damage response—events that share some similarities to crucial steps in the complex CSR process. Transcripts of *hMSH5* are present in human spleen and peripheral blood B cells (Her & Doggett 1998; Sekine *et al.* 2007). Association studies have linked one of the non-synonymous alleles of *hMSH5* to IgAD and CVID, two syndromes that are attributable to abnormal CSR. The allele encoding the hMSH5$^{L85F/P786S}$ variant is significantly more frequent in IgAD patients and with borderline significance in CVID patients. One *hMSH5* SNP (rs3131378), located within intron 12, is also tightly associated with IgAD and CVID. Furthermore, CVID patients carrying the *hMSH5*$^{L85F/P786S}$ allele display increased microhomology at Sμ-Sα1 joints, which commonly associate with far fewer mutations (Sekine *et al.* 2007). The L85F and P786S alterations, located within the hMSH4-interacting domain, significantly compromise the protein interaction between hMSH5 and hMSH4, suggesting both hMSH5 and hMSH4 are required for efficient CSR (Sekine *et al.* 2007).

In mice, however, the effects of Msh5 on CSR seem to be strain-specific. In an earlier study, most of the congenic H-2$^{b/b}$ MRL/*lpr* mice (introgression of H-2^{b} MHC haplotype from129/Sv onto a MRL/*lpr* background) show undetectable serum IgG3, reduced levels of serum IgA and elevated levels of serum IgM and IgG2a in older mice, suggesting impaired CSR in these animals. Microarray analysis of gene expression reveals a hypomorphic allele of *Msh5* on the H-2^{b} haplotype. Comparing to controls, H-2$^{b/b}$ MRL/*lpr* mice without serum IgG3 (IgG3^{neg}) exhibit significantly increased microhomology at Sμ-Sγ3 (*i.e.* IgM to IgG3 switch) and Sμ-Sα (*i.e.* IgM to IgA switch) joints in splenic B cells (Sekine *et al.* 2007). This phenotype of increased microhomology is also observed in B cells from *Msh5*-null FVB mice (de Vries *et al.* 1999) and *Msh4* knockout mice on C57BL/6 background (Sekine *et al.* 2007). These studies indicate that both MSH5 and MSH4 are involved in CSR and may function as a heterodimer. Interestingly, studies performed with *Msh5*-null C57BL/6 mice show no detectable alterations in the length of microhomology (Guikema *et al.* 2008). It is conceivable that the different effects of Msh5 deficiency on CSR in these two mouse strains might be attributable to different levels of *Msh5* expression, of which MRL/lpr is a high *Msh5* expresser, whereas C57BL/6 expresses very low levels of Msh5, and the difference between them is about 100-fold (Sekine *et al.* 2007; Sekine *et al.* 2009). It is also important to note that these two *Msh5*-null mouse lines have been reported to display different degrees of meiotic chromosome pairing defects (de Vries *et al.* 1999; Edelmann *et al.* 1999), suggesting that the role of *Msh5* might be influenced by its associated genetic backgrounds.

3. Conclusion

The MMR system has received a considerable amount of attention over the last decade. It is now clear that the MMR system is multifaceted and participates in several different pathways of DNA metabolism. Among all MMR components, the MutS family of proteins plays critical and conserved functions during the initiation phase of mismatch recognition. In contrast to those MutS homologues involved in MMR, the functions of MSH4 and MSH5 are still not fully understood. These two MutS homologues share similar structure and sequence features with the other members of the MutS family. Present evidence suggests that MSH4 and MSH5 have evolved to function in recombinational DSB repair, DNA damage signaling, and immunoglobulin class switch recombination. Although the mechanistic details of their involvement in these processes have yet to be elucidated, it is conceivable that the actions of hMSH5 in recombinational DSB repair is both hMSH4-independent and hMSH4-dependent, presumably coordinating with their functions in homology searching and the resolution of recombination intermediate structures. Available evidence supports a scenario that the expression of hMSH5 is maintained at a low level under normal conditions, whereas DNA damage-elicited hMSH5 induction can promote c-Abl activation and the initiation of a p73-mediated caspase 3-dependent apoptotic response. On the contrary, moderate hMSH5 induction, caused by less severe DNA damage, is expected to facilitate recombinational DSB repair. It is plausible that hMSH4 and hMSH5 may also play a role in CSR, in particular, through manipulating the process of MMEJ.

The current and emerging evidence has lent support to the idea that MSH4 and MSH5 are involved in diverse functions by engaging different pathways through various interactions with different proteins. Undoubtedly, the current knowledge about these two MutS homologues has created a solid steppingstone for future exploration of their biological functions and potential association with disease conditions in humans.

4. Acknowledgment

We would like to take this opportunity to thank all previous and current members of the Her laboratory at Washington State University, particularly, for their contributions to our current understanding of the role of hMSH4 and hMSH5 proteins in various cellular processes in human cells. The work conducted in the Her laboratory is generously supported by research grants from the National Institutes of Health, U.S. Department of Health and Human Services.

5. References

Adamo, A., Montemauri, P., Silva, N., Ward, J. D., Boulton, S. J., & La Volpe A. (2008). BRC-1 acts in the inter-sister pathway of meiotic double-strand break repair. *EMBO Rep*, Vol. 9, No. 3, (March 2008), pp. 287-292, ISSN 1469-221X.

Akimoto, C., Kitagawa, H., Matsumoto, A., & Kato, S. (2008). Spermatogenesis-specific association of SMCY and MSH5. *Genes Cells*, Vol. 13, No. 6, (June 2008), pp. 623-633, ISSN 1356-9597.

Ataian, Y. & Krebs, J. E. (2006). Five repair pathways in one context: chromatin modification during DNA repair. *Biochem Cell Biol*, Vol. 84, No. 4, (August 2006), pp. 490-504, ISSN 0829-8211.

Baudat, F. & de Massy, B. (2007). Regulating double-stranded DNA break repair towards crossover or non-crossover during mammalian meiosis. *Chromosome Res*, Vol. 15, No. 5, (2007), pp. 565-577, ISSN 0967-3849.

Bawa, S. & Xiao, W. (1997). A mutation in the MSH5 gene results in alkylation tolerance. *Cancer Res*, Vol. 57, No. 13, (July 1997), pp. 2715-2720, ISSN 0008-5472.

Bawa, S. & Xiao, W. (2003). A single amino acid substitution in MSH5 results in DNA alkylation tolerance. *Gene*, Vol. 315, (October 2003), pp. 177-182, ISSN 0378-1119.

Bemark, M., Sale, J. E., Kim, H. J., Berek, C., Cosgrove, R. A., & Neuberger, M. S. (2000). Somatic hypermutation in the absence of DNA-dependent protein kinase catalytic subunit (DNA-PK(cs)) or recombination-activating gene (RAG)1 activity. *J Exp Med*, Vol. 192, No. 10, (November 2000), pp. 1509-1514, ISSN 0022-1007.

Bishop, D. K. (1994). RecA homologs Dmc1 and Rad51 interact to form multiple nuclear complexes prior to meiotic chromosome synapsis. *Cell*, Vol. 79, No. 6, (December 1994), pp. 1081-1092, ISSN 0092-8674.

Bocker, T., Barusevicius, A., Snowden, T., Rasio, D., Guerrette, S., Robbins, D., Schmidt, C., Burczak, J., Croce, C. M., Copeland, T., Kovatich, A. J., & Fishel, R. (1999). hMSH5: a human MutS homologue that forms a novel heterodimer with hMSH4 and is expressed during spermatogenesis. *Cancer Res*, Vol. 59, No. 4, (February 1999), pp. 816-822, ISSN 0008-5472.

Bouquet, F., Muller, C., & Salles, B. (2006). The loss of gammaH2AX signal is a marker of DNA double strand breaks repair only at low levels of DNA damage. *Cell Cycle*, Vol. 5, No. 10, (May 2006), pp. 1116-1122, ISSN 1538-4101.

Burns, N., Grimwade, B., Ross-Macdonald, P. B., Choi, E. Y., Finberg, K., Roeder, G. S., & Snyder, M. (1994). Large-scale analysis of gene expression, protein localization, and gene disruption in Saccharomyces cerevisiae. *Genes Dev*, Vol. 8, No. 9, (May 1994), pp. 1087-1105, ISSN 0890-9369.

Casellas, R., Nussenzweig, A., Wuerffel, R., Pelanda, R., Reichlin, A., Suh, H., Qin, X. F., Besmer, E., Kenter, A., Rajewsky, K., & Nussenzweig, M. C. (1998). Ku80 is required for immunoglobulin isotype switching. *EMBO J*, Vol. 17, No. 8, (April 1998), pp. 2404-2411, ISSN 0261-4189.

Crul, M., van Waardenburg, R. C., Bocxe, S., van Eijindhoven, M. A., Pluim, D., Beijnen, J. H., & Schellens, J. H. (2003). DNA repair mechanisms involved in gemcitabine cytotoxicity and in the interaction between gemcitabine and cisplatin. *Biochem Pharmacol*, Vol. 65, No. 2, (January 2003), pp. 275-282, ISSN 0006-2952.

Culligan, K. M. & Hays, J. B. (1997). DNA mismatch repair in plants. An Arabidopsis thaliana gene that predicts a protein belonging to the MSH2 subfamily of eukaryotic MutS homologs. *Plant Physiol*, Vol. 115, No. 2, (October 1997), pp. 833-839, ISSN 0032-0889.

de Vries, S. S., Baart, E. B., Dekker, M., Siezen, A., de Rooij, D. G., de Boer, P., & te Riele, H. (1999). Mouse MutS-like protein Msh5 is required for proper chromosome synapsis in male and female meiosis. *Genes Dev*, Vol. 13, No. 5, (March 1999), pp. 523-531, ISSN 0890-9369.

Dery, U. & Masson, J. Y. (2007). Twists and turns in the function of DNA damage signaling and repair proteins by post-translational modifications. *DNA Repair (Amst)*, Vol. 6, No. 5, (May 2007), pp. 561-577, ISSN 1568-7864.

Di Noia, J. & Neuberger, M. S. (2002). Altering the pathway of immunoglobulin hypermutation by inhibiting uracil-DNA glycosylase. *Nature*, Vol. 419, No. 6902, (September 2002), pp. 43-48, ISSN 0028-0836.

Edelmann, W., Cohen, P. E., Kneitz, B., Winand, N., Lia, M., Heyer, J., Kolodner, R., Pollard, J. W., & Kucherlapati, R. (1999). Mammalian MutS homologue 5 is required for chromosome pairing in meiosis. *Nat Genet*, Vol. 21, No. 1, (January 1999), pp. 123-127, ISSN 1061-4036.

Ehrenstein, M. R. & Neuberger M. S. (1999). Deficiency in Msh2 affects the efficiency and local sequence specificity of immunoglobulin class-switch recombination: parallels with somatic hypermutation. *EMBO J*, Vol. 18, No. 12, (June 1999), pp. 3484-3490, ISSN 0261-4189.

Ehrenstein, M. R., Rada, C, Jones, A. M., Milstein, C., & Neuberger, M. S. (2001). Switch junction sequences in PMS2-deficient mice reveal a microhomology-mediated mechanism of Ig class switch recombination. *Proc Natl Acad Sci U S A*, Vol. 98, No. 25, (December 2001), pp. 14553-14558, ISSN 0027-8424.

Fishel, R. & Wilson, T. (1997). MutS homologs in mammalian cells. *Curr Opin Genet Dev*, Vol. 7, No. 1, (February 1997), pp. 105-113, ISSN 0959-437X.

Guikema, J. E., Linehan, E. K., Tsuchimoto, D., Nakabeppu, Y., Strauss, P. R., Stavnezer, J., & Schrader, C. E. (2007). APE1- and APE2-dependent DNA breaks in immunoglobulin class switch recombination. *J Exp Med*, Vol. 204, No. 12, (November 2007), pp. 3017-3026, ISSN 0022-1007.

Guikema, J. E., Schrader, C. E., Leus, N. G., Ucher, A., Linehan, E. K., Werling, U., Edelmann, W., & Stavnezer, J. (2008). Reassessment of the role of Mut S homolog 5 in Ig class switch recombination shows lack of involvement in cis- and trans-switching. *J Immunol*, Vol. 181, No. 12, (December 2008), pp. 8450-8459, ISSN 0022-1767.

Harfe, B. D. & Jinks-Robertson, S. (2000). DNA mismatch repair and genetic instability. *Annu Rev Genet*, Vol. 34, (December 2000), pp. 359-399, ISSN 0066-4197.

Helleday, T., Lo, J., van Gent, D. C., & Engelward, B. P. (2007). DNA double-strand break repair: from mechanistic understanding to cancer treatment. *DNA Repair (Amst)*, Vol. 6, No. 7, (July 2007), pp. 923-935, ISSN 1568-7864.

Her, C. & Doggett, N. A. (1998). Cloning, structural characterization, and chromosomal localization of the human orthologue of Saccharomyces cerevisiae MSH5 gene. *Genomics*, Vol. 52, No. 1, (August 1998), pp. 50-61, ISSN 0888-7543.

Her, C., Wu, X., Wan, W., & Doggett, N. A. (1999). Identification and characterization of the mouse MutS homolog 5: Msh5. *Mamm Genome*, Vol. 10, No. 11, (November 1999), pp. 1054-1061, ISSN 0938-8990.

Her, C., Wu, X., Bailey, S. M., & Doggett, N. A. (2001). Mouse MutS homolog 4 is predominantly expressed in testis and interacts with MutS homolog 5. *Mamm Genome*, Vol. 12, No. 1, (January 2001), pp. 73-76, ISSN 0938-8990.

Her, C., Wu, X., Griswold, M. D., & Zhou, F. (2003). Human MutS homologue MSH4 physically interacts with von Hippel-Lindau tumor suppressor-binding protein 1. *Cancer Res*, Vol. 63, No. 4, (February 2003), pp. 865-872, ISSN 0008-5472.

Her, C., Zhao, N., Wu, X., & Tompkins, J. D. (2007). MutS homologues hMSH4 and hMSH5: diverse functional implications in humans. *Front Biosci*, Vol. 12 (January 2007), pp. 905-911, ISSN 1093-9946.

Hollingsworth, N. M., Ponte, L., & Halsey, C. (1995). MSH5, a novel MutS homolog, facilitates meiotic reciprocal recombination between homologs in Saccharomyces cerevisiae but not mismatch repair. *Genes Dev*, Vol. 9, No. 14, (July 1995), pp. 1728-1739, ISSN 0890-9369.

Hung, S. I., Chung, W. H., Liou, L. B., Chu, C. C., Lin, M., Huang, H. P., Lin, Y. L., Lan, J. L., Yang, L. C., Hong, H. S., Chen, M. J., Lai, P. C., Wu, M. S., Chu, C. Y., Wang, K. H., Chen, C. H., Fann, C. S., Wu, J. Y., & Chen, Y. T. (2005). HLA-B*5801 allele as a genetic marker for severe cutaneous adverse reactions caused by allopurinol. *Proc Natl Acad Sci U S A*, Vol. 102, No. 11, (March 2005), pp. 4134-4139, ISSN 0027-8424.

Imai, K., Slupphaug, G., Lee, W. I., Revy, P., Nonoyama, S., Catalan, N., Yel, L., Forveille, M., Kavli, B., Krokan, H. E., Ochs, H. D., Fischer, A., & Durandy, A. (2003). Human uracil-DNA glycosylase deficiency associated with profoundly impaired immunoglobulin class-switch recombination. *Nat Immunol*, Vol. 4, No. 10, (October 2003), pp. 1023-1028, ISSN 1529- 2908.

Iyer, R. R., Pluciennik, A., Burdett, V., & Modrich, P. L. (2006). DNA mismatch repair: functions and mechanisms. *Chem Rev*, Vol. 106, No. 2, (February 2006), pp. 302-323, ISSN 0009-2665.

Jin, D. Y., Teramoto, H., Giam, C. Z., Chun, R. F., Gutkind, J. S., & Jeang, K. T. (1997). A human suppressor of c-Jun N-terminal kinase 1 activation by tumor necrosis factor alpha. *J Biol Chem*, Vol. 272, No. 41, (October 1997), pp. 25816-25823, ISSN 0021-9258.

Jiricny, J. (2006). The multifaceted mismatch-repair system. *Nat Rev Mol Cell Biol*, Vol. 7, No. 5, (May 2006), pp. 335-346, ISSN 1471-0072.

Junop, M. S., Obmolova, G., Rausch, K., Hsieh, P., & Yang, W. (2001). Composite active site of an ABC ATPase: MutS uses ATP to verify mismatch recognition and authorize DNA repair. *Mol Cell*, Vol. 7, No. 1, (January 2001), pp. 1-12, ISSN 1097-2765.

Kato, T., Sato, N., Hayama, S., Yamabuki, T., Ito, T., Miyamoto, M., Kondo, S., Nakamura, Y., & Daigo, Y. (2007). Activation of Holliday junction recognizing protein involved in the chromosomal stability and immortality of cancer cells. *Cancer Res*, Vol. 67, No. 18, (September 2007), pp. 8544-8553, ISSN 0008-5472.

Keeney, S., Giroux, C. N., & Kleckner, N. (1997). Meiosis-specific DNA double-strand breaks are catalyzed by Spo11, a member of a widely conserved protein family. *Cell*, Vol. 88, No. 3, (February 1997), pp. 375-384, ISSN 0092-8674.

Kelly, K. O., Dernburg, A. F., Stanfield, G. M., & Villeneuve, A. M. (2000). Caenorhabditis elegans msh-5 is required for both normal and radiation-induced meiotic crossing over but not for completion of meiosis. *Genetics*, Vol. 156, No. 2, (October 2000), pp. 617-630, ISSN 0016-6731.

Kenter, A. L. (1999). The liaison of isotype class switch and mismatch repair: an illegitimate affair. *J Exp Med*, Vol. 190, No. 3, (August 1999), pp. 307-310, ISSN 0022-1007.

Khanna, K. K., & Jackson, S. P. (2001). DNA double-strand breaks: signaling, repair and the cancer connection. *Nat Genet,* Vol. 27, No. 3, (March 2001), pp. 247-254, ISSN 1061-4036.

Kneitz, B., Cohen, P. E., Avdievich, E., Zhu, L., Kane, M. F., Hou, H. Jr., Kolodner, R. D., Kucherlapati, R., Pollard, J. W., & Edelmann, W. (2000). MutS homolog 4 localization to meiotic chromosomes is required for chromosome pairing during meiosis in male and female mice. *Genes Dev,* Vol. 14, No. 9, (May 2000), pp. 1085-1097, ISSN 0890-9369.

Kolodner, R. (1996). Biochemistry and genetics of eukaryotic mismatch repair. *Genes Dev,* Vol. 10, No. 12, (June 1996), pp. 1433-1442, ISSN 0890-9369.

Kramer, W., Kramer, B., Williamson, M. S., & Fogel, S. (1989). Cloning and nucleotide sequence of DNA mismatch repair gene PMS1 from Saccharomyces cerevisiae: homology of PMS1 to procaryotic MutL and HexB. *J Bacteriol,* Vol. 171, No. 10, (October 1989), pp. 5339-5346, ISSN 0021-9193.

Kunkel, T. A. & Erie, D. A. (2005). DNA mismatch repair. *Annu Rev Biochem,* Vol. 74, (July 2005), pp. 681-710, ISSN 0066-4154. Lahaye, F., Lespinasse, F., Staccini, P., Palin, L., Paquis-Flucklinger, V., & Santucci-Darmanin, S. (2010). hMSH5 is a nucleocytoplasmic shuttling protein whose stability depends on its subcellular localization. *Nucleic Acids Res,* Vol. 38, No. 11m (June 2010), pp. 3655-3671, ISSN 0305-1048.

Lamers, M. H., Perrakis, A., Enzlin, J. H., Winterwerp, H. H., de Wind, N, & Sixma, T. K. (2000). The crystal structure of DNA mismatch repair protein MutS binding to a G x T mismatch. *Nature,* Vol. 407, No. 6805, (October 2000), pp. 711-717, ISSN 0028-0836.

Lamers, M. H., Winterwerp, H. H., & Sixma, T. K. (2003). The alternating ATPase domains of MutS control DNA mismatch repair. *EMBO J,* Vol. 22, No. 3, (February 2003), pp. 746-756, ISSN 0261-4189.

Lamers, M. H., Georgijevic, D., Lebbink, J. H., Winterwerp, H. H., Agianian, B., de Wind, N., & Sixma, T. K. (2004). ATP increases the affinity between MutS ATPase domains. Implications for ATP hydrolysis and conformational changes. *J Biol Chem,* Vol. 279, No. 42, (October 2004), pp. 43879-43885, ISSN 0021-9258.

Lee, T. H., Yi, W., Griswold, M. D., Zhu, F., & Her, C. (2006). Formation of hMSH4-hMSH5 heterocomplex is a prerequisite for subsequent GPS2 recruitment. *DNA Repair (Amst),* Vol. 5, No. 1, (January 2006), pp. 32-42, ISSN 1568-7864.

Lenzi, M. L., Smith, J., Snowden, T., Kim, M., Fishel, R., Poulos, B. K., & Cohen, P. E. (2005). Extreme heterogeneity in the molecular events leading to the establishment of chiasmata during meiosis i in human oocytes. *Am J Hum Genet,* Vol. 76, No. 1, (January 2005), pp. 112-127, ISSN 0002-9297.

Li, Z., Scherer, S. J., Ronai, D., Iglesias-Ussel, M. D., Peled, J. U., Bardwell, P. D., Zhuang, M., Lee, K., Martin, A., Edelmann, W., & Scharff, M. D. (2004a). Examination of Msh6- and Msh3-deficient mice in class switching reveals overlapping and distinct roles of MutS homologues in antibody diversification. *J Exp Med,* Vol. 200, No. 1, (July 2004), pp. 47-59, ISSN 0022-1007.

Li, Z., Woo, C. J., Iglesias-Ussel, M. D., Ronai, D., & Scharff, M. D. (2004b). The generation of antibody diversity through somatic hypermutation and class switch recombination. *Genes Dev,* Vol. 18, No. 1, (January 2004), pp. 1-11, ISSN 0890-9369.

Lipkin, S. M., Wang, V., Jacoby, R., Banerjee-Basu, S., Baxevanis, A. D., Lynch, H. T., Elliott, R. M., & Collins, F. S. (2000). MLH3: a DNA mismatch repair gene associated with mammalian microsatellite instability. *Nat Genet*, Vol. 24, No. 1, (January 2000), pp. 27-35, ISSN 1061-4036.

Lynn, A., Ashley, T., Hassold, T. (2004). Variation in human meiotic recombination. *Annu Rev Genomics Hum Genet*, Vol. 5. (September 2004), pp. 317-349, ISSN 1527-8204.

Mahadevaiah, S. K., Turner, J. M., Baudat, F., Rogakou, E. P., de Boer, P., Blanco-Rodriguez, J., Jasin, M., Keeney, S., Bonner, W. M., & Burgoyne, P. S. (2001). Recombinational DNA double-strand breaks in mice precede synapsis. *Nat Genet*, Vol. 27, No. 3, (March 2001), pp. 271-276, ISSN 1061-4036.

Manis, J. P., Gu, Y., Lansford, R., Sonoda, E., Ferrini, R., Davidson, L., Rajewsky, K., & Alt, F. W. (1998). Ku70 is required for late B cell development and immunoglobulin heavy chain class switching. *J Exp Med*, Vol. 187, No. 12, (June 1998), pp. 2081-2089, ISSN 0022-1007.

Manis, J. P., Dudley, D., Kaylor, L., & Alt, F. W. (2002). IgH class switch recombination to IgG1 in DNA-PKcs-deficient B cells. *Immunity*, Vol. 16, No. 4, (April 2002), pp. 607-617, ISSN 1074-7613.

Martin, A. & Scharff, M. D. (2002). AID and mismatch repair in antibody diversification. *Nat Rev Immunol*, Vol. 2, No. 8, (August 2002), pp. 605-614, ISSN 1474-1733.

Modrich, P. (1991). Mechanisms and biological effects of mismatch repair. *Annu Rev Genet*, Vol. 25 (December 1991), pp. 229-253, ISSN 0066-4197.

Moens, P. B., Kolas, N. K., Tarsounas, M., Marcon, E., Cohen, P. E., & Spyropoulos, B. (2002). The time course and chromosomal localization of recombination-related proteins at meiosis in the mouse are compatible with models that can resolve the early DNA-DNA interactions without reciprocal recombination. *J Cell Sci*, Vol. 115, No. Pt. 8, (April 2002), pp.1611-1622, ISSN 0021-9533.

Muramatsu, M., Sankaranand, V. S., Anant, S., Sugai, M., Kinoshita, K., Davidson, N. O., & Honjo, T. (1999). Specific expression of activation-induced cytidine deaminase (AID), a novel member of the RNA-editing deaminase family in germinal center B cells. *J Biol Chem*, Vol. 274, No. 26, (June 1999), pp. 18470-18476, ISSN 0021-9258.

Muramatsu, M., Kinoshita, K., Fagarasan, S., Yamada, S., Shinkai, Y., & Honjo, T. (2000). Class switch recombination and hypermutation require activation-induced cytidine deaminase (AID), a potential RNA editing enzyme. *Cell*, Vol. 102, No. 5, (September 2000), pp. 553-563, ISSN 0092-8674.

Neyton, S., Lespinasse, F., Moens, P. B., Paul, R., Gaudray, P., Paquis-Flucklinger, V., & Santucci-Darmanin, S. (2004). Association between MSH4 (MutS homologue 4) and the DNA strand-exchange RAD51 and DMC1 proteins during mammalian meiosis. *Mol Hum Reprod*, Vol. 10, No. 12, (December 2004), pp. 917-924, ISSN 1360-9947.

Neyton, S., Lespinasse, F., Lahaye, F. Staccini, P., Paquis-Flucklinger, V., & Santucci-Darmannin, S. (2007). CRM1-dependent nuclear export and dimerization with hMSH5 contribute to the regulation of hMSH4 subcellular localization. *Exp Cell Res*, Vol. 313, No. 17, (October 2007), pp. 3680-3693, ISSN 0014-4827.

Novak, J. E., Ross-Macdonald, P. B., & Roeder, G. S. (2001). The budding yeast Msh4 protein functions in chromosome synapsis and the regulation of crossover distribution. *Genetics*, Vol. 158, No. 3, (July 2001), pp. 1013-1025, ISSN 0016-6731.

Obmolova, G., Ban, C. Hsieh, P., & Yang, W. (2000). Crystal structures of mismatch repair protein MutS and its complex with a substrate DNA. *Nature*. Vol. 407, No. 6805, (October 2000), pp. 703-710, ISSN 0028-0836.

Paquis-Flucklinger, V., Santucci-Darmanin, S., Paul, R., Saunieres, A., Turc-Carel, C., & Desnuelle, C. (1997). Cloning and expression analysis of a meiosis-specific MutS homolog: the human MSH4 gene. *Genomics*, Vol. 44, No. 2, (September 1997), pp. 188-194, ISSN 0888-7543.

Peng, Y. C., Kuo, F., Breiding, D. E. Wang, Y. F., Mansur, C. P., & Androphy, E. J. (2001). AMF1 (GPS2) modulates p53 transactivation. *Mol Cell Biol*, Vol. 21, No. 17, (September 2001), pp. 5913-5924, ISSN 0270- 7306.

Pochart, P., Woltering, D., & Hollingsworth, N. M. (1997). Conserved properties between functionally distinct MutS homologs in yeast. *J Biol Chem*, Vol. 272, No. 48, (November 1997), pp. 30345-30349, ISSN 0021-9258.

Rada, C., Williams, G. T., Nilsen, H., Barnes, D. E., Lindahl, T., & Neuberger, M. S. (2002). Immunoglobulin isotype switching is inhibited and somatic hypermutation perturbed in UNG-deficient mice. *Curr Biol*, Vol. 12, No. 20, (October 2002), pp. 1748-1755, ISSN 0960-9822.

Reenan, R. A. & Kolodner, R. D. (1992). Characterization of insertion mutations in the Saccharomyces cerevisiae MSH1 and MSH2 genes: evidence for separate mitochondrial and nuclear functions. *Genetics*, Vol. 132, No. 4, (December 1992), pp. 975-985, ISSN 0016-6731.

Reina-San-Martin, B., Difilippantonio, S., Hanitsch, L., Masilamani, R. F., Nussenzweig, A., & Nussenzweig, M. C. (2003). H2AX is required for recombination between immunoglobulin switch regions but not for intra-switch region recombination or somatic hypermutation. *J Exp Med*, Vol. 197, No. 12, (June 2003), pp. 1767-1778, ISSN 0022-1007.

Reina-San-Martin, B., Chen, H. T., Nussenzweig, A., & Nussenzweig, M. C. (2004). ATM is required for efficient recombination between immunoglobulin switch regions. *J Exp Med*, Vol. 200, No. 9, (November 2004), pp. 1103-1110, ISSN 0022-1007.

Rinaldo, C., Bazzicalupo, P., Ederle, S., Hilliard, M., La Volpe, A. (2002). Roles for Caenorhabditis elegans rad-51 in meiosis and in resistance to ionizing radiation during development. *Genetics*, Vol. 160, No. 2, (February 2002), pp. 471-479, ISSN 0016-6731.

Ross-Macdonald, P. & Roeder, G. S. (1994). Mutation of a meiosis-specific MutS homolog decreases crossing over but not mismatch correction. *Cell*, Vol. 79, No. 6, (December 1994), pp. 1069-1080, ISSN 0092-8674.

Saleh-Gohari, N. & Helleday, T. (2004). Conservative homologous recombination preferentially repairs DNA double-strand breaks in the S phase of the cell cycle in human cells. *Nucleic Acids Res*, Vol. 32, No. 12, (July 2004), pp. 3683-3688, ISSN 0305-1048.

Santucci-Darmanin, S., Paul, R., Michiels, J. F., Saunieres, A., Desnuelle, C., & Paquis-Flucklinger, V. (1999). Alternative splicing of hMSH4: two isoforms in testis and abnormal transcripts in somatic tissues. *Mamm Genome*, Vol. 10, No. 4, (April 1999), pp. 423-427, ISSN 0938-8990.

Santucci-Darmanin, S., Walpita, D., Lespinasse, F., Desnuelle, C., Ashley, T., & Paquis-Flucklinger, V. (2000). MSH4 acts in conjunction with MLH1 during mammalian meiosis. *FASEB J*, Vol. 14, No. 11, (August 2000), pp. 1539-1547, ISSN 0892-6638.

Santucci-Darmanin, S., Neyton, S., Lespinasse, F., Saunieres, A., Gaudray, P., & Paquis-Flucklinger, V. (2002). The DNA mismatch-repair MLH3 protein interacts with MSH4 in meiotic cells, supporting a role for this MutL homolog in mammalian meiotic recombination. *Hum Mol Genet*, Vol. 11, No. 15, (July 2002), pp. 1697-1706, ISSN 0964-6906.

Schrader, C. E., Edelmann, W., Kucherlapati, R., & Stavnezer, J. (1999). Reduced isotype switching in splenic B cells from mice deficient in mismatch repair enzymes. *J Exp Med*, Vol. 190, No. 3, (August 1999), pp. 323-330, ISSN 0022-1007.

Schrader, C. E., Vardo, J., & Stavnezer, J. (2002). Role for mismatch repair proteins Msh2, Mlh1, and Pms2 in immunoglobulin class switching shown by sequence analysis of recombination junctions. *J Exp Med*, Vol. 195, No. 3, (February 2002), pp. 367-373, ISSN 0022-1007.

Schroeder, H. W., Jr., & Cavacini, L. (2010). Structure and function of immunoglobulins. *J Allergy Clin Immunol*, Vol. 125, No. 2, Suppl. 2, (February 2010), pp. S41-S52, ISSN 0091-6749.

Sekine, H., Ferreira, R. C., Pan-Hammarstrom, Q., Graham, R. R., Ziemba, B., de Vries, S. S., Liu, J., Hippen, K., Koeuth, T., Ortmann, W., Iwahori, A., Elliott, M. K., Offer, S., Skon, C., Du, L., Novitzke, J., Lee, A. T., Zhao, N., Tompkins, J. D., Altshuler, D., Gregersen, P. K., Cunningham-Rundles, C., Harris, R. S., Her, C., Nelson, D. L., Hammarstrom, L., Gilkeson, G. S., & Behrens, T. W. (2007). Role for Msh5 in the regulation of Ig class switch recombination. *Proc Natl Acad Sci U S A*, Vol. 104, No. 17, (April 2007), pp. 7193-7198, ISSN 0027-8424.

Sekine, H., Ferreira, R. C., Pan-Hammarstrom, Q., Hammarstrom, L., Gilkeson, G. S., & Behrens, T. W. (2009). Comment on "Reassessment of the role of mut S homolog 5 in Ig class switch recombination shows lack of involvement in cis- and trans-switching. *J Immunol*, Vol. 182, No. 8, (April 2009), pp. 4495-4496, ISSN 0022-1767.

Snowden, T., Acharya, S., Butz, C., Berardini, M., & Fishel, R. (2004). hMSH4-hMSH5 recognizes Holliday Junctions and forms a meiosis-specific sliding clamp that embraces homologous chromosomes. *Mol Cell*, Vol. 15, No. 3, (August 2004), pp. 437-451, ISSN 1097-2765.

Spain, B. H., Bowdish, K. S., Pacal, A. R., Staub, S. F., Koo, D., Chang, C. Y., Xie, W., & Colicelli, J. (1996). Two human cDNAs, including a homolog of Arabidopsis FUS6 (COP11), suppress G-protein- and mitogen-activated protein kinase-mediated signal transduction in yeast and mammalian cells. *Mol Cell Biol*, Vol. 16, No. 12, (December 1996), pp. 6698-6706, ISSN 0270- 7306.

Stavnezer, J. (2000). Molecular processes that regulate class switching. *Curr Top Microbiol Immunol*, Vol. 245, No. 2, (2000) pp. 127-168, ISSN 0070-217X.

Szostak, J. W., Orr-Weaver, T. L., Rothstein, R. J., & Stahl, F. W. (1983). The double-strand-break repair model for recombination. *Cell*, Vol. 33, No. 1, (May 1983), pp. 25-35, ISSN 0092-8674.

Takata, M., Sasaki, M. S., Tachiiri, S., Fukushima, T., Sonoda, E., Schild, D., Thompson, L. H., & Takeda, S. (2001). Chromosome instability and defective recombinational repair in knockout mutants of the five Rad51 paralogs. *Mol Cell Biol*, Vol. 21, No. 8, (April 2001), pp. 2858-2866, ISSN 0270-7306.

Tompkins, J. D., Wu, X., Chu, Y. L., & Her, C. (2009). Evidence for a direct involvement of hMSH5 in promoting ionizing radiation induced apoptosis. *Exp Cell Res*, Vol. 315, No. 14, (August 2009), pp. 2420-2432, ISSN 0014-4827.

van Waardenburg, R. C., de Jong, L. A., van Delft, F., van Eijindhoven, M. A., Bohlander, M., Bjornsti, M. A., Brouwer, J., & Schellens, J. H. (2004). Homologous recombination is a highly conserved determinant of the synergistic cytotoxicity between cisplatin and DNA topoisomerase I poisons. *Mol Cancer Ther*, Vol. 3, No. 4, (April 2004), pp. 393-402, ISSN 1535-7163.

Wang, Y., Broderick, P., Webb, E., Wu, X., Vijayakrishnan, J., Matakidou, A., Qureshi, M. Dong, Q., Gu, X., Chen, W. V., Spitz, M. R., Eisen, T., Amos, C. I. & Houlston, R. S. (2008). Common 5p15.33 and 6p21.33 variants influence lung cancer risk. *Nat Genet*, Vol. 40, No. 12, (December 2008), pp. 1407-1409, ISSN 1061-4036.

Wang, Y., Cortez, D., Yazdi, P., Neff, N., Elledge, S. J., & Qin, J. (2000). BASC, a super complex of BRCA1-associated proteins involved in the recognition and repair of aberrant DNA structures. *Genes Dev*, Vol. 14, No. 8, (April 2000), pp. 927-939, ISSN 0890-9369.

Winand, N. J., Panzer, J. A., & Kolodner, R. D. (1998). Cloning and characterization of the human and Caenorhabditis elegans homologs of the Saccharomyces cerevisiae MSH5 gene. *Genomics*, Vol. 53, No. 1, (October 1998), pp. 69-80, ISSN 0888-7543.

Wu, X., Tsai, C. Y., Patam, M. B., Zan, H., Chen, J. P., Lipkin, S. M., & Casali, P. (2006). A role for the MutL mismatch repair Mlh3 protein in immunoglobulin class switch DNA recombination and somatic hypermutation. *J Immunol*, Vol. 176, No. 9, (May 2006), pp. 5426-5437, ISSN 0022-1767.

Wuerffel, R. A., Du, J., Thompson, R. J., & Kenter, A. L. (1997). Ig Sgamma3 DNA-specifc double strand breaks are induced in mitogen-activated B cells and are implicated in switch recombination. *J Immunol*, Vol. 159, No. 9, (November 1997), pp. 4139-4144, ISSN 0022-1767.

Xu, K., Lu, T., Zhou, H., Bai, L., & Xiang, Y. (2010). The role of MSH5 C85T and MLH3 C2531T polymorphisms in the risk of male infertility with azoospermia or severe oligozoospermia. *Clin Chim Acta*, Vol. 411, No. 1-2, (January 2010), pp. 49-52, ISSN 0009-8981.

Yi, W., Lee, T. H., Tompkins, J. D., Zhu, F., Wu, X., & Her, C. (2006). Physical and functional interaction between hMSH5 and c-Abl. *Cancer Res*, Vol. 66, No. 1, (January 2006), pp. 151-158, ISSN 0008-5472.

Yi, W., Wu, X., Lee, T. H., Doggett, N. A., & Her, C. (2005). Two variants of MutS homolog hMSH5: prevalence in humans and effects on protein interaction. *Biochem Biophys Res Commun*, Vol. 332, No. 2, (July 2005), pp. 524-532, ISSN 0006-291X.

Youds, J. L. & Boulton, S. J. (2011). The choice in meiosis - defining the factors that influence crossover or non-crossover formation. *J Cell Sci*, Vol. 124, No. Pt. 4, (February 2011), pp. 501-513, ISSN 0021-9533.

Zalevsky, J., MacQueen, A. J.. Duffy, J. B., Kemphues, K. J., & Villeneuve, A. M. (1999). Crossing over during Caenorhabditis elegans meiosis requires a conserved MutS-based pathway that is partially dispensable in budding yeast. *Genetics*, Vol. 153, No. 3, (November 1999), pp. 1271-1283, ISSN 0016-6731.

Zdraveski, Z. Z., Mello, J. A., Marinus, M. G., & Essigmann, J. M. (2000). Multiple pathways of recombination define cellular responses to cisplatin. *Chem Biol*, Vol. 7, No. 1, (January 2000), pp. 39-50, ISSN 1074-5521.

Zetka, M. C. & Rose, A. M. (1995). Mutant rec-1 eliminates the meiotic pattern of crossing over in Caenorhabditis elegans. *Genetics*, Vol. 141, No. 4, (December 1995), pp. 1339-1349, ISSN 0016-6731.

6

Reverse Transcriptase and Retroviral Replication

T. Matamoros, M. Álvarez, V. Barrioluengo, G. Betancor and L. Menéndez-Arias
Centro de Biología Molecular "Severo Ochoa" (Consejo Superior de Investigaciones Científicas – Universidad Autónoma de Madrid), Campus de Cantoblanco, Madrid Spain

1. Introduction

Within each viral particle, retroviruses package two copies of a single-stranded RNA genome of about 10 kb. All of the viral genomes contain three major genes, arranged in the order: 5′-*gag–pol–env*-3′, and some retroviruses may also have accessory genes (*e.g. vif, vpr, tax,* etc…). Structural proteins such as MA (matrix protein), CA (capsid protein) and NC (nucleocapsid protein) are encoded within *gag*. Envelope proteins that mediate viral entry (surface and transmembrane glycoproteins) derive from expression of the *env* gene. Virus-encoded enzymes such as the protease, the reverse transcriptase (RT) and the integrase, required to complete the viral life cycle, usually derive from the expression of *pol*. The reverse transcription of the viral single-stranded (+) RNA genome into double-stranded DNA is an essential step in retroviral replication and an important target for therapeutic intervention (for reviews, see Telesnitsky & Goff, 1997; Abbink & Berkhout, 2008; Sarafianos et al., 2009). Reverse transcription is a relatively complex process that requires the intervention of at least three elements: (i) the viral genomic RNA (that serves as template); (ii) a specific primer (*i.e.* a transfer RNA); and (iii) the viral RT. Retroviral RTs are enzymes that possess two activities: (i) a DNA polymerase activity that uses either RNA or DNA as template, and (ii) an RNase H activity, which degrades RNA from RNA/DNA hybrids.
Unlike eukaryotic DNA polymerases, retroviral RTs are devoid of 3′→ 5′ exonucleolytic proofreading and show intrinsic error frequencies of around 10^{-4} to 10^{-5}, well above the values reported for cellular DNA polymerases. Their lower accuracy together with their ability to switch templates during reverse transcription are major contributors to the extensive genetic variability observed in many retroviruses including human immuno-deficiency virus type 1 and type 2 (HIV-1 and HIV-2). The diversification of retroviral genomes, based on the sequence of the *pol* gene (encoding for viral enzymes including RT) is illustrated in Fig. 1. Environmental factors as well as the molecular structure of retroviral RTs modulate their fidelity. In addition, retrovirus genetic variability can be affected by viral and cellular proteins. In this review, studies dealing with the molecular basis of fidelity of HIV-1 RT are summarized and discussed in the light of crystal structures of the enzyme. Structural information has been most useful in the design of antiretroviral drugs targeting the DNA polymerase activity of the RT. The last sections of this chapter summarize current

knowledge on the molecular basis of antiretroviral drug resistance and the mechanisms leading to selection of drug-resistant HIV.

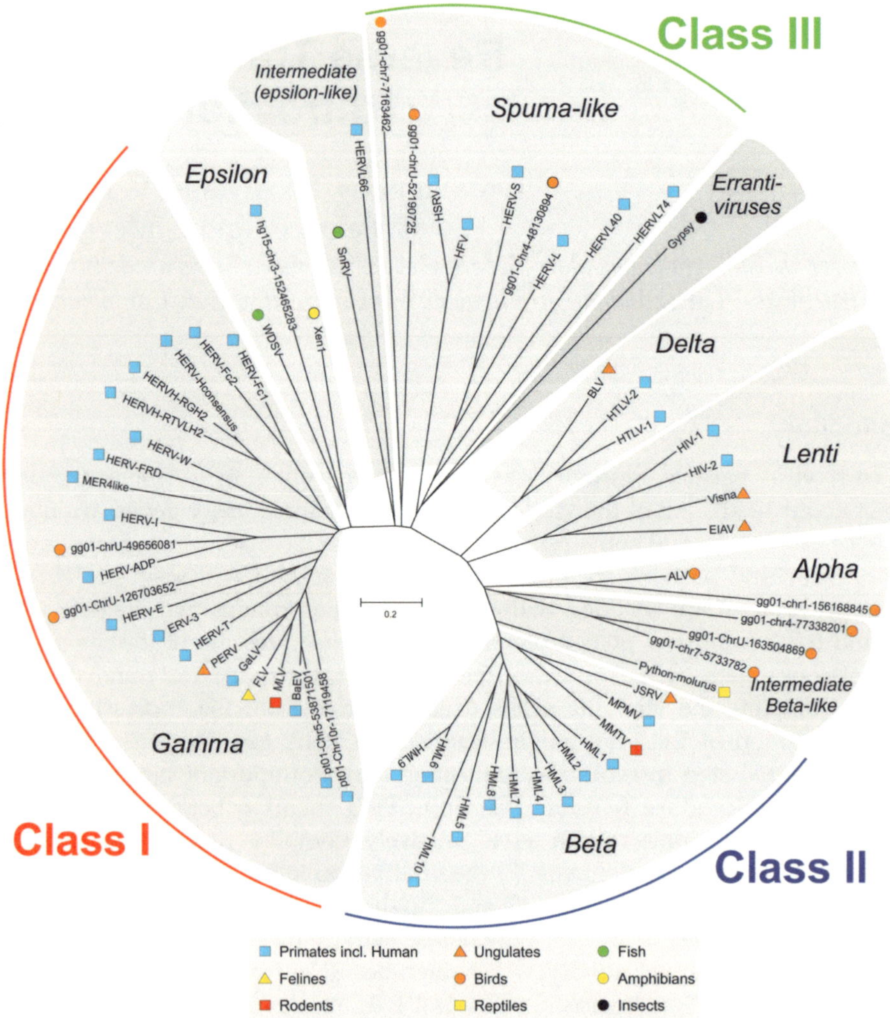

Fig. 1. Dendrogram representing phylogenetic relationships between retroviruses. The unrooted neighbour joining dendrogram is based on *pol* sequences of seven retroviral genera (alpha-, beta-, gamma-, delta-, epsilon-, lenti- and spuma-like retroviruses). Reproduced from Jern et al. (2005); originally published by BioMed Central.

2. The process of reverse transcription

An overview of the reverse transcription process is shown in Fig. 2. Reverse transcription initiates after binding of a cellular tRNA primer (in HIV-1, $tRNA^{Lys,3}$), to the primer binding site (PBS). The PBS is a sequence of 18 nucleotides, located downstream of the 5′-end of the genomic RNA. The viral RNA that serves as template for reverse transcription is flanked by repeat (R) sequences at its 5′ and 3′ termini. Upon annealing, the tRNA primer is extended up to the 5′ end of the genome, generating an intermediate which is known as the minus-strand strong-stop DNA ((-)ssDNA). Simultaneously, the RNase H activity of the RT degrades the RNA strand annealed to (-)ssDNA, and the (-)ssDNA is released to hybridize with the R sequence located at the 3′-end of the same RNA (intra-molecular jump) or with an R sequence located at a different viral genome (inter-molecular jump). This step is referred to as the first strand-transfer.

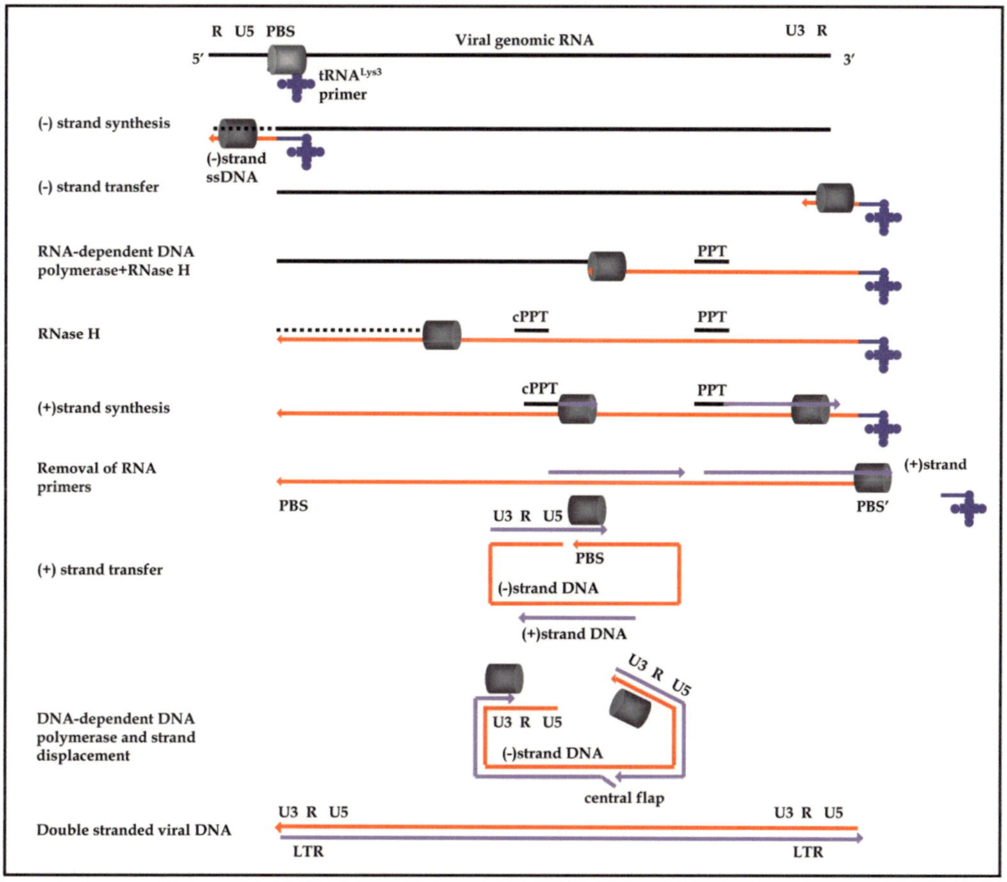

Fig. 2. Overview of the reverse transcription process.

After binding of the (-)ssDNA molecule to the R sequence, synthesis of the minus-strand DNA continues along the viral RNA together with simultaneous degradation of the template RNA. Polypurine tracts at the U3 region (3′-PPT) and in some retroviruses, at the centre of the genomic RNA (cPPT) resist degradation. These sequences serve as primers for synthesis of plus-strand DNA. Plus-strand DNA synthesis originating from the 3′-PPT continues to the 5′-end of the minus-strand until it reaches the 18th nucleotide in the tRNA where further synthesis is blocked by a methylated base. Priming from both PPTs involves discontinuous DNA synthesis that generates a 99-nucleotide DNA "flap" in the centre of the molecule. This product is referred to as plus strong-stop DNA ((+)ssDNA). The second strand transfer reaction involves the annealing of the (+)ssDNA to the 3′-end of the full-

length (-)strand DNA, through base pairing of the complementary PBS and PBS′ sequences. This strand transfer reaction is usually intra-molecular (Yu et al., 1998), and renders a circular intermediate.
The strand displacement activity of the RT is required to complete DNA synthesis and for the generation of a proviral DNA with duplicated long terminal repeats (LTR) at both ends. In the case of HIV-1 and other lentiviruses a "flap" appears in the centre of the DNA. This structure is eliminated by the activities of a cellular endonuclease that removes the "flap" and a ligase that joins the DNA ends to render the complete provirus that can eventually integrate in the host cell genome.

2.1 Role of the NC protein in reverse transcription

In most retroviruses, NC is a small nucleic-acid binding protein that derives from cleavage of the Gag polyprotein. In HIV-1, it has 55 amino acid residues and contains two conserved zinc fingers with the sequence $\mathbf{C}X_2\mathbf{C}X_4\mathbf{H}X_4\mathbf{C}$ (CCHC) connected by a short basic peptide linker. NC functions mainly as a nucleic acid chaperone (Levin et al., 2010), but it also contributes to packaging and dimerization of genomic RNAs, virus assembly, integration and reverse transcription.
NC influences almost every step in the reverse transcription process: (i) it facilitates annealing of the $tRNA^{Lys,3}$ to the viral genomic RNA; (ii) basic residues of NC bring the complementary tRNA and PBS sequences together, while its zinc fingers destabilize secondary structures in the 5′ LTR to prevent pausing of RT during reverse transcription; (iii) NC enhances minus strand transfer, by accelerating the annealing of 5′ repeat cDNA to the 3′ repeat sequence of the viral RNA genome; and (iv) NC increases RNase H activity, thereby enhancing cleavage of the donor template and promoting strand transfer by creating free cDNA available for interaction with the acceptor (Thomas & Gorelick, 2008). The ability of NC to destabilize secondary structures alleviates pausing and enhances RT processivity, leading to the generation of a greater proportion of full-length DNA products. NC is also important for removal of non-PPT RNAs, since it inhibits elongation of these primers without affecting extension of genuine polypurine tracts (Jacob & DeStefano, 2008).

2.2 Host and viral factors controlling reverse transcription

Interactions between RT and other viral proteins and/or cellular factors are likely to occur during early and late phases of viral replication. The formation of the reverse transcription complex involves packaging of tRNA in virions. This is possible because during assembly, Gag and Gag-Pol precursors interact with the aminoacyl-$tRNA^{Lys,3}$ synthetase (LysRS) which has bound $tRNA^{Lys,3}$ (reviewed in Abbink & Berkhout, 2008). RNA helicase A is a cellular protein that is able to rearrange RNA structures due to its unwinding activity on RNA secondary structures. RNA helicase A activity promotes viral reverse transcription by facilitating the accessibility of the RT to the viral RNA (Roy et al., 2006). Other cellular proteins such as HuR, AKAP149 and DNA topoisomerase I have been shown to interact with retroviral RTs (for a review, see Warren et al., 2009).
In addition, several factors have shown an influence on the integrity of the viral genome. Thus, in HIV-1, the accessory protein Vif (viral infectivity factor) promotes reverse transcription while increasing viral infectivity (Carr et al., 2008). In the absence of NC, Vif promotes annealing of $tRNA^{Lys,3}$, decreases pausing of the RT, destabilizes nucleic acid secondary structures, stimulates ssDNA synthesis and increases the efficiency of the first

strand transfer event during reverse transcription. Moreover, Vif is also an RNA chaperone. In the presence of NC, Vif inhibits NC-induced $tRNA^{Lys,3}$ annealing, RNA dimerization and reverse transcription initiation. Taken together, those results suggest that Vif could prevent premature initiation of reverse transcription (Henriet et al., 2007).

Through the expression of Vif, HIV-1 counteracts the antiviral effect of apolipoprotein B mRNA-editing, catalytic polypeptide enzymes (APOBEC3). APOBEC3 family members are cellular proteins with cytidine deaminase activity that have anti-HIV-1 activity (Sheehy et al., 2002; reviewed in Aguiar & Peterlin, 2008). APOBEC3F and APOBEC3G are encapsidated into budding virions. In the absence of Vif, APOBEC3F/G induce hypermutation of the HIV-1 genome. *In vitro* studies have also shown that in the presence of NC, APOBEC3G affects $tRNA^{Lys,3}$ annealing (Guo et al., 2007), and reduces strand transfer and integration (Mbisa et al., 2007).

2.3 RNase H activity and dynamics of RT/nucleic acid interactions

As mentioned earlier, retroviral RTs have an endonuclease activity that hydrolyzes the RNA strand in RNA/DNA hybrids to generate 5′-phosphate and 3′-hydroxyl ends. Retroviral RNase H has two major distinct modes of activity: (i) polymerase-dependent (DNA 3′-end-directed cleavage), and (ii) polymerase-independent (RNA 5′-end-directed cleavage). In addition, internal cleavage of RNA on RNA/DNA hybrids can also occur in the absence of 5′ or 3′ ends. The efficiency of this cleavage depends on the specific nucleotide sequence in the vicinity of the cleavage site (for a review, see Schultz & Champoux, 2008) (Fig. 3).

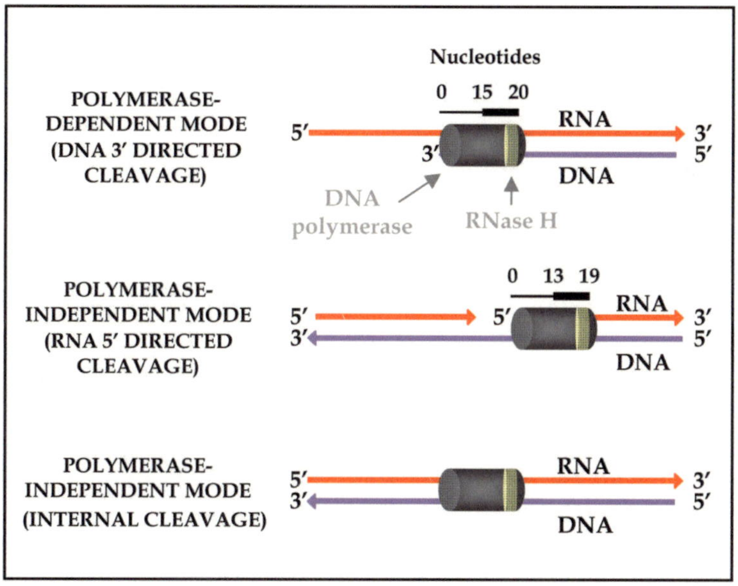

Fig. 3. Retroviral RT binding modes to RNA/DNA hybrids and effects on RNase H cleavage. The polymerase-dependent mode is characterized by the polymerase active site being in contact with the 3′ DNA primer terminus. The polymerase-independent mode depends on the position of 5′-end of RNA fragments relative to the polymerase active site. Nucleotides 15-20 and 13-19, numbered from the 3′-end of DNA and the 5′-end of the RNA, respectively, are those susceptible to RNase H cleavage in the proposed models.

In the polymerase-dependent mode, the polymerase active site of the RT locates at the 3′-end of DNA primer, while the RNase H domain is positioned 15-20 nucleotides away from the DNA primer terminus. In this situation, the RNase H makes primary cuts and then slides forward to make the secondary cuts 5-8 nucleotides from the 3′-end of DNA primer. These cleavages can occur during DNA synthesis and in the absence of dNTPs. Factors that decrease the rate of DNA polymerization result in an increased number of RNase H cuts, due to RT pausing. The distance from the recessed DNA 3′ and the nucleotide sequence in the vicinity of the cleavage site are important factors that contribute to the frequency of DNA 3′-end-directed cleavages (Basu et al., 2008; Schultz & Champoux, 2008).
Polymerase-independent cleavages depend on the precise position of the 5′-end of RNA fragments relative to the polymerase active site. In this mode, the polymerase domain of the RT binds the DNA strand in a site that is near the RNA 5′-end. The RNase H domain is positioned 13-19 nucleotides away from the 5′-end of the RNA. The distance from the recessed end, the nucleotide sequence in the vicinity of the cleavage site and the accessibility of the 5′-end (a gap of 2 or more bases is sufficient for such recognition) are important factors influencing RNA 5′-end-directed cleavages (Schultz & Champoux, 2008; Champoux & Schultz, 2009; Herschhorn & Hizi, 2010).
During reverse transcription, the polymerase-dependent mode is used during minus-strand DNA synthesis to cleave the RNA strand of the hybrid. However, the rate of DNA polymerization is about 10 times faster than the RNase H cleavage rate and therefore, insufficient for total RNA degradation and DNA release. Polymerase-independent RNase H activity is required to complete the process. Cleavages to generate the PPT primer are sequence-specific and can occur internally on RNA/DNA hybrids, without DNA synthesis. Polymerization-independent RNase H activity also appears to be important for removal of extended tRNA and PPT primers.
PPT primer removal could occur by an internal cleavage event at the RNA-DNA junction, or alternatively by an RNA 5′-end-directed cleavage after extension (Schultz & Champoux, 2008; Champoux & Schultz, 2009). However, molecular details underlying these events are largely unknown. Chemical probing, NMR spectroscopy and single-molecule fluorescence resonance energy transfer (FRET) have been recently used to explore molecular aspects involved in the communication between RT and the RNA/DNA hybrid (Liu et al., 2008; Abbondanzieri et al., 2008; reviewed in Fabris et al., 2009; Götte et al., 2010). These studies revealed that an important factor determining enzyme binding orientation is the backbone composition of nucleotides at the 5′-end of the primer. These nucleotides make specific contacts with RNase H primer grip residues, and thereby regulate the DNA polymerase activity of the RT (Abbondanzieri et al., 2008). These studies also showed that during reverse transcription, the RT could alternate binding modes (*i.e.* polymerase-dependent or independent) in the presence of PPT. The switching kinetics can be regulated. Thus, in the presence of dNTP, the polymerization binding mode predominates and flipping between both orientations decreases (Liu et al., 2008; reviewed in Götte et al., 2010).

2.4 Recombination and strand transfer

Recombination is the major source of genetic variability in retrovirus. Recombination can mediate the repair of defective retroviral genomes, increase viral diversity and accelerate the spread of beneficial mutations. In HIV-1, recombinant genetic forms derived from virus of different subtypes emerged in individuals infected with viruses of two or more different subtypes. Inter-subtype recombination allowed the generation of around 50 different well-characterized circulating recombinant forms (CRFs) (for an update, see http://www.hiv.lanl.gov/content/sequence/HIV/CRFs/CRFs.html).

Two relevant properties of retroviral reverse transcription contribute to the high frequency of recombination. First, retroviral genomic RNAs are encapsidated in pairs. Second, the replication machinery is prone to recombination, since template switching is required to complete proviral DNA synthesis (Yu et al, 1998; Ramírez et al., 2008; Onafuwa-Nuga & Telesnitsky, 2009). Recent studies have shown that the HIV-1 RT can stabilize short (2-nucleotide) duplexes of 3'-overhangs of the primer strand that are annealed to complementary dinucleotide tails of DNA or RNA template strands. This RT "clamping" activity that anneals RNA and DNA strands could have a role in strand transfer (Oz-Gleenberg et al., 2011).

3. The crystal structures of retroviral RTs

Although all retroviral RTs share similar activities and derive from expression of the viral *pol* gene, they differ in size and subunit composition (Herschhorn & Hizi, 2010). Lentiviral RTs are asymmetric heterodimeric enzymes, as shown for HIV-1 and equine infectious anemia virus (with subunits of 66 and 51 kDa), feline immunodeficiency virus RTs (67 and 54 kDa) and HIV-2 RT (68 and 55 kDa). Viral RTs arise from processing of the Gag-Pol precursor and contain DNA polymerase and RNase H domains in the large subunit and the DNA polymerase domain alone in the smaller subunit. The function of the small subunit is mainly structural. The bovine immunodeficiency virus RT has been expressed in bacteria as a 64/51-kDa heterodimer. A similar structure is shared by the human T cell lymphotropic virus type I RT that contains subunits of 62 and 49 kDa. The RTs of alpharetroviruses (*e.g.* avian sarcoma leukaemia virus) are larger heterodimers composed of subunits of 94 and 62 kDa, where the 94-kDa subunit also contains the viral integrase protein (Hizi & Joklik, 1977). On the other hand, the RT of the murine leukaemia virus (MLV) (a gammaretrovirus) is a monomer of 75 kDa, containing both DNA polymerase and RNase H domains. Less-studied recombinant RTs from mouse mammary tumour virus (66 kDa), bovine leukaemia virus (64-80 kDa) and prototype foamy virus (80 kDa) appear to be active as monomers or homodimers, although their subunit composition in the virion is unknown.

Our current knowledge on the structure of retroviral RTs is essentially based on many crystal structures of HIV-1 RT alone or in complex with nucleic acid or inhibitors, as well as additional information on a few crystal structures of HIV-2 RT and MLV RT. These studies have revealed the structure of the two catalytic domains of the RTs (DNA polymerase and RNase H), which are separated by a connection subdomain. As found in other DNA polymerases, RTs have a structure that resembles a right hand (Fig. 4), with three subdomains in the DNA polymerase domain, designated as fingers, palm and thumb.

3.1 HIV-1 RT

HIV-1 RT is a heterodimer composed of two subunits known as p66 (560 amino acids) and p51 (440 amino acids). The DNA polymerase active site residues (Asp110, Asp185 and Asp186) are located in the palm subdomain of p66 (Fig. 4). In p66, the palm and connection subdomains consist of five stranded β sheets with two α helices on one side, while the thumb subdomain is composed of a bundle of four helices (Kohlstaedt et al., 1992; Jacobo

Molina et al., 1993). The fingers subdomain contains a mixed β sheet and three α helices. The RNase H domain consists of five β sheets flanked by four α helices (Fig. 4). The p66 and p51 subunits have similar folds but p51 is more tightly packaged. Fingers, palm, thumb and connection subdomains fold similarly in both subunits, but their spatial organization changes due to the different positioning of the fingers, thumb and palm subdomains. Both HIV-1 RT subunits form a large cleft, where the thumb subdomain of p51 and the connection subdomains of p66 and p51 form the "floor", and fingers, palm and thumb subdomains of p66 provide lateral and apical interactions with the nucleic acid substrate (Jacobo-Molina et al., 1993). Active site residues in p66 are exposed to the cleft, but they are buried in the 51-kDa subunit (Rodgers et al., 1995).

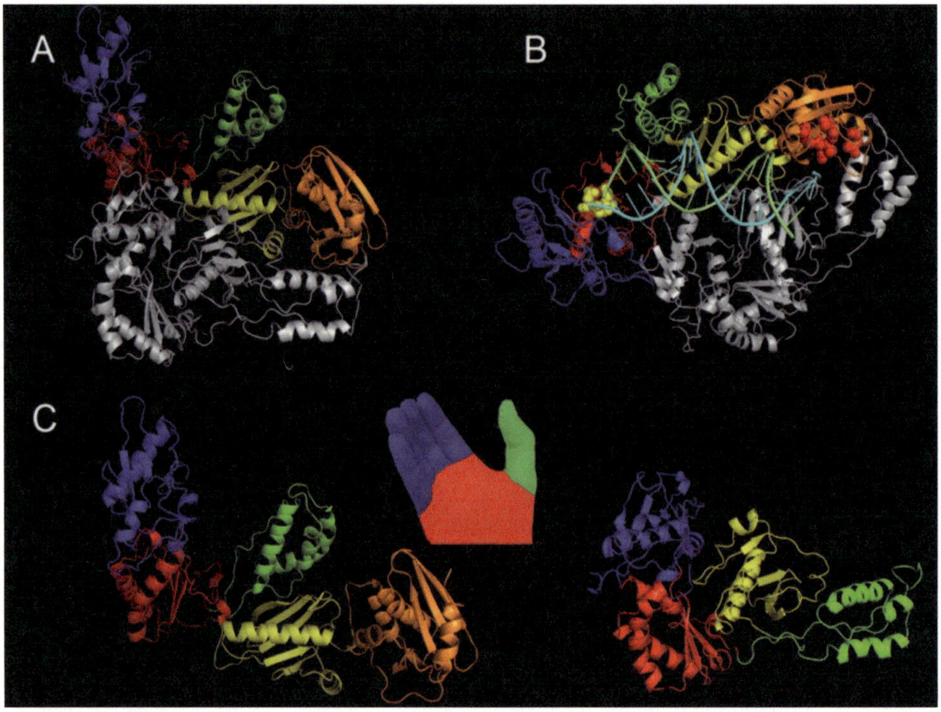

Fig. 4. Crystal structure of HIV-1 RT. (A) Ribbon representation of the structure of HIV-1 RT showing the fingers, palm and thumb subdomains of p66 in blue, red and green, respectively, the connection subdomain in yellow, the RNAse H domain in orange, and p51 in grey. (B) Ribbon representation of HIV-1 RT bound to a double stranded DNA. The template is shown in cyan and the primer in pale green. Catalytic Asp residues in the DNA polymerase domain are shown as yellow spheres and RNase H catalytic residues (Asp443, Glu478, Asp498 and Asp549) are represented as red spheres. (C) Individual structures of p66 (left) and p51 (right). Color codes are the same as in panels (A) and (B). Shown structures were all obtained with the PyMol molecular viewer (http://www.pymol.org) and Protein Data Bank coordinates 2HMI (Ding et al., 1998).

The structure of the binary complex of HIV-1 RT and double-stranded DNA (Jacobo-Molina et al., 1993; Ding et al., 1998) showed that the nucleic acid binding cleft can accommodate 17 nucleotides between the active sites of the DNA polymerase and the RNase H. Major interactions between the RT and the template-primer are indicated in Table 1. The comparison of crystal structures of binary complexes with those obtained with unliganded RTs showed conformational changes involving the movement of the p66 thumb subdomain away from the fingers subdomain (Jacobo-Molina et al., 1993, Rodgers et al., 1995). In addition, the bound DNA adopts an A-type conformation in the vicinity of the DNA polymerase active site, but a B-like conformation near the RNase H domain. These changes in orientation involve a 40° bend of the DNA/DNA complex, near α-helix H in the thumb subdomain of p66 (Jacobo-Molina et al., 1993).

Motif	RT subdomain	Residues involved
Primer grip	p66 palm (β12-β13)	227-235
Helix clamp	p66 thumb (αH-αI)	255-268 (αH)/278-286 (αI)
RNase H primer grip	p66 connection, p51 connection, p66 RNase H	358-361 (p66 connection), 395-396 (p51 connection), 473-476, 501, 505 (p66 RNase H)
Template grip	p66 fingers, p66 palm (β4, αB, β5, β8-αE)	73-77 (β4), 78-83 (αE), 86-90 (β5), 141-174 (β8-αE)

Table 1. HIV-1 RT residues and subdomains interacting with nucleic acid in the binary complex (Ding et al., 1998).

The crystal structure of a binary complex of HIV-1 RT and an RNA/DNA hybrid revealed only small differences in comparison with the HIV-1 RT/double-stranded DNA complex (Sarafianos et al., 2001). Thus, the distance between the DNA polymerase and RNase H active sites is slightly larger (18 nucleotides) in the RNA/DNA complex, with most of the contacts between RT and template-primer being maintained. However, the RNA/DNA hybrid makes more contacts with the p66 subunit of the RT at α-helix I (thumb subdomain), β-sheet 5 (palm subdomain) and with residues of the RNase H domain (Sarafianos et al., 2001; Tuske et al., 2004). Also, a number of contacts between the p51 subunit and the RNA template were not detected in the structure having the DNA/DNA substrate (Sarafianos et al., 2001). Nucleic acids have similar A-like/B-like conformations in complexes containing DNA/DNA or RNA/DNA. However, the transition from the A- to the B-forms generates a wider minor groove in the RNA/DNA complex, which together with additional contacts between the RNase H primer grip and the RNA template seem to be determinant for the RNase H catalytic activity.

An important milestone towards understanding the mechanisms and nucleotide specificity in DNA polymerization by retroviral RTs was the determination of the crystal structure of a ternary complex of HIV-1 RT bound to double-stranded DNA and an incoming dNTP (Huang et al., 1998). Nucleotide binding facilitates transition from an "open" conformation of the fingers subdomain in p66 (as observed in the structure of RT/DNA binary complexes) to a "closed" conformation where the β3-β4 hairpin loop in the fingers subdomain moves towards the p66 palm subdomain (see review by Sarafianos et al., 2009). This movement in the fingers subdomain is known to be the rate-limiting step in the polymerization reaction (Sarafianos et al., 2009), and brings amino acid residues Lys65 and Arg72 into close proximity with the incoming nucleotide (Tuske et al., 2004). Apart from these two residues, other important interactions in the nucleotide binding site are those established between the incoming dNTP and RT residues Asp113-Ala114-Tyr115-Phe116 and Gln151, as well as with the two divalent cations (probably Mg^{2+}); and between RT residues Tyr183 and Met184 and the DNA primer terminus (Huang et al., 1998). Binding of the incoming dNTP also produces a movement of the YMDD motif (including catalytic residues Asp185 and Asp186) that allows proper coordination of the catalytic aspartates with the metal cofactors, and triggers the nucleophilic attack of the 3′OH of the primer terminus on the α phosphorous of the incoming dNTP (Huang et al., 1998; Mendieta et al., 2008). This polymerization event renders an elongated DNA primer and a pyrophosphate molecule that is released in the reaction. Structural data suggest that the YMDD motif acts as a "springboard" supplying some of the energy required for translocation (Sarafianos et al., 2002).

3.2 HIV-2 RT

HIV-2 RT shares around 60% sequence identity with HIV-1 RT. Despite conservation of the cleavage site at the N-terminus of the RNase H domain, the size of the small HIV-2 RT subunit is uncertain (for a review, see Herschhorn & Hizi, 2010). There is only one crystal structure of HIV-2 RT available, and this was obtained as an unliganded form using the complete p68 subunit (559 residues) bound to a smaller subunit that contained only 427 residues due to degradation of the p68 polypeptide by bacterial proteases (Ren et al., 2002). The crystal structure of unliganded HIV-2 RT is similar to that of the HIV-1 RT, but the p68 thumb subdomain is rotated by 8° relative to the unliganded HIV-1 RT p66 subunit. HIV-2 RT heterodimers are also more stable than HIV-1 RT heterodimers (Divita et al., 1995).

3.3 MLV RT

Although MLV RT is quite different from HIV-1 and HIV-2 RTs (MLV RT is a monomer), the basic structure is the same: a right hand conformation with fingers, palm, thumb and connection subdomains and a C-terminal RNase H domain (Das & Georgiadis, 2004; Lim et al., 2006). Structural analysis revealed that HIV-1 and MLV RTs are rather different at their thumb and connection subdomains, while their fingers and palm subdomains show significant homology (for a review, see Coté & Roth, 2008). MLV RT is 111 amino acids longer than the p66 subunit of HIV-1 RT. Major differences are found at the N-terminus which is about 40 amino acids longer in MLV RT, and between the connection subdomain and the RNase H domain that contains 32 extra residues in the MLV RT. In the RNase H domain of this enzyme, there is a C-helix motif followed by a loop region of 11 amino acids, absent from HIV-1 RT. This structure is present in *Escherichia coli* RNase H.

4. The copying fidelity of RTs

The intrinsic fidelity of RTs has a major role in retroviral variability (for a recent review, see Menéndez-Arias, 2009), although cellular polymerases (*e.g.* replicative eukaryotic DNA polymerases α/β/δ/ε and RNA polymerase II) may also modulate the mutation rate in retroviruses. Other viral and host factors influencing the retroviral mutation rate include the cellular transcriptional machinery, physiological fluctuations of dNTP pools and asymmetric error repair. Several retroviruses (*e.g.* feline immunodeficiency virus, mouse mammary tumour virus, etc…) encode a dUTP pyrophosphatase (dUTPase) that prevents the incorporation of uracil into the viral genome. This protein is not present in HIV-1, but this virus contains a protein (Vpr) that allows for the encapsidation of isoforms of uracil DNA glycosylase. This cellular enzyme could contribute to reducing uracil content in the nascent viral DNA. In HIV, the virally encoded Vif protein overcomes the activity of APOBEC proteins, thereby contributing to maintain a non-lethal level of G→A mutations.

The intrinsic fidelity of purified retroviral RTs has been analyzed *in vitro* by using enzymatic (gel-based) or genetic assays (for a review, see Menéndez-Arias, 2002). Gel-based assays are based on the determination of kinetic parameters for the incorporation of correct and incorrect nucleotides on specific template-primers, and provide an estimate of the nucleotide selectivity of the DNA polymerase. The relevant kinetic parameters are the k_{pol} (nucleotide incorporation rate constant) and the K_d (equilibrium dissociation constant for dNTP) (Fig. 5). Their determination should be done under pre-steady-state conditions to avoid the contribution of the template-primer dissociation rate (Kellinger & Johnson, 2010). Since the fixation of a mutation involves nucleotide misincorporation followed by extension of the mismatched primer, similar assays should be carried out with template-primers having a mismatch at the 3′-end of the DNA primer, in order to have a better estimate of the intrinsic fidelity of RTs. These assays have demonstrated that HIV-1 RT, MLV RT and RTs of other retroviruses are one to three orders of magnitude faster in extending mispaired template-primers than the dissociation of the retroviral RT from DNA. Reported mispair extension efficiencies for HIV-1 and MLV RTs are usually within the range of 10^{-2} to 10^{-4}, while misinsertion ratios range from 10^{-3} to 10^{-6} (Menéndez-Arias, 2002; Matamoros et al., 2008; Álvarez et al., 2009).

$$T/P_n + dNTP \underset{}{\overset{K_d}{\rightleftharpoons}} T/P_n\,dNTP \underset{}{\overset{k_{pol}}{\rightleftharpoons}} T/P_{n+1}\,PP_i \xrightarrow{\text{fast}} T/P_{n+1} + PP_i$$

$$k_{obs} = \frac{k_{pol} \times [dNTP]}{K_d + [dNTP]}$$

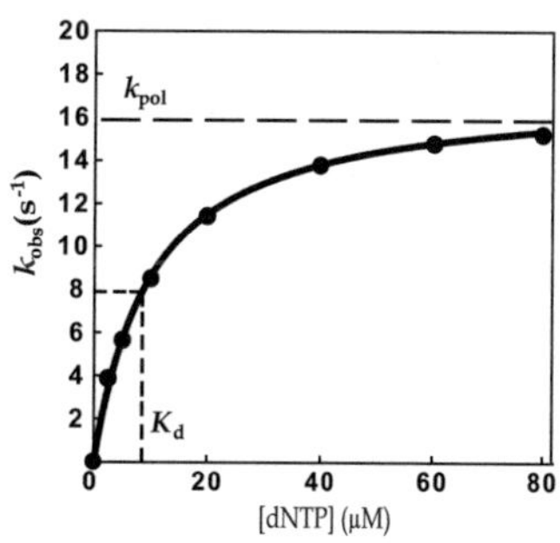

Fig. 5. Nucleotide incorporation reaction and example of the determination of kinetic parameters k_{pol} and K_d under pre-steady-state conditions. T/P_n represents the template-primer with *n* being the nucleotide length, and T/P_{n+1} represents the same template-primer after the incorporation of one nucleotide. PPi stands for pyrophosphate.

Genetic assays are based on the expression of reporter genes. The most popular assay is probably the one based on the use as substrate of a gapped doubled-stranded M13mp2 DNA duplex that contains the *lacZα* gene (Bebenek & Kunkel, 1995). A gap-filling reaction is carried out in the presence of RT and dNTPs, and mutants are identified after transformation of appropriate bacteria by the white/blue color of M13 plaques revealed using X-Gal indicator plates. Nucleotide sequence analysis of the M13 DNA obtained from white and pale blue plaques allows for the identification of base substitutions, insertions, deletions, etc… These assays have shown that the HIV-1 RT is 10 to 20 times less faithful than the MLV and avian myeloblastosis virus RTs (Roberts et al, 1989). Since the crystal structure of HIV-1 RT is known and this enzyme is an important target of antiretroviral therapy, there have been many studies on the effects of amino acid substitutions on the copying fidelity of this enzyme. A summary is presented in Table 2. Major structural determinants of the accuracy of DNA synthesis by the HIV-1 RT involve dNTP binding residues, amino acids that interact with the template-primer or the primer strand, minor groove binding track residues and amino acids located at the RNase H primer grip.

RT location	Residue	Amino acid substitution	Effect on fidelity		References
			Enzymatic assays	Genetic assays	
Nucleotide binding site residues	Lys65	K65R	▲	▲ (8.1)	1-3
		K65A	▲	ND	1
	Arg72	R72A	▼/▲	▲ (1.6)	4
	Ala114	A114S	≈	≈	5
		A114G	≈	≈	5
	Tyr115	Y115A	▼	▼ (4.0)	2, 6-8
		Y115F/V	▼	≈	7-10
		Y115L/I/N	▼	ND	8
		Y115M/H/G	▼	ND	8
		Y115C/S/W	▼	ND	7, 8, 10
	Gln151	Q151M	≈	▲ (1.2)	11, 12
		Q151N	▲	▲ (13.1)	12-14
	Phe160	F160Y	≈	ND	15
		F160W	≈	ND	15
	Met184	M184I	▲	▲ (4.0)	16-18
		M184A	▼	ND	6, 19
		M184V	▲/▼	≈	6, 17, 20-22
		M184L	▲	ND	6, 23
Located in the RT palm subdomain, close to the dNTP binding site	Val148	V148I	ND	▲ (8.7)	24
	Tyr183	Y183F	▲	▼ (1.6)	6, 23
Residues that interact with the template strand	Trp24	W24G	▲	ND	25
	Phe61	F61A	ND	▲ (11.7)	26
		F61G	≈	ND	25
	Leu74	L74V	▲	▲ (1.7-3.5)	2, 3, 6, 27
	Val75	V75A	▼	▼ (1.4)	28
		V75F	▲	▲ (1.8)	28
		V75I	▲	▲ (1.8-3.0)	28, 29
	Asp76	D76V	▲	▲ (8.8)	2, 30, 31
	Arg78	R78A	ND	▲ (8.9)	2, 30
	Glu89	E89G	▼/▲	▲ (1.4-2.0)	2, 6, 20, 21
		E89K	ND	▲ (1.2)	32
		E89S	ND	▲ (1.6)	32
		E89V	ND	▲ (1.3)	32
Residues that interact with the primer strand (β2- β3 hairpin)	Phe227	F227A	▲	ND	33
	Trp229	W229A	▲	ND	33
	Met230	M230L	ND	▼	34
		M230I	▼	▼	10, 34
	Gly231	G231A	▼	ND	35
	Tyr232	Y232A	▼	ND	35

RT location	Residue	Amino acid substitution	Effect on fidelity		References
			Enzymatic assays	Genetic assays	
Minor groove binding track residues	Gln258	Q258A	**ND**	▼ (2.0)	36
	Gly262	G262A	**ND**	▼ (4.1)	36, 37
	Trp266	W266A	**ND**	▼ (3.0)	36, 37
	Gln269	Q269A	**ND**	▼ (2.6)	36
α-Helices H and I (additional thumb subdomain residues)	Asp256	D256A	**ND**	▼ (1.2)	36
	Lys259	K259A	**ND**	▼ (1.5)	36
	Leu260	L260A	**ND**	▼ (1.2)	36
	Lys263	K263A	**ND**	▼ (1.5)	36
	Arg277	R277A	≈	▲ (1.1)	38
	Gln278	Q278A	≈	▼ (1.2)	38
	Leu279	L279A	≈	▲ (1.1)	38
	Cys280	C280A	≈	▼ (1.9)	38
	Lys281	K281A	≈	▲ (1.1)	38
	Leu282	L282A	≈	▲ (1.3)	38
	Arg284	R284A	≈	▼ (1.1)	38
	Gly285	G285A	≈	≈	38
	Lys287	K287A	≈	▲ (1.3)	38

Symbols: ▼ and ▲ indicate a decrease or an increase in RT's accuracy, respectively, ≈ indicates that the fidelity of the enzyme is not affected by the mutation. Numbers between parentheses represent the fold-change in mutant frequency as determined with the M13mp2 *lacZα* forward mutation assay. ND, not determined. References: (1) Garforth et al., 2010; (2) Mansky et al., 2003; (3) Shah et al., 2000; (4) Lewis et al., 1999; (5) Cases-González & Menéndez-Arias, 2005; (6) Jonckheere et al., 2000; (7) Martín-Hernández et al., 1996; (8) Martín-Hernández et al., 1997; (9) Boyer & Hughes, 2000; (10) Gutiérrez-Rivas & Menéndez-Arias, 2001; (11) Rezende et al., 1998a; (12) Weiss et al., 2002; (13) Weiss et al., 2000; (14) Jamburuthugoda et al., 2005; (15) Gutiérrez-Rivas et al., 1999; (16) Rezende et al., 1998b; (17) Hsu et al., 1997; (18) Oude Essink et al., 1997; (19) Pandey et al., 1996; (20) Hamburg et al., 1998; (21) Drosopoulos & Prasad, 1998; (22) Wainberg et al., 1996; (23) Bakhanashvili et al., 1996; (24) Weiss et al., 2004; (25) Agopian et al., 2007; (26) Fisher & Prasad, 2002; (27) Rubinek et al., 1997; (28) Matamoros et al., 2008; (29) Álvarez et al., 2009; (30) Kim et al., 1998; (31) Kim et al., 1999; (32) Hamburg et al., 2006; (33) Wisniewski et al., 1999; (34) Cases-González & Menéndez-Arias, 2004; (35) Wöhrl et al., 1997; (36) Beard et al., 1994; (37) Bebenek et al., 1995; (38) Beard et al., 1996.

Table 2. Effect of amino acid substitutions on the copying fidelity of HIV-1 RT.

5. HIV-1 RT as a drug target

Despite the contribution of other RTs to our general understanding of their biochemistry and role in retroviral replication, HIV-1 RT has been the most widely studied enzyme due to its relevance as a target for the development of antiretroviral drugs. Around half of the currently licensed drugs for treatment of HIV-1 infection are RT inhibitors. These drugs can be classified into nucleoside RT inhibitors (NRTIs) (Fig. 6) and non-nucleoside RT inhibitors (NNRTIs) (Fig. 7).

5.1 Inhibitors of the DNA polymerase activity of HIV-1 RT
5.1.1 Nucleoside RT inhibitors (NRTIs)
Currently, there are seven NRTIs approved for treatment of HIV-1-infected patients, as well as a nucleotide analogue inhibitor, tenofovir disoproxil fumarate, which is a precursor of an acyclic nucleoside phosphonate known as tenofovir (Fig. 6). Newly developed NRTIs are currently at different stages of drug development (for recent reviews, see Jochmans, 2008; Menéndez-Arias, 2008; Cahn & Wainberg, 2010).

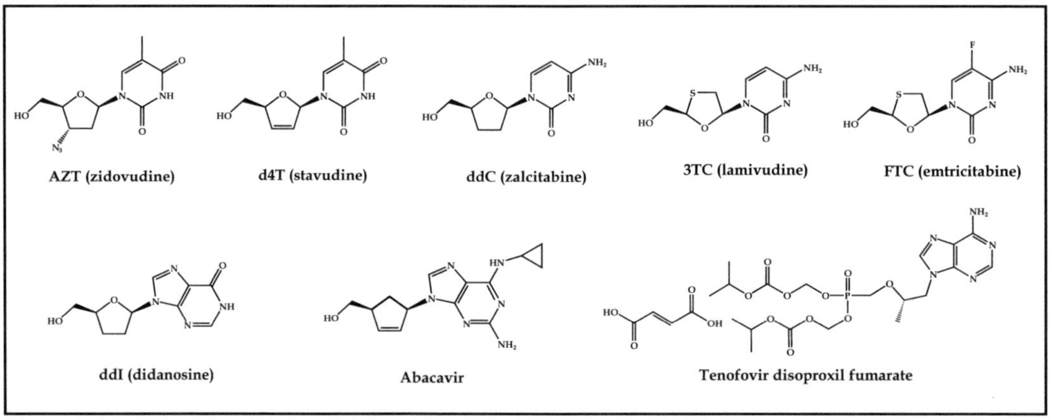

Fig. 6. Chemical structures of approved NRTIs: β-D-(+)-3′-azido-3′-deoxythymidine (zidovudine, AZT), β-D-(+)-2′,3′-didehydro-2′,3′dideoxythymidine (stavudine, d4T), β-D-(+)-2′,3′-dideoxyinosine (didanosine, ddI), β-D-(+)-2′,3′-dideoxycytidine (zalcitabine, ddC), β-L-(-)-2′,3′-dideoxy-3′-thiacytidine, (lamivudine, 3TC), (-)-(1S,4R)-4-[2-amino-6-(cyclo-propylamino)-9H-purin-9-yl]-2-cyclopentene-1-methanol (abacavir), β-L-(-)-2′,3′-dideoxy-5-fluoro-3′-thiacytidine (emtricitabine, FTC), and R-9-(2-phosphonomethoxy-propyl)adenine disoproxil fumarate (tenofovir disoproxil fumarate).

NRTIs are prodrugs that inside the cell will be phosphorylated by cellular kinases to their triphosphate forms. The resulting triphosphate derivatives are used as substrates by HIV-1 RT and incorporated at the 3′-end of the elongating DNA primer. Once incorporated, NRTIs act as chain terminators, blocking further DNA synthesis since these inhibitors lack the catalytically essential 3′OH group in the ribose ring. The therapeutic efficacy of NRTIs is determined by the efficiency of the activation process by cellular kinases (for a review, see Bazzoli et al., 2010). The long-term use of those drugs has been associated with a number of clinically relevant toxicities such as hyperlactatemia and lactic acidosis, lipoatrophy, etc. (Nolan & Mallal, 2004; Hammond et al., 2010). Some of those adverse effects appear to be related to the low specificity of the NRTIs, which do not markedly discriminate between RTs from different origins (HIV-1, HIV-2, SIV, MLV, etc) or cellular DNA polymerases. Most of these toxic effects are related to the inhibition of mitochondrial DNA polymerase γ (reviewed in Kohler & Lewis, 2007).

5.1.2 Non-nucleoside RT inhibitors (NNRTIs)
There are five NNRTIs that are currently approved for treating HIV-1 infections: nevirapine, delavirdine, efavirenz, etravirine and rilpivirine (Fig. 7), and others are currently in clinical trials (for a recent review, see Jochmans, 2008). Unlike NRTIs, these inhibitors do not need

intracellular metabolic activation to inhibit the viral replication. The interaction of these compounds with the RT induces conformational changes that impact the catalytic activities of the enzyme (Sluis-Cremer et al., 2004).

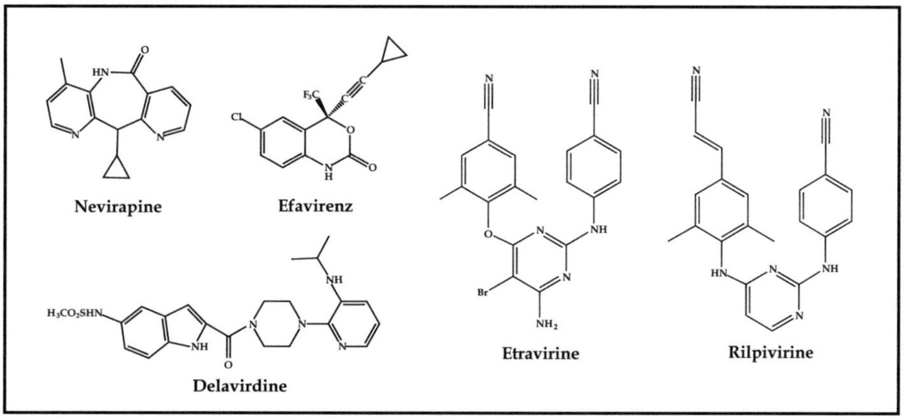

Fig. 7. Chemical structures of approved NNRTIs.

NNRTIs inhibit RT through binding to a hydrophobic pocket, located in the palm subdomain of the p66 subunit, at a distance of around 10 Å from the DNA polymerase catalytic site. The hydrophobic pocket is lined by aromatic residues Tyr181, Tyr188, Phe227, Trp229 and Tyr232, hydrophobic amino acids Pro59, Leu100, Val106, Val179 Leu234, and Pro236, and hydrophilic residues Lys101, Lys103, Ser105, Asp132 and Glu224, all of them in p66. In addition, two residues in p51 (Ile135 and Glu138) contribute to NNRTI binding. In the crystal structures of unliganded RT, there is no NNRTI binding pocket, but this pocket is formed when the inhibitor binds to the RT (Das et al., 2005). These drugs act as non-competitive inhibitors, binding to an allosteric site and interfering with dNTP incorporation, probably by altering the conformation of residues in the vicinity of the active site (Xia et al., 2007), rather than having a direct effect on phosphodiester bond formation (Spence et al., 1995).

5.2 Molecular mechanisms of HIV-1 RT resistance

Currently, most HIV-infected patients are treated with so-called "highly active antiretroviral therapy" (HAART), which consists of combinations of three or more inhibitors usually acting on two or more targets (*e.g.* RT DNA polymerase, NNRTI binding pocket, viral protease, etc.). One of the most successful combinations is made of three RT inhibitors: tenofovir, emtricitabine and efavirenz (see Figs. 6 and 7 for chemical structures). HAART can efficiently block viral replication, but modest levels of replication can lead to development of drug resistance. Although drug-resistant variants may have an overall rate of replication lower than the wild-type viruses in the absence of drugs; compensatory mutations may emerge to improve the viral replication capacity of these viruses (for reviews, see Menéndez-Arias et al., 2003; Martinez-Picado & Martínez, 2008).

5.2.1 Resistance to NRTIs

Zidovudine (AZT) was the first drug approved by the U.S. Food and Drug Administration (FDA), in 1987. Resistance to AZT was soon detected in patients under monotherapy for 6 months or longer (Larder et al., 1989a,b). The first AZT resistance mutations identified were M41L, D67N, K70R, L210W, T215F/Y and K219Q (Larder and Kemp, 1989). After the incorporation of new drugs into anti-HIV therapies, such as zalcitabine (ddC), didanosine (ddI) or stavudine (d4T), many other resistance mutations were identified. Interestingly, AZT resistance mutations were also found in patients under d4T therapy. These mutations were called "thymidine analogue resistance mutations" (TAMs). TAMs reside primarily in the palm and fingers subdomain of the RT, relatively far away from dNTP binding site. However, several NRTIs resistance mutations affect residues located at the nucleotide binding site (*e.g.* K65R, Q151M, M184V, etc.) or at residues that interact with the 5′ single-stranded template overhang (*e.g.* L74V, V75I, V75T, etc) (Huang et al., 1998).

HIV-1 becomes resistant to NRTIs by two different mechanisms: (i) by increasing discrimination against the triphosphate forms of the drug, or (ii) by increasing the RT's ability to remove the NRTIs from blocked DNA primers, through phosphorolysis mediated by ATP or pyrophosphate (PPi). These two mechanisms are not mutually exclusive.

i. Resistance by NRTI discrimination during DNA polymerization

Mutations that confer resistance through this mechanism reduce the incorporation of the NRTI-triphosphate while the RT retains the ability to incorporate natural dNTPs. In these cases, resistance is usually associated with a decrease of the catalytic efficiency (k_{pol}/K_d) for NRTI-triphosphate incorporation, through the loss of affinity for the inhibitor (increase of its K_d) and/or by a reduction in the NRTI incorporation rate (reduced k_{pol}). A number of single amino acid substitutions found *in vivo* were associated with this mechanism (Table 3). A representative example is M184V/I, which confers high-level resistance to lamivudine (3TC) and emtricitabine (FTC). Met184 is within the highly conserved YXDD motif, and its substitution to Val or Ile causes a steric hindrance between the side-chain of these residues and the sulfur atom present in the ribose ring of 3TC and FTC (Sarafianos et al., 1999; Kellinger & Johnson, 2010).

Combination therapies can select for mutational patterns that confer multidrug resistance. Thus, NRTI-resistant viruses containing amino acid changes A62V, V75I, F77L, F116Y and Q151M were initially observed in virus isolated from patients receiving AZT and ddI (Shirasaka et al., 1995). These mutants exhibited high-level resistance to AZT, ddI and d4T, and low-level resistance to abacavir, 3TC, FTC and tenofovir in phenotypic assays. This multidrug resistance pattern is known as the "Q151M pathway". Gln151 interacts with the ribose moiety and the nitrogen base of the incoming dNTP (Huang et al., 1998). Q151M and the accompanying mutations affect the hydrogen bonding network between the nucleotide deoxyribose and the RT, while increasing the relevance of the interaction between the enzyme and the 3′OH of the nucleotide (Deval et al., 2002). This allows the mutant RT to better discriminate between normal dNTPs (with 3′-OH) and triphosphate derivatives of NRTIs (without 3′-OH).

ii. Excision-mediated resistance.

The NRTI excision reaction is one of the most important pathways towards the acquisition of resistance to antiretroviral drugs. Early biochemical studies revealed that nucleotide discrimination was not impaired in AZT-resistant HIV-1 RTs (*e.g.* in the quadruple mutant D67N/K70R/T215F/K219Q) (Carroll et al., 1994; Krebs et al., 1997). However, in the presence of a PPi donor, AZT-resistant RTs were able to remove the inhibitor from the 3′-end of the primer, thereby allowing DNA synthesis to proceed through phosphorolysis

Mutation	Subdomain	Resistance	Mechanism	Comments	Ref.
K65R	fingers	ddA, 3TC, FTC, tenofovir, ddI, abacavir	k_{pol}	Suppresses AZT resistance.	1-6
		ddC	k_{pol}-K_d		
K70E	fingers	Tenofovir	k_{pol}	Mixed mechanism of resistance: discrimination and excision.	6, 7
L74V	fingers	Abacavir, ddI	k_{pol}-K_d	Impairs viral replication. Antagonizes the effect of TAMs on AZT resistance.	2, 8, 9
V75I	fingers	acyclovir	K_d	Accessory mutation of the Q151 complex. Antagonizes the effect of TAMs on AZT resistance.	10-12
V75T	fingers	d4T	K_d	Mixed mechanism of resistance: discrimination and excision.	1, 13, 14
Q151M	palm	Multidrug-resistance	k_{pol}	Associated with 4 mutations: A62V, V75I, F77L and F116Y.	3, 15-18
M184V	palm	3TC, FTC, Abacavir	k_{pol}-K_d	It can suppress AZT resistance.	2, 3, 19, 20

References: (1) Selmi et al., 2001; (2) Deval et al., 2004; (3) Deval et al., 2005; (4) Feng et al., 2006; (5) White et al., 2006; (6) Sluis-Cremer et al., 2007; (7) Kagan et al., 2007; (8) Miranda et al., 2005; (9) Frankel et al., 2005; (10) McMahon et al., 2008; (11) Matamoros et al., 2009; (12) Tchesnokov et al., 2009; (13) Petropoulos et al., 2000; (14) Lennerstrand et al., 2001; (15) Kaushik et al., 2000; (16) Deval et al., 2002; (17) Ray et al., 2002; (18) Frangeul et al., 2008; (19) Sarafianos et al., 1999; (20) Kellinger & Johnson, 2010. For additional references, see Menéndez-Arias, 2010. Acyclovir is a guanosine nucleoside analogue that inhibits herpes simplex virus replication. In patients co-infected with herpes simplex virus, it can inhibit HIV replication. Phosphorylated acyclovir inhibits HIV-1 RT, by terminating DNA chain elongation (Lisco et al., 2008).

Table 3. NRTI resistance mutations which increase the discrimination capacity.

mediated by ATP or PPi (Arion et al., 1998; Meyer et al., 1999; reviewed in Menéndez-Arias, 2008, 2010). The excision reaction involves a nucleophilic attack of the hydroxyl group substituent at the γ-phosphorous of ATP (the PPi donor) on the terminal phosphodiester bond of the blocked DNA primer (Matamoros et al., 2005).

The efficiency of the excision reaction is influenced by several factors such as the nature of the template strand, the sequence context in which chain termination occurs, the Mg^{2+} concentration, or the specific nucleoside analogue that blocks the 3′ end of the primer. Thymidine analogues (AZT, d4T and ddT) and tenofovir are the best substrates of the reaction, while cytidine analogues (3TC and ddC) are removed very inefficiently (Mas et al., 2002; White et al., 2004; Marchand et al., 2007; Sluis-Cremer et al., 2007). Another important parameter for the excision reaction is the positioning of the 3′ end of the blocked primer. Newly incorporated NRTI, present at the primer site (P) (post-tranlocational complex) makes the terminal primer unavailable for excision. Nucleotide excision occurs if the 3′ end of the primer is located in the nucleotide binding site (N) (pre-translocational complex) (Fig. 8). The efficiency of this reaction also depends on the presence of a dNTP complementary to the next position on the template, that leads to the formation of a "dead-end complex" that blocks the excision reaction by forcing the equilibrium towards the post-translocational status (for a review, see Götte, 2006).

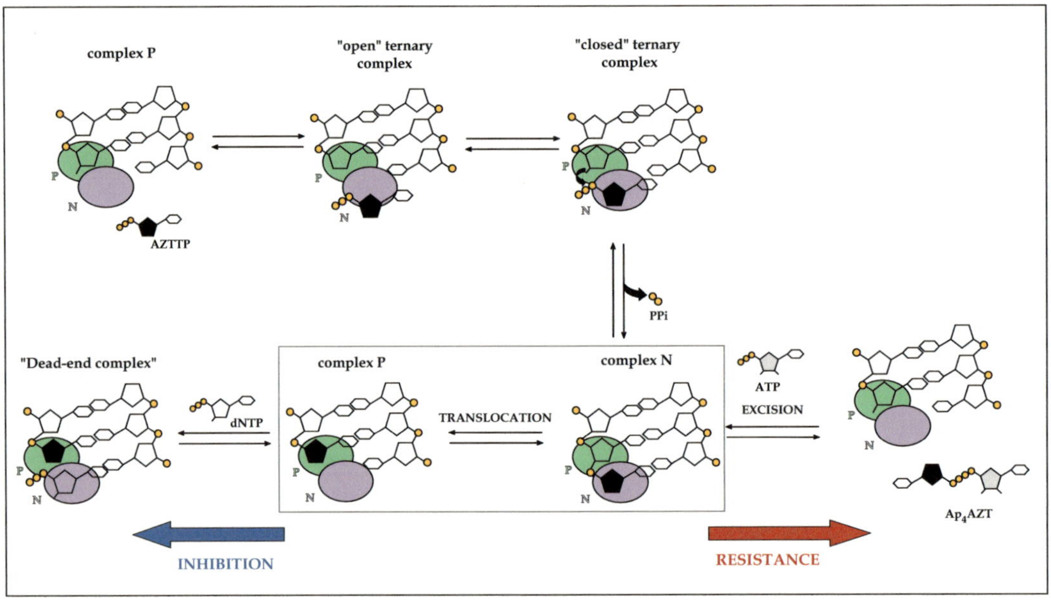

Fig. 8. Model showing the equilibrium between AZTTP incorporation and AZT excision from chain-terminated primers. The inhibition of DNA polymerization is favoured when the AZT moiety is at the P site (in green) and the next dNTP complementary is able to occupy the N site (in purple) to form a "dead-end" complex. Resistance occurs when the PPi donor (usually ATP) is able to excise the inhibitor when this is positioned at the N site.

The recently solved crystal structures of complexes of wild-type and mutant M41L/D67N/K70R/T215Y/K219Q HIV-1 RTs bound to double-stranded DNA and the product of the excision reaction, AZT adenosine dinucleoside tetraphosphate (Ap_4AZT, Fig. 8) have revealed different orientations for the adenosine-monophosphate moiety of Ap_4AZT in the wild-type and mutant RT complexes (Tu et al., 2010). The structures are consistent with an important role of π-π stacking interactions between the adenine ring of Ap_4AZT and the side-chain of Tyr215, while phosphate portions of the excision product seem to be stabilized by the side-chain of Arg70 in the mutant enzyme. Secondary TAMs such as D67N and K219Q would enhance the ability of the adenosine-monophosphate moiety to interact with Tyr215, while contributing to the proper alignment of the phosphates during the excision reaction.

The emergence of HIV variants containing insertions or deletions in the fingers subdomain of the RT has been facilitated by the extensive use of NRTIs in the treatment of HIV-infected individuals (for review, see Menéndez-Arias et al., 2006). HIV-1 RT mutants with a dipeptide insertion (usually Ser–Ser, Ser–Gly or Ser–Ala) between codons 69 and 70 and additional TAMs such as M41L, A62V, T69S, K70R and T215Y showed very high levels of excision activity with primers terminated with AZT and d4T (Mas et al., 2000; Matamoros et al., 2004; Cases-González et al., 2007). In addition, deletions of residues at positions 67 or 69 of the RT have been associated with AZT resistance or hypersusceptibility (Imamichi et al., 2000; Villena et al., 2007; Kisic et al., 2008).

A number of mutations have been reported to reduce ATP-mediated excision activity in the presence of TAMs. Examples are K65R (White et al., 2006), L74V (Frankel et al., 2005; Miranda et al., 2005), V75I (Matamoros et al., 2009), Y181C (Selmi et al., 2003) or M184V (Götte et al., 2000; for a review, see Menéndez-Arias, 2008). Finally, mutations in the connection subdomain (for example, E312Q, G335C/D, N348I, A360I/V, V365I and A376S) or in the RNase H domain of RT (such a Q509L, H539N and D549N) can enhance resistance to AZT by altering the balance between excision and template RNA degradation (Nikolenko et al., 2005, 2007; Delviks-Frankenberry et al., 2007, 2008; Yap et al., 2007; Ehteshami et al., 2008), while thumb subdomain polymorphisms (P272A/R277K/T286A) could also modulate excision by affecting the interaction of the RT with the RNA/DNA hybrid, without involvement of the RNase H activity of the RT (Betancor et al., 2010).

5.2.2 Resistance to NNRTIs

More than 40 NNRTIs resistance mutations have been identified *in vitro* or *in vivo* (Tambuyzer et al., 2009; reviewed in Clotet et al., 2009). Nearly all of these mutations occur at the NNRTI binding site and lead to the loss of NNRTI binding affinity by the HIV-1 RT. In many cases, the rigid structure of the inhibitors decreases their ability to accommodate themselves inside the hydrophobic pocket of the mutated RT. This could be the result of a loss of key hydrophobic interactions. For example, mutations involved in resistance to delavirdine or nevirapine (*e.g.* Y181C, Y188L or F227L) affect interactions between aromatic residues in the RT and the NNRTIs. Rigid molecules such as nevirapine or efavirenz are prone to development of NNRTI resistance through single amino acid substitutions (*e.g.* K103N). Novel inhibitors (*e.g.* etravirine) have been designed as more flexible molecules that are more resilient to resistance since their binding to the RT is compromised only when two or more resistance mutations appear (for recent reviews, see Sluis-Cremer and Tachedjian, 2008; Sarafianos et al., 2009; de Béthune, 2010). Mutations outside the NNRTI binding site (*e.g.* N348I or A376S in the connection subdomain) have been recently associated with NNRTI resistance (Nikolenko et al., 2007; Yap et al., 2007; Schuckmann et al., 2010; Paredes et al., 2011). Their mechanism of action is indirect and relates to their effects on RT dimerization and interaction with the template-primer.

5.3 Inhibition of the RNase H activity of HIV-1 RT

RNase H activity offers an additional target for the development of antiretroviral drugs due to its essential role in HIV-1 replication. Unfortunately, progress in the development of RNase H inhibitors has been relatively slow, due to problems of citotoxycity or limited cell uptake, as well as an interest in exploiting other viral targets. As of today, there are no drugs of this kind approved for clinical use. RNase H inhibitors that interfere with metal cofactor binding include N-hydroxymides, hydroxylated tropolones and diketo acids (for reviews, see Jochmans, 2008; Adamson & Freed, 2010; Beilhartz & Götte, 2010). The interference with metal-ion coordination has been demonstrated by the structure of HIV-1 RT complexed with β-thujaplicinol (Himmel et al., 2009), a hydroxylated tropolone. Other RNase H inhibitors such as napthoquinones, vinologous ureas, small nucleic acid fragments (aptamers) and hydrazones show different mechanisms of action (Chung et al., 2010; Gong et al., 2011; reviewed in Jochmans, 2008; Beilhartz & Götte, 2010). For example, the crystal structure of HIV-1 RT complexed with an N-acyl hydrazone analogue shows that this drug binds more than 50 Å away from the RNase H domain, at a novel site between the polymerase active site and the NNRTI binding pocket (Himmel et al., 2006). This study suggests that these compounds may alter the trajectory of the template-primer inducing structural changes at the DNA polymerase primer grip and at the thumb subdomain, thereby preventing RNase H-catalyzed cleavage.

6. Conclusions

The discovery of reverse transcription forty years ago constituted a major breakthrough leading to the birth of modern retrovirology. With the identification of pathogenic human retroviruses and most notably HIV-1, the study of reverse transcription has devoted a lot of attention. These investigations have led to the development and clinical use of about a dozen compounds targeting HIV-1 RT that play a major role in the control of the disease. However, further studies should help us to find other targets in the reverse transcription process. Novel inhibitors targeting RNase H activity would be a valuable addition to the antiretroviral drug armamentarium, and experimental therapeutic approaches such as viral decay acceleration induced by mutagenic nucleosides could be promising if they prove to be efficient *in vivo*. In addition, there are important aspects related to retroviral replication that should be further studied. Namely, the contribution of viral and cellular proteins to the reverse transcription process; how reverse transcription is regulated inside the cell (or in virions); how cellular factors associate and control the reverse transcription complex after entering the cell and prior to proviral DNA synthesis; and also the dynamics of strand transfer that seem to be basic for understanding recombination in retroviruses.

7. Acknowledgments

This work was supported by grants of the Ministry of Science and Innovation of Spain (BIO2010/15542), Fundación para la Investigación y Prevención del SIDA en España (FIPSE) (grant 36771/08), Fondo de Investigación Sanitaria (through the "Red Temática de Investigación Cooperativa en SIDA" RD06/006), and an institutional grant from the Fundación Ramón Areces.

8. References

Abbink, T.E.M. & Berkhout, B. (2008). HIV-1 reverse transcription initiation: A potential target for novel antivirals?. *Virus Res.*, 134, 4-18.

Abbondanzieri, E.A., Bokinsky, G., Rausch, J.W., Zhang, J.X., Le Grice, S.F.J. & Zhuang, X. (2008). Dynamic binding orientations direct activity of HIV reverse transcriptase. *Nature*, 453, 184-189.

Adamson C.S. & Freed E.O. (2010). Novel approaches to inhibiting HIV-1 replication. *Antiviral Res.*, 85, 119-141.

Agopian, A., Depollier, J., Lionne, C. & Divita, G. (2007). p66 Trp24 and Phe61 are essential for accurate association of HIV-1 reverse transcriptase with primer/template. *J. Mol. Biol.*, 373, 127-140.

Aguiar, R.S. & Peterlin, B.M. (2008). APOBEC3 proteins and reverse transcription. *Virus Res.*, 134, 74-85.

Álvarez, M., Matamoros, T. & Menéndez-Arias, L. (2009). Increased thermostability and fidelity of DNA synthesis of wild-type and mutant HIV-1 group O reverse transcriptases. *J. Mol. Biol.*, 392, 872-884.

Arion, D., Kaushik, N., McCormick, S., Borkow, G. & Parniak, M.A. (1998). Phenotypic mechanism of HIV-1 resistance to 3′-azido-3′-deoxythymidine (AZT): Increased polymerization processivity and enhanced sensitivity to pyrophosphate of the mutant viral reverse transcriptase. *Biochemistry*, 37, 15908-15917.

Bakhanashvili, M., Avidan, O. & Hizi, A. (1996). Mutational studies of human immunodeficiency virus type 1 reverse transcriptase: the involvement of residues 183 and 184 in the fidelity of DNA synthesis. *FEBS Lett.*, 391, 257-262.

Basu, V.P., Song, M., Gao, L., Rigby, S.T., Hanson, M.N. & Bambara, R.A. (2008). Strand transfer events during HIV-1 reverse transcription. *Virus Res.*, 134, 19-38.

Bazzoli, C., Jullien, V., Le Tiec, C., Rey, E., Mentre, F. & Taburet, A.M. (2010). Intracellular pharmacokinetics of antiretroviral drugs in HIV-infected patients, and their correlation with drug action. *Clin. Pharmacokinet.*, 49, 17-45.

Beard, W.A., Stahl, S.J., Kim, H.R., Bebenek, K., Kumar, A., Strub, M.P., Becerra, S.P., Kunkel, T.A. & Wilson, S.H. (1994). Structure/function studies of human immunodeficiency virus type 1 reverse transcriptase. Alanine scanning mutagenesis of an α-helix in the thumb subdomain. *J. Biol. Chem.*, 269, 28091-28097.

Beard, W.A., Minnick, D.T., Wade, C.L., Prasad, R., Won, R.L., Kumar, A., Kunkel, T.A. & Wilson, S.H. (1996). Role of the "helix clamp" in HIV-1 reverse transcriptase catalytic cycling as revealed by alanine-scanning mutagenesis. *J. Biol. Chem.*, 271, 12213-12220.

Bebenek, K., Beard, W.A., Casas-Finet, J.R., Kim, H.R., Darden, T.A., Wilson, S.H. & Kunkel, T.A. (1995). Reduced frameshift fidelity and processivity of HIV-1 reverse transcriptase mutants containing alanine substitutions in helix H of the thumb subdomain. *J. Biol. Chem.*, 270, 19516-19523.

Bebenek, K. & Kunkel, T.A. (1995). Analyzing fidelity of DNA polymerases. *Methods Enzymol.*, 262, 217-232.

Betancor, G., Puertas, M.C., Nevot, M., Garriga, C., Martínez, M.A., Martinez-Picado, J. & Menéndez-Arias, L. (2010). Mechanisms involved in the selection of HIV-1 reverse transcriptase thumb subdomain polymorphisms associated with nucleoside analogue therapy failure. *Antimicrob. Agents Chemother.*, 54, 4799-4811.

Beilhartz, G.L. & Götte, M. (2010). HIV-1 ribonuclease H: Structure, catalytic mechanism and inhibitors. *Viruses*, 2, 900-926.

Boyer, P.L. & Hughes, S.H. (2000). Effects of amino acid substitutions at position 115 on the fidelity of human immunodeficiency virus type 1 reverse transcriptase. *J. Virol.*, 74, 6494-6500.

Cahn, P. & Wainberg, M.A. (2010). Resistance profile of the new nucleoside reverse transcriptase inhibitor apricitabine. *J. Antimicrob. Chemother.*, 65, 213-217.

Carr, J.M., Coolen, C., Davis, A.J., Burrell, C.J. & Li, P. (2008). Human immunodeficiency virus 1 (HIV-1) virion infectivity factor (Vif) is part of reverse transcription complexes and acts as an accessory factor for reverse transcription. *Virology*, 372, 147-156.

Carroll, S.S., Geib, J., Olsen, D.B., Stahlhut, M., Shafer, J.A. & Kuo, L.C. (1994). Sensitivity of HIV-1 reverse transcriptase and its mutants to inhibition by azidothymidine triphosphate. *Biochemistry*, 33, 2113-2120.

Cases-González, C.E. & Menéndez-Arias, L. (2004). Increased G $\rightarrow$ A transition frequencies displayed by primer grip mutants of human immunodeficiency virus type 1 reverse transcriptase. *J. Virol.*, 78, 1012-1019.

Cases-González, C.E. & Menéndez-Arias, L. (2005). Nucleotide specificity of HIV-1 reverse transcriptases with amino acid substitutions affecting Ala-114. *Biochem. J.*, 387, 221-229.

Cases-González, C.E., Franco, S., Martínez, M.A. & Menéndez-Arias, L. (2007). Mutational patterns associated with the 69 insertion complex in multi-drug-resistant HIV-1 reverse transcriptase that confer increased excision activity and high-level resistance to zidovudine. *J. Mol. Biol.*, 365, 298-309.

Champoux, J.J. & Schultz, S.J. (2009). Ribonuclease H: Properties, substrate specificity and roles in retroviral reverse transcription. *FEBS J.*, 276, 1506-1516.

Chung, S., Wendeler, M., Rausch, J.W., Beilhartz, G., Gotte, M., O'Keefe, B.R., Bermingham, A., Beutler, J.A., Liu, S., Zhuang, X. & Le Grice, S.F.J. (2010). Structure-activity analysis of vinylogous urea inhibitors of human immunodeficiency virus-encoded ribonuclease H. *Antimicrob. Agents Chemother.*, 54, 3913-3921.

Clotet, B., Menéndez-Arias, L., Schapiro, J.M., Kuritzkes, D., Burger, D., Telenti, A., Brun-Vézinet, F., Geretti, A.M., Boucher, C.A. & Richman, D.D. (eds) (2009). *Guide to management of HIV drug resistance, antiretrovirals pharmacokinetics and viral hepatitis in HIV infected subjects*, Fundació de Lluita contra la SIDA, ISBN: 978-692-5025-9, Barcelona, Spain.

Coté, M. & Roth, M. (2008). Murine leukemia virus reverse transcriptase: Structural comparision with HIV-1 reverse transcriptase. *Viruses*, 134, 186-202.

Das, D. & Georgiadis M. (2004). The crystal structure of the monomeric reverse transcriptase from Moloney murine leukemia virus. *Structure*, 12, 819-829.

Das, K., Lewi, P.J., Hughes, S.H. & Arnold, E. (2005). Crystallography and the design of anti-AIDS drugs: conformational flexibility and positional adaptability are important in the design of non-nucleoside HIV-1 reverse transcriptase inhibitors. *Prog. Biophys. Mol. Biol.*, 88, 209-231.

De Béthune, M.P. (2010). Non-nucleoside reverse transcriptase inhibitors (NNRTIs), their discovery, development, and use in the treatment of HIV-1 infection: a review of the last 20 years (1989-2009). *Antiviral Res.*, 85, 75-90.

Delviks-Frankenberry, K.A., Nikolenko, G.N., Barr, R. & Pathak, V.K. (2007). Mutations in human immunodeficiency virus type 1 RNase H primer grip enhance 3′-azido- 3′-deoxythymidine resistance. *J. Virol.*, 81, 6837–6845.

Delviks-Frankenberry, K.A., Nikolenko, G.N., Boyer, P.L., Hughes, S.H., Coffin, J.M., Jere, A., & Pathak, V.K. (2008). HIV-1 reverse transcriptase connection subdomain mutations reduce template RNA degradation and enhance AZT excision. *Proc. Natl. Acad. Sci. U.S.A.*, 105, 10943–10948.

Deval, J., Selmi, B., Boretto, J., Egloff, M.P., Guerreiro, C., Sarfati, S. & Canard, B. (2002). The molecular mechanism of multidrug resistance by the Q151M human immunodeficiency virus type 1 reverse transcriptase and its suppression using α-boranophosphate nucleotide analogues. *J. Biol. Chem.*, 277, 42097-42104.

Deval, J., White, K.L., Miller, M.D., Parkin, N.T., Courcambeck, J., Halfon, P., Selmi, B., Boretto, J. & Canard, B. (2004). Mechanistic basis for reduced viral and enzymatic fitness of HIV-1 reverse transcriptase containing both K65R and M184V mutations. *J. Biol. Chem.*, 279, 509-516.

Deval, J., Alvarez, K., Selmi, B., Bermond, M., Boretto, J., Guerreiro, C., Mulard, L. & Canard, B. (2005). Mechanistic insights into the suppression of drug resistance by human immunodeficiency virus type 1 reverse transcriptase using α-boranophosphate nucleoside analogs. *J. Biol. Chem.*, 280, 3838-3846.

Ding, J., Das, K., Hsiou, Y., Sarafianos, S., Clark, A., Jacobo-Molina, A., Tantillo, C., Hughes, S. & Arnold, E. (1998). Structure and functional implications of the polymerase active site region in a complex of HIV-1 RT with a double-stranded DNA template-primer and an antibody Fab fragment at 2.8 Å resolution. *J. Mol. Biol.*, 284, 1095-1111.

Divita, G., Rittinger, K., Restle, T., Immendorfer, U. & Goody, R.S. (1995). Conformational stability of dimeric HIV-1 and HIV-2 reverse transcriptases. *Biochemistry*, 34, 16337-16346.

Drosopoulos, W.C. & Prasad, V.R. (1998). Increased misincorporation fidelity observed for nucleoside analog resistance mutations M184V and E89G in human immunodeficiency virus type 1 reverse transcriptase does not correlate with the overall error rate measured *in vitro*. *J. Virol.*, 72, 4224-4230.

Ehteshami, M., Beilhartz, G.L., Scarth, B.J., Tchesnokov, E.P., McCormick, S., Wynhoven, B., Harrigan, P.R. & Götte, M. (2008). Connection domain mutations N348I and A360V in HIV-1 reverse transcriptase enhance resistance to 3′-azido-3′-deoxythymidine through both RNase H-dependent and –independent mechanisms. *J. Biol. Chem.*, 283, 22222–22232.

Fabris, D., Marino, J.P. & Le Grice, S.F.J. (2009). Revisiting plus-strand DNA synthesis in retroviruses and long terminal repeat retrotransposons: Dynamics of enzyme: substrate interactions. *Viruses*, 1, 657-677.

Feng, J.Y., Myrick, F.T., Margot, N.A., Mulamba, G.B., Rimsky, L., Borroto-Esoda, K., Selmi, B. & Canard, B. (2006). Virologic and enzymatic studies revealing the mechanism of K65R- and Q151M-associated HIV-1 drug resistance towards emtricitabine and lamivudine. *Nucleosides Nucleotides Nucleic Acids*, 25, 89-107.

Fisher, T.S. & Prasad, V.R. (2002). Substitutions of Phe61 located in the vicinity of template 5'-overhang influence polymerase fidelity and nucleoside analog sensitivity of HIV-1 reverse transcriptase. *J. Biol. Chem.*, 277, 22345-22352.

Frangeul, A., Bussetta, C., Deval, J., Barral, K., Alvarez, K. & Canard, B. (2008). Gln151 of HIV-1 reverse transcriptase acts as a steric gate towards clinically relevant acyclic phosphonate nucleotide analogues. *Antivir. Ther.*, 13, 115-124.

Frankel, F.A., Marchand, B., Turner, D., Götte, M. & Wainberg, M.A. (2005). Impaired rescue of chain-terminated DNA synthesis associated with the L74V mutation in human immunodeficiency virus type 1 reverse transcriptase. *Antimicrob. Agents Chemother.*, 49, 2657-2664.

Garforth, S.J., Domaoal, R.A., Lwatula, C., Landau, M.J., Meyer, A.J., Anderson, K.S. & Prasad, V.R. (2010). K65R and K65A substitutions in HIV-1 reverse transcriptase enhance polymerase fidelity by decreasing both dNTP misinsertion and mispaired primer extension efficiencies. *J. Mol. Biol.*, 401, 33-44.

Gong, Q., Menon, L., Ilina, T., Miller, L.G., Ahn, J., Parniak, M.A. & Ishima, R. (2011). Interaction of HIV-1 reverse transcriptase ribonuclease H with an acylhydrazone inhibitor. *Chem. Biol. Drug Des.*, 77, 39-47.

Götte, M. (2006). Effects of nucleotides and nucleotide analogue inhibitors of HIV-1 reverse transcriptase in a ratchet model of polymerase translocation. *Curr. Pharm. Des.*, 12, 1867-1877.

Götte, M., Arion, D., Parniak, M.A. & Wainberg, M.A. (2000). The M184V mutation in the reverse transcriptase of human immunodeficiency virus type 1 impairs rescue of chain-terminated DNA synthesis. *J. Virol.*, 74, 3579–3585.

Götte, M., Rausch, J.W., Marchand, B., Sarafianos, S. & Le Grice, S.F.J. (2010). Reverse transcriptase in motion: conformational dynamics of enzyme-substrate interactions. *Biochim. Biophys. Acta*, 1804, 1202-1212.

Guo, F., Cen, S., Niu, M., Yang, Y., Gorelick, R.J. & Kleiman, L. (2007). The interaction of APOBEC3G with HIV-1 nucleocapsid inhibits $tRNA^{Lys3}$ annealing to viral RNA. *J Virol.*, 81, 11322-11331.

Gutiérrez-Rivas, M., Ibáñez, A., Martínez, M.A., Domingo, E. & Menéndez-Arias, L. (1999). Mutational analysis of Phe160 within the "palm" subdomain of human immunodeficiency virus type 1 reverse transcriptase. *J. Mol. Biol.*, 290, 615-625.

Gutiérrez-Rivas, M. & Menéndez-Arias, L. (2001). A mutation in the primer grip region of HIV-1 reverse transcriptase that confers reduced fidelity of DNA synthesis. *Nucleic Acids Res.*, 29, 4963-4972.

Hamburgh, M.E., Drosopoulos, W.C. & Prasad, V.R. (1998). The influence of 3TC-resistance mutations E89G and M184V in the human immunodeficiency virus reverse transcriptase on mispair extension efficiency. *Nucleic Acids Res.*, 26, 4389-4394.

Hamburgh, M.E., Curr, K.A., Monaghan, M., Rao, V.R., Tripathi, S., Preston, B.D., Sarafianos, S., Arnold, E., Darden, T. & Prasad, V.R. (2006). Structural determinants of slippage-mediated mutations by human immunodeficiency virus type 1 reverse transcriptase. *J. Biol. Chem.*, 281, 7421-7428.

Hammond, E., McKinnon, E. & Nolan, D. (2010). Human immunodeficiency virus treatment-induced adipose tissue pathology and lipoatrophy: prevalence and metabolic consequences. *Clin. Infect. Dis.*, 51, 591-599.

Henriet, S., Sinck, L., Bec, G., Gorelick, R.J., Marquet, R. & Paillart J.C. (2007). Vif is a RNA chaperone that could temporally regulate RNA dimerization and the early steps of HIV-1 reverse transcription. *Nucleic Acids Res.*, 35, 5141-5153.

Herschhorn, A. & Hizi, A. (2010). Retroviral reverse transcriptases. *Cell. Mol. Life Sci.*, 67, 2717-2747.

Himmel, D.M., Sarafianos, S.G., Dharmasena, S., Hossain, M.M., McCoy-Simandle, K., Ilina, T., Clark A.D. Jr., Knight, J.L., Julias, J.G., Clark, P.K., Krogh-Jespersen, K., Levy, R.M., Hughes, S.H., Parniak, M.A. & Arnold, E. (2006). HIV-1 reverse transcriptase structure with RNase H inhibitor dihydroxy benzoyl naphthyl hydrazone bound at a novel site. *ACS Chem. Biol.*, 1, 702–712.

Himmel, D.M., Maegley, K.A., Pauly, T.A., Bauman, J.D., Das, K., Dharia, C., Clark, A.D. Jr., Ryan, K., Hickey, M.J., Love, R.A., Hughes, S.H., Bergqvist, S. & Arnold, E. (2009). Structure of HIV-1 reverse transcriptase with the inhibitor β-thujaplicinol bound at the RNase H active site. *Structure*, 17, 1625-1635.

Hizi, A. & Joklik, W.K. (1977). RNA-dependent DNA polymerase of avian sarcoma virus B77. I. Isolation and partial characterization of the α, β_2, and αβ forms of the enzyme. *J. Biol. Chem.*, 252, 2290-2295.

Hsu, M., Inouye, P., Rezende, L., Richard, N., Li, Z., Prasad, V.R. & Wainberg, M.A. (1997). Higher fidelity of RNA-dependent DNA mispair extension by M184V drug-resistant than wild-type reverse transcriptase of human immunodeficiency virus type 1. *Nucleic Acids Res.*, *25*, 4532-4536.

Huang, H., Chopra, R., Verdine, G. & Harrison, S. (1998). Structure of a covalently trapped catalytic complex of HIV-1 reverse transcriptase: Implications for drug resistance. *Science*, 282, 1669-1675.

Imamichi, T., Berg, S.C., Imamichi, H., Lopez, J.C., Metcalf, J.A., Falloon, J. & Lane, H.C. (2000). Relative replication fitness of a high-level 3'-azido-3'-deoxythymidine-resistant variant of human immunodeficiency virus type 1 possessing an amino acid deletion at codon 67 and a novel substitution (Thr→Gly) at codon 69. *J. Virol.*, 74, 10958-10964.

Jacob, D.T. & DeStefano, J.J. (2008). A new role for HIV nucleocapsid protein in modulating the specificity of plus strand priming. *Virology*, 378, 385-396.

Jacobo-Molina A., Ding, J., Nanni, R., Clark, A., Lu, X., Tantillo, C., Williams, R., Kamer, G., Ferris, A., Clark, P., Hizi, A., Hughes, S. & Arnold, E. (1993). Crystal structure of human immunodefiency virus type 1 reverse transcriptase complexed with double-stranded DNA at 3.0 Å resolution shows bent DNA. *Proc. Natl. Acad. Sci. USA*, 90, 6320-6324.

Jamburuthugoda, V.K., Guo, D., Wedekind, J.E. & Kim, B. (2005). Kinetic evidence for interaction of human immunodeficiency virus type 1 reverse transcriptase with the 3'-OH of the incoming dTTP substrate. *Biochemistry*, 44, 10635-10643.

Jern, P., Sperber, G.O. & Blomberg, J. (2005). Use of endogenous retroviral sequences (ERVs) and structural markers for retroviral phylogenetic inference and taxonomy. *Retrovirology*, 2, 50.

Jochmans, D. (2008). Novel HIV-1 reverse transcriptase inhibitors. *Virus Res.*, 134, 171-185.

Jonckheere, H., De Clercq, E. & Anne, J. (2000). Fidelity analysis of HIV-1 reverse transcriptase mutants with an altered amino-acid sequence at residues Leu74, Glu89, Tyr115, Tyr183 and Met184. *Eur. J. Biochem.*, 267, 2658-2665.

Kagan, R.M., Lee, T.S., Ross, L., Lloyd, R.M., Jr., Lewinski, M.A. & Potts, S.J. (2007). Molecular basis of antagonism between K70E and K65R tenofovir-associated mutations in HIV-1 reverse transcriptase. *Antiviral Res.*, 75, 210-218.

Kaushik, N., Talele, T.T., Pandey, P.K., Harris, D., Yadav, P.N. & Pandey, V.N. (2000). Role of glutamine 151 of human immunodeficiency virus type-1 reverse transcriptase in substrate selection as assessed by site-directed mutagenesis. *Biochemistry*, 39, 2912-2920.

Kellinger, M.W. & Johnson, K.A. (2010). Nucleotide-dependent conformational change governs specificity and analog discrimination by HIV reverse transcriptase. *Proc. Natl. Acad. Sci. USA*, 107, 7734-7739.

Kim, B., Hathaway, T.R. & Loeb, L.A. (1998). Fidelity of mutant HIV-1 reverse transcriptases: interaction with the single-stranded template influences the accuracy of DNA synthesis. *Biochemistry*, 37, 5831-5839.

Kim, B., Ayran, J.C., Sagar, S.G., Adman, E.T., Fuller, S.M., Tran, N.H. & Horrigan, J. (1999). New human immunodeficiency virus, type 1 reverse transcriptase (HIV-1 RT) mutants with increased fidelity of DNA synthesis. Accuracy, template binding, and processivity. *J. Biol. Chem.*, 274, 27666-27673.

Kisic, M., Mendieta, J., Puertas, M.C., Parera, M., Martínez, M.A., Martinez-Picado, J. & Menéndez-Arias, L. (2008). Mechanistic basis of zidovudine hypersusceptibility and lamivudine resistance conferred by the deletion of codon 69 in the HIV-1 reverse transcriptase coding region. *J. Mol. Biol.*, 382, 327–341.

Kohler, J.J. & Lewis, W. (2007). A brief overview of mechanisms of mitochondrial toxicity from NRTIs. *Environ. Mol. Mutagen*, 48, 166-172.

Kohlstaedt, L., Wang, J., Friedman, J., Rice, P. & Steitz, T. (1992). Crystal structure at 3.5Å resolution of HIV-1 reverse transcriptase complexed with an inhibitor. *Science*, 256, 1783-1790.

Krebs, R., Immendorfer, U., Thrall, S.H., Wohrl, B.M. & Goody, R.S. (1997). Single-step kinetics of HIV-1 reverse transcriptase mutants responsible for virus resistance to nucleoside inhibitors zidovudine and 3-TC. *Biochemistry*, 36, 10292-10300.

Larder, B.A. & Kemp, S.D. (1989). Multiple mutations in HIV-1 reverse transcriptase confer high-level resistance to zidovudine (AZT). *Science*, 246, 1155-1158.

Larder, B.A., Darby, G. & Richman, D.D. (1989a). HIV with reduced sensitivity to zidovudine (AZT) isolated during prolonged therapy. *Science*, 243, 1731-1734.

Larder, B.A., Kemp, S.D. & Purifoy, D.J. (1989b) Infectious potential of human immunodeficiency virus type 1 reverse transcriptase mutants with altered inhibitor sensitivity. *Proc. Natl. Acad. Sci. USA*, 86, 4803-4807.

Lennerstrand, J., Stammers, D.K. & Larder, B.A. (2001). Biochemical mechanism of human immunodeficiency virus type 1 reverse transcriptase resistance to stavudine. *Antimicrob. Agents Chemother.*, 45, 2144-2146.

Levin, J.G., Mitra, M., Mascarenhas, A. & Musier-Forsyth, K. (2010). Role of HIV-1 nucleocapsid protein in HIV-1 reverse transcription. *RNA Biology*, 7, 754-774.

Lewis, D. A., Bebenek, K., Beard, W. A., Wilson, S. H. & Kunkel, T. A. (1999). Uniquely altered DNA replication fidelity conferred by an amino acid change in the nucleotide binding pocket of human immunodeficiency virus type 1 reverse transcriptase. *J. Biol. Chem.*, 274, 32924-32930.

Lim, D., Gregorio, G.G., Bingman, C., Martinez-Hackert, E., Hendrickson, W.A. & Goff, S.P. (2006). Crystal structure of the Moloney murine leukemia virus RNase H domain. *J. Virol.*, 80, 8379-8389.

Lisco, A., Vanpouille, C., Tchesnokov, E.P., Grivel, J.C., Biancotto, A., Brichacek, B., Elliott, J., Fromentin, E., Shattock, R., Anton, P., Gorelick, R., Balzarini, J., McGuigan, C., Derudas, M., Götte, M., Schinazi, R.F. & Margolis, L. (2008). Acyclovir is activated into a HIV-1 reverse transcriptase inhibitor in herpesvirus-infected human tissues. *Cell Host Microbe,* 4, 260-270.

Liu, S., Abbondanzieri, E.A., Rausch J.W., Le Grice S.F.J. & Zhuang, X. (2008). Slide into action: dynamic shuttling of HIV reverse transcriptase on nucleic acid substrates. *Science,* 322, 1092-1097.

Mansky, L.M., Le Rouzic, E., Benichou, S. & Gajary, L.C. (2003). Influence of reverse transcriptase variants, drugs, and Vpr on human immunodeficiency virus type 1 mutant frequencies. *J. Virol.,* 77, 2071-2080.

Marchand, B., Tchesnokov, E.P. & Götte, M. (2007). The pyrophosphate analogue foscarnet traps the pre-translocational state of HIV-1 reverse transcriptase in a Brownian ratchet model of polymerase translocation. *J. Biol. Chem.,* 282, 3337-3346.

Martín-Hernández, A.M., Domingo, E. & Menéndez-Arias, L. (1996). Human immunodeficiency virus type 1 reverse transcriptase: role of Tyr115 in deoxynucleotide binding and misinsertion fidelity of DNA synthesis. *EMBO J.,* 15, 4434-4442.

Martín-Hernández, A.M., Gutiérrez-Rivas, M., Domingo, E. & Menéndez-Arias, L. (1997). Mispair extension fidelity of human immunodeficiency virus type 1 reverse transcriptases with amino acid substitutions affecting Tyr115. *Nucleic Acids Res.,* 25, 1383-1389.

Martinez-Picado, J. & Martínez, M. A. (2008). HIV-1 reverse transcriptase inhibitor resistance mutations and fitness: a view from the clinic and *ex vivo*. *Virus Res.,* 134, 104-123.

Mas, A., Parera, M., Briones, C., Soriano, V., Martínez, M.A., Domingo, E. & Menéndez-Arias, L. (2000). Role of a dipeptide insertion between codons 69 and 70 of HIV-1 reverse transcriptase in the mechanism of AZT resistance. *EMBO J.,* 19, 5752-5761.

Mas, A., Vázquez-Álvarez, B.M., Domingo, E. & Menéndez-Arias, L. (2002). Multidrug-resistant HIV-1 reverse transcriptase: involvement of ribonucleotide-dependent phosphorolysis in cross-resistance to nucleoside analogue inhibitors. *J. Mol. Biol.,* 323, 181-197.

Matamoros, T., Franco, S., Vázquez-Álvarez, B.M., Mas, A., Martínez, M.A. & Menéndez-Arias, L. (2004). Molecular determinants of multi-nucleoside analogue resistance in HIV-1 reverse transcriptases containing a dipeptide insertion in the fingers subdomain – Effect of mutations D67N and T215Y on removal of thymidine nucleotide analogues from blocked DNA primers. *J. Biol. Chem.,* 279, 24569-24577.

Matamoros, T., Deval, J., Guerreiro, C., Mulard, L., Canard, B. & Menéndez-Arias, L. (2005). Suppression of multidrug-resistant HIV-1 reverse transcriptase primer unblocking activity by α-phosphate-modified thymidine analogues. *J. Mol. Biol.,* 349, 451-463.

Matamoros, T., Kim, B. & Menéndez-Arias, L. (2008). Mechanistic insights into the role of Val75 of HIV-1 reverse transcriptase in misinsertion and mispair extension fidelity of DNA synthesis. *J. Mol. Biol.,* 375, 1234-1248.

Matamoros, T., Nevot, M., Martínez, M.A. & Menéndez-Arias, L. (2009). Thymidine analogue resistance suppression by V75I of HIV-1 reverse transcriptase: effects of substituting valine 75 on stavudine excision and discrimination. *J. Biol. Chem.,* 284, 32792-32802.

Mbisa, J.L., Barr, R., Thomas, J.A., Vandegraaff, N., Dorweiler, I.J., Svarovskaia, E.S., Brown, W.L., Mansky, L.M., Gorelick, R.J., Harris, R.S., Engelman, A. & Pathak, V.K. (2007). Human immunodeficiency virus tipe 1 cDNAs produced in the presence of APOBEC3G exhibit defects in plus-strand DNA transfer and integration. *J. Virol.,* 81, 7099-7110.

McMahon, M.A., Siliciano, J.D., Lai, J., Liu, J.O., Stivers, J.T., Siliciano, R.F. & Kohli, R.M. (2008). The antiherpetic drug acyclovir inhibits HIV replication and selects the V75I reverse transcriptase multidrug resistance mutation. *J. Biol. Chem.,* 283, 31289-31293.

Mendieta, J., Cases-González, C.E., Matamoros, T., Ramírez, G. & Menéndez-Arias, L. (2008). A Mg^{2+}-induced conformational switch rendering a competent DNA polymerase catalytic complex. *Proteins,* 71, 565-574.

Menéndez-Arias, L. (2002). Molecular basis of fidelity of DNA synthesis and nucleotide specificity of retroviral reverse transcriptases. *Progr. Nucleic Acid Res. Mol. Biol.,* 71, 91-147.

Menéndez-Arias, L. (2008). Mechanisms of resistance to nucleoside analogue inhibitors of HIV-1 reverse transcriptase. *Virus Res.,* 134, 124-146.

Menéndez-Arias, L. (2009) Mutation rate and intrisic fidelity of retroviral reverse transcriptases. *Viruses,* 1, 1137-1165.

Menéndez-Arias, L. (2010) Molecular basis of human immunodeficiency virus drug resistance: an update. *Antiviral Res.,* 85, 210-231.

Menéndez-Arias, L., Martínez, M. A., Quiñones-Mateu, M. E. & Martínez-Picado, J. (2003). Fitness variations and their impact on the evolution of antiretroviral drug resistance. *Curr. Drug Targets Infect. Disord.,* 3, 355-371.

Menéndez-Arias, L., Matamoros, T. & Cases-González, C.E. (2006). Insertions and deletions in HIV-1 reverse transcriptase: consequences for drug resistance and viral fitness. *Curr. Pharm. Des.,* 12, 1811-1825.

Meyer, P.R., Matsuura, S.E., Mian, A.M., So, A.G. & Scott, W.A. (1999). A mechanism of AZT resistance: An increase in nucleotide-dependent primer unblocking by mutant HIV-1 reverse transcriptase. *Mol. Cell,* 4, 35-43.

Miranda, L.R., Götte, M., Liang, F. & Kuritzkes, D.R. (2005). The L74V mutation in human immunodeficiency virus type 1 reverse transcriptase counteracts enhanced excision of zidovudine monophosphate associated with thymidine analog resistance mutations. *Antimicrob. Agents Chemother.,* 49, 2648-2656.

Nikolenko, G.N., Palmer, S., Maldarelli, F., Mellors, J.W., Coffin, J.M. & Pathak, V.K. (2005). Mechanism for nucleoside analog-mediated abrogation of HIV-1 replication: balance between RNase H activity and nucleotide excision. *Proc. Natl. Acad. Sci. USA,* 102, 2093-2098.

Nikolenko, G.N., Delviks-Frankenberry, K.A., Palmer, S., Maldarelli, F., Fivash, M.J., Jr., Coffin, J.M. & Pathak, V.K. (2007). Mutations in the connection domain of HIV-1 reverse transcriptase increase 3'-azido-3'-deoxythymidine resistance. *Proc. Natl. Acad. Sci. USA,* 104, 317-322.

Nolan, D. & Mallal, S. (2004). Complications associated with NRTI therapy: update on clinical features and possible pathogenic mechanisms. *Antivir. Ther.,* 9, 849-863.

Onafuwa-Nuga, A. & Telesnitsky, A. (2009). The remarkable frequency of human immuno-deficiency virus type 1 genetic recombination. *Microbiol. Mol. Biol. Rev.,* 73, 451-480.

Oude Essink, B.B., Back, N.K.T. & Berkhout, B. (1997). Increased polymerase fidelity of the 3TC-resistant variants of HIV-1 reverse transcriptase. *Nucleic Acids Res., 25,* 3212-3217.

Oz-Gleenberg, I., Herschhorn, A. & Hizi, A. (2011). Reverse transcriptases can clamp together nucleic acids strands with two complementary bases at their 3'-termini for initiating DNA synthesis. *Nucleic Acids. Res.,* 39, 1042-1053.

Pandey, V.N., Kaushik, N., Rege, N., Sarafianos, S.G., Yadav, P.N. & Modak, M.J. (1996). Role of methionine 184 of human immunodeficiency virus type-1 reverse transcriptase in the polymerase function and fidelity of DNA synthesis. *Biochemistry* 35, 2168-2179.

Paredes, R., Puertas, M.C., Bannister, W., Kisic, M., Cozzi-Lepri, A., Pou, C., Bellido, R., Betancor, G., Bogner, J., Gargalianos, P., Bánhegyi, D., Clotet, B., Lundgren, J., Menéndez-Arias, L., Martinez-Picado, J. & The EuroSIDA Study Group (2011) A376S in the connection subdomain of HIV-1 reverse transcriptase confers increased risk of virological failure to nevirapine therapy. *J. Infect. Dis.,* in press.

Petropoulos, C.J., Parkin, N.T., Limoli, K.L., Lie, Y.S., Wrin, T., Huang, W., Tian, H., Smith, D., Winslow, G.A., Capon, D.J. & Whitcomb, J.M. (2000). A novel phenotypic drug susceptibility assay for human immunodeficiency virus type 1. *Antimicrob. Agents Chemother.,* 44, 920-928.

Ramirez, B.C., Simon-Loriere, E., Galetto, R. & Negroni, M. (2008). Implications of recombination for HIV diversity. *Virus Res.,* 134, 64-73.

Ray, A.S., Basavapathruni, A. & Anderson, K.S. (2002). Mechanistic studies to understand the progressive development of resistance in human immunodeficiency virus type 1 reverse transcriptase to abacavir. *J. Biol. Chem.,* 277, 40479-40490.

Ren, J., Bird, L., Chamberlain, P., Stewart-Jones, G., Stuart, D. & Stammers, D. (2002). Structure of HIV-2 reverse transcriptase at 2.35 Å resolution and the mechanism of resistance to non-nucleoside inhibitors. *Proc. Natl. Acad. Sci. USA,* 99, 14410-14415.

Rezende, L.F., Curr, K., Ueno, T., Mitsuya, H. & Prasad, V.R. (1998a). The impact of multidideoxynucleoside resistance-conferring mutations in human immuno-deficiency virus type 1 reverse transcriptase on polymerase fidelity and error specificity. *J. Virol.,* 72, 2890-2895.

Rezende, L.F., Drosopoulos, W.C. & Prasad, V.R. (1998b). The influence of 3TC resistance mutation M184I on the fidelity and error specificity of human immunodeficiency virus type 1 reverse transcriptase. *Nucleic Acids Res.,* 26, 3066-3072.

Roberts, J.D., Preston, B.D., Johnston, L.A., Soni, A., Loeb, L.A. & Kunkel, T.A. (1989). Fidelity of two retroviral reverse transcriptases during DNA-dependent DNA synthesis *in vitro. Mol. Cell. Biol.,* 9, 469-476.

Rodgers, D., Gamblin, S., Harris, B., Ray, S., Culp, J., Hellmig, B., Woolf, D., Debouck, C. & Harrison, S. (1995). The structure of unliganded reverse transcriptase from the human immunodefiency virus type 1. *Proc. Natl. Acad. Sci. USA,* 92, 1222-1226.

Roy, B.B., Hu, J., Guo, X., Russel, R.S., Guo, F., Kleiman, L. & Liang, C. (2006). Association of RNA Helicase A with human immunodeficiency virus type 1 particles. *J. Biol. Chem.,* 281, 12625-12635.

Rubinek, T., Bakhanashvili, M., Taube, R., Avidan, O. & Hizi, A. (1997). The fidelity of 3′ misinsertion and mispair extension during RNA synthesis exhibited by two drug-resistant mutants of the reverse transcriptase of human immunodeficiency virus type 1 with Leu74→Val and Glu89→Gly. *Eur. J. Biochem.*, 247, 238-247.

Sarafianos, S.G., Das, K., Clark, A.D., Jr., Ding, J., Boyer, P.L., Hughes, S.H. & Arnold, E. (1999). Lamivudine (3TC) resistance in HIV-1 reverse transcriptase involves steric hindrance with β-branched amino acids. *Proc. Natl. Acad. Sci. USA*, 96, 10027-10032.

Sarafianos, S., Das, K., Tantillo, C., Clark, A., Ding, J., Whitcomb, J., Boyer, P., Hughes, S. & Arnold, E. (2001). Crystal structure of HIV-1 reverse transcriptase in complex with a polypurine tract RNA:DNA. *EMBO J.*, 20, 1449-1461.

Sarafianos, S., Clark, A., Das, K., Tuske, S., Birktoft, J., Ilankuraman, P., Ramesha, A., Sayer, J., Jerina, D., Boyer, P., Hughes, S. & Arnold, E. (2002). Structures of HIV-1 reverse transcriptase with pre- and post-translocation AZTMP-terminated DNA. *EMBO J.*, 21, 6614-6624.

Sarafianos, S.G., Marchand, B., Das, K., Himmel, D., Parniak, M.A., Hughes, S.H. & Arnold, E. (2009). Structure and function of HIV-1 reverse transcriptase: molecular mechanisms of polymerization and inhibition. *J. Mol. Biol.*, 385, 693-713.

Schuckmann, M.M., Marchand, B., Hachiya, A., Kodama, E.N., Kirby, K.A., Singh, K. & Sarafianos, S.G. (2010). The N348I mutation at the connection subdomain of HIV-1 reverse transcriptase decreases binding to nevirapine. *J. Biol. Chem.*, 285, 38700-38709.

Schultz, S.J. & Champoux, J.J. (2008). RNase H activity: Structure, specificity, and function in reverse transcription. *Virus Res.*, 134, 86-103.

Selmi, B., Boretto, J., Sarfati, S.R., Guerreiro, C. & Canard, B. (2001). Mechanism-based suppression of dideoxynucleotide resistance by K65R human immunodeficiency virus reverse transcriptase using an α-boranophosphate nucleoside analogue. *J. Biol. Chem.*, 276, 48466-48472.

Selmi, B., Deval, J., Alvarez, K., Boretto, J., Sarfati, S., Guerreiro, C. & Canard, B. (2003). The Y181C substitution in 3'-azido-3'-deoxythymidine-resistant human immunodeficiency virus, type 1, reverse transcriptase suppresses the ATP-mediated repair of the 3'-azido-3'-deoxythymidine 5'-monophosphate-terminated primer. *J. Biol. Chem.*, 278, 40464-40472.

Shah, F.S., Curr, K.A., Hamburgh, M.E., Parniak, M., Mitsuya, H., Arnez, J.G. & Prasad, V.R. (2000). Differential influence of nucleoside analog-resistance mutations K65R and L74V on the overall mutation rate and error specificity of human immunodeficiency virus type 1 reverse transcriptase. *J. Biol. Chem.*, 275, 27037-27044.

Sheehy, A.M., Gaddis, N.C., Choi, J.D. & Malim, M.H. (2002). Isolation of a human gene that inhibits HIV infection and is suppressed by the viral Vif protein. *Nature*, 418, 646-650.

Shirasaka, T., Kavlick, M.F., Ueno, T., Gao, W.Y., Kojima, E., Alcaide, M.L., Chokekijchai, S., Roy, B.M., Arnold, E., Yarchoan, R. & Mitsuya, H. (1995). Emergence of human immunodeficiency virus type 1 variants with resistance to multiple dideoxynucleosides in patients receiving therapy with dideoxynucleosides. *Proc. Natl. Acad. Sci. USA*, 92, 2398-2402.

Sluis-Cremer, N., Temiz, N.A. & Bahar, I. (2004). Conformational changes in HIV-1 reverse transcriptase induced by nonnucleoside reverse transcriptase inhibitor binding. *Curr. HIV Res.*, 2, 323-332.

Sluis-Cremer, N., Sheen, C.W., Zelina, S., Torres, P.S., Parikh, U.M. & Mellors, J.W. (2007). Molecular mechanism by which the K70E mutation in human immunodeficiency virus type 1 reverse transcriptase confers resistance to nucleoside reverse transcriptase inhibitors. *Antimicrob. Agents Chemother.*, 51, 48-53.

Sluis-Cremer, N. & Tachedjian, G. (2008). Mechanisms of inhibition of HIV replication by non-nucleoside reverse transcriptase inhibitors. *Virus Res.*, 134, 147-156.

Spence, R.A., Kati, W.M., Anderson, K.S. & Johnson, K.A. (1995). Mechanism of inhibition of HIV-1 reverse transcriptase by nonnucleoside inhibitors. *Science*, 267, 988-993.

Tambuyzer, L., Azijn, H., Rimsky, L.T., Vingerhoets, J., Lecocq, P., Kraus, G., Picchio, G. & de Bethune, M. P. (2009). Compilation and prevalence of mutations associated with resistance to non-nucleoside reverse transcriptase inhibitors. *Antivir. Ther.*, 14, 103-109.

Tchesnokov, E.P., Obikhod, A., Massud, I., Lisco, A., Vanpouille, C., Brichacek, B., Balzarini, J., McGuigan, C., Derudas, M., Margolis, L., Schinazi, R.F. & Götte, M. (2009). Mechanisms associated with HIV-1 resistance to acyclovir by the V75I mutation in reverse transcriptase. *J. Biol. Chem.*, 284, 21496-21504.

Telesnitsky, A. & Goff, S.P. (1997). Reverse transcriptase and the generation of retroviral DNA. In *Retroviruses* (J.M, Coffin, S.H. Hughes, H.E. Varmus, eds), pp. 121-160. Cold Spring Harbor Laboratory Press, Plainview, NY.

Thomas, J.A. & Gorelick, R.J. (2008). Nucleocapsid protein function in early infection processes. (2008). *Virus Res.*, 134, 39-63.

Tu., X., Das, K., Han, Q., Bauman, J., Clark, A., Hou, X., Frenkel, Y., Gaffney, B., Jones, R., Boyer, P., Hughes, S. & Arnold, E. (2010). Structural basis of HIV-1 resistance to AZT by excision. *Nature Struct. Mol. Biol.*, 17, 1202-1209.

Tuske, S., Sarafianos, S., Clark, A., Ding, J., Naeger, L., White, K., Miller, M., Gibbs, C., Boyer, P., Clark, P., Wang, G., Gaffney, B., Jones, R., Jerina, D., Hughes, S. & Arnold, E. (2004). Structures of HIV-1 RT-DNA complexes before and after incorporation of the anti-AIDS drug tenofovir. *Nature Struct. Mol. Biol.*, 11, 469-474.

Villena, C., Prado, J.G., Puertas, M.C., Martínez, M.A., Clotet, B., Ruiz, L., Parkin, N.T., Menéndez-Arias, L. & Martinez-Picado, J. (2007). Relative fitness and replication capacity of a multinucleoside analogue-resistant clinical human immunodeficiency virus type 1 isolate with a deletion of codon 69 in the reverse transcriptase coding region. *J. Virol.*, 81, 4713-4721.

Wainberg, M.A., Drosopoulos, W.C., Salomon, H., Hsu, M., Borkow, G., Parniak, M.A., Gu, Z., Song, Q., Manne, J., Islam, S., Castriota, G. & Prasad, V.R. (1996). Enhanced fidelity of 3TC-selected mutant HIV-1 reverse transcriptase. *Science*, *271*, 1282-1285.

Warren, K., Warrilow, D., Meredith, L. & Harrich, D. (2009). Reverse transcriptase and cellular factors: Regulators of HIV-1 reverse transcription. *Viruses*, 1, 873-894.

Weiss, K.K., Isaacs, S. J., Tran, N.H., Adman, E.T. & Kim, B. (2000). Molecular architecture of the mutagenic active site of human immunodeficiency virus type 1 reverse transcriptase: roles of the β8-αE loop in fidelity, processivity, and substrate interactions. *Biochemistry*, 39, 10684-10694.

Weiss, K.K., Bambara, R.A. & Kim, B. (2002). Mechanistic role of residue Gln151 in error prone DNA synthesis by human immunodeficiency virus type 1 (HIV-1) reverse transcriptase (RT). Pre-steady state kinetic study of the Q151N HIV-1 RT mutant with increased fidelity. *J. Biol. Chem.*, 277, 22662-22669.

Weiss, K.K., Chen, R., Skasko, M., Reynolds, H.M., Lee, K., Bambara, R.A., Mansky, L.M. & Kim, B. (2004). A role for dNTP binding of human immunodeficiency virus type 1 reverse transcriptase in viral mutagenesis. *Biochemistry*, 43, 4490-4500.

White, K.L., Chen, J.M., Margot, N.A., Wrin, T., Petropoulos, C.J., Naeger, L.K., Swaminathan, S. & Miller, M.D. (2004). Molecular mechanisms of tenofovir resistance conferred by human immunodeficiency virus type 1 reverse transcriptase containing a diserine insertion after residue 69 and multiple thymidine analog-associated mutations. *Antimicrob. Agents Chemother.*, 48, 992-1003.

White, K.L., Chen, J.M., Feng, J.Y., Margot, N.A., Ly, J.K., Ray, A.S., Macarthur, H.L., McDermott, M.J., Swaminathan, S. & Miller, M.D. (2006). The K65R reverse transcriptase mutation in HIV-1 reverses the excision phenotype of zidovudine resistance mutations. *Antivir. Ther.*, 11, 155-163.

Wisniewski, M., Palaniappan, C., Fu, Z., Le Grice, S.F., Fay, P. & Bambara, R.A. (1999). Mutations in the primer grip region of HIV reverse transcriptase can increase replication fidelity. *J. Biol. Chem.*, 274, 28175-28184.

Wöhrl, B.M., Krebs, R., Thrall, S.H., Le Grice, S.F., Scheidig, A.J. & Goody, R.S. (1997). Kinetic analysis of four HIV-1 reverse transcriptase enzymes mutated in the primer grip region of p66. Implications for DNA synthesis and dimerization. *J. Biol. Chem.*, 272, 17581-17587.

Xia, Q., Radzio, J., Anderson, K.S. & Sluis-Cremer, N. (2007). Probing nonnucleoside inhibitor-induced active-site distortion in HIV-1 reverse transcriptase by transient kinetic analyses. *Protein Sci.*, 16, 1728-1737.

Yap, S.-H., Sheen, C.-W., Fahey, J., Zanin, M., Tyssen, D., Lima, V.D., Wynhoven, B., Kuiper, M., Sluis-Cremer, N., Harrigan, P.R. & Tachedjian, G. (2007). N348I in the connection domain of HIV-1 reverse transcriptase confers zidovudine and nevirapine resistance. *PLoS Med.*, 4, e335.

Yu, H., Jetzt, A.E., Ron, Y., Preston, B.D. & Dougherty, J.P. (1998). The nature of human immunodeficiency virus type 1 strand transfers. *J. Biol. Chem.*, 273, 28384-28391.

7

DNA Replication Fidelity of Herpes Simplex Virus

Charles Bih-Chen Hwang
Upstate Medical University, Syracuse, NY
U.S.A.

1. Introduction

The role of DNA replication is to successfully transfer all genetic information from parental to daughter cells. While this process requires faithful DNA duplication to maintain genome integrity, certain errors during DNA replication, coupled with selection and fitness, are critical for evolutionary events. Therefore, regulatory mechanisms are involved in achieving a certain degree of DNA replication fidelity and satisfying these diverse needs. It is reasonable to predict that microorganisms also replicate under tight regulations to accomplish the required DNA replication fidelity for selection and fitness. This notion also applies to herpes simplex virus type 1 (HSV-1), which replicates DNA with a genomic mutation rate similar to those of other DNA-based microbes examined (Drake and Hwang, 2005). Since the HSV-1 genome can be easily manipulated, it offers a good model for a variety of studies, including the study of DNA replication (reviewed in (Coen, 1996)). This review discusses the current knowledge of HSV-1 DNA replication fidelity with an emphasis on the role of DNA polymerase and other replicative proteins in regulating replication fidelity.

2. Antiviral therapy and emergence of resistant mutants

HSVs are ubiquitous human pathogens, causing significant public health issues. Although current antiviral drugs can effectively inhibit HSV replication, the increasing number of drug-resistance mutants is becoming a major problem in successful treatment of HSV diseases. Resistance to antiviral drugs arises from the development of mutations in viral genes that encode the antiviral target proteins. Antiviral drug treatment may provide an environment suitable for the emergence of resistant mutants, especially in immunocompromised patients, which confer the advantage to survive under antiviral drug pressure. Alternatively, spontaneous mutations may arise during drug treatment (reviewed in Kimberlin and Whitley, 1996). Although it can be debated that antiviral drugs may induce and/or enhance the selection and growth of drug-resistant mutants, it is generally believed that replication errors (spontaneous mutations) play a role in the development of mutations. Therefore, it is important to understand the regulatory mechanisms, including the replication errors and the subsequent repair processes, leading to the development of mutations during HSV DNA replication. This information can also be applied to understand the general mechanisms of how a cell controls and maintains certain degrees of DNA replication fidelity.

3. HSV-1 as a model for studying DNA replication fidelity

HSV-1 contains a linear double-stranded DNA genome with a size of 152 kbp, coding for approximately 80 open reading frames. HSV can be amended to delete or modify the genetic components, regardless of whether the gene is essential or non-essential for growth in cultured cells. This offers the advantage that the virus can be modified for a variety of biological, biochemical and genetic studies of each gene. For example, recombinant virus HP66, which is a HSV-1 polymerase catalytic subunit (*pol*) null mutant and contains a reporter gene, β-galactosidase, replaced parts of the *pol* sequences, had been constructed (Marcy, Yager, and Coen, 1990). Since Pol is essential for viral replication, such a recombinant virus can only be propagated in cells containing the integrated *pol* gene and expressing the Pol proteins, such as DP6 or Pol A5 cells (Hwang et al., 1997; Marcy, Yager, and Coen, 1990). Using this approach various *pol* mutant viruses, including the lethal mutants (Gibbs et al., 1991; Marcy, Yager, and Coen, 1990), can be constructed, propagated, and characterized.

3.1 HSV-1 for the study of DNA replication fidelity

While biochemical assays can measure the enzyme kinetics and the fidelity of the Pol *in vitro*, examination of the *in vivo* fidelity of DNA replication is more complicated than the *in vitro* enzymatic studies. Nonetheless molecular biological assays have been developed to examine DNA replication fidelity of HSV-1 in infected cells. The information obtained by the *in vivo* experiments together with kinetic data is invaluable for understanding the mechanisms regulating the fidelity of DNA replication. Three *in vivo* mutagenesis assays are discussed below.

3.1.1 TK mutagenesis assay

The TK (thymidine kinase) mutagenesis assay applies the principle that HSV-1 encoded TK enzyme is not essential for virus growth in proliferating cells in cultures and that it can specifically activate certain antiviral drugs, leading to the inhibition of viral growth. In another words, *tk* mutants that do not express the TK enzyme or express TK with altered substrate specificity can grow and form plaques in the presence of antiviral drug while those with functional TK that can activate the drugs fail to form plaques in plaque assay. Based on the unique property of the TK enzyme, Hall et al. (Hall et al., 1984) devised the TK mutagenesis assay to examine the mutation frequency of HSV-1.

For example, HSV-1 TK can induce the phosphorylation of the antiviral drug acyclovir (ACV), a guanosine analog. Following phosphorylation by TK enzyme, the mono-phosphate form of ACV is converted to di- and tri-phosphate ACV by cellular enzymes, allowing its incorporation into newly synthesized DNA by HSV Pol. Since ACV lacks the 3′-OH group on the acyclic ribose structure, its incorporation into nascent DNA blocks further extension from the 3′-terminus and inhibits viral DNA replication. Thus, HSV TK plays an essential role in activation of the antiviral drug, and HSV TK mutants that fail to activate ACV will become resistance and form plaques on cultured cells in the presence of ACV.

It is worth noting that the inhibitory effect of ACV triphosphate (ACV-TP) on viral Pol is mediated by a three-step mechanism (Reardon and Spector, 1989). In the first step, ACV-TP binds to Pol and acts as a competitive inhibitor of dGTP. The interaction between Pol and ACV-TP results in the incorporation of ACV monophosphate (ACV-MP) into the growing DNA chain, leading to chain termination. However, the inhibitory effect on Pol is dependent on the presence of the next nucleotide complementary to the next template base, which freezes the ACV-MP on the primer/template to form the dead-end complex (Reardon and Spector, 1989). Examination of certain Pol mutants containing mutations within the conserved Pol domain further demonstrate that a Pol resistance to ACV-TP can be due to the altered enzyme kinetics of K_m or K_{cat}, or both. Further information is discussed in (Huang et al., 1999). Furthermore, HSV Pol exhibits a much greater affinity for ACV-TP than does cellular Pol, which offers the specificity of inhibiting viral DNA replication with the very low toxicity of normal host cells (Furman et al., 1979).

Although *tk* mutants are easily identified in a simple plaque assay, this method may not be sensitive enough to detect all mutants, such as silent mutations and mutations that maintain enzyme activity. It is estimated that the TK mutagenesis assay can detect less than 50% of all possible substitutions of *tk* mutations (Hwang, Liu, and Hwang, 2002). Despite this, an extensive study (Lu, Hwang, and Hwang, 2002a) of *tk* mutants derived from wild-type HSV-1 strain KOS found that HSV replicates DNA with a genomic mutation rate similar to those of other DNA-based microbes (Drake and Hwang, 2005). However, earlier studies (Hall et al., 1984; Hall et al., 1985; Parris and Harrington, 1982; Hwang and Chen, 1995) demonstrated a roughly 10-fold higher mutation frequency than those (Hwang et al., 1997; Lu, Hwang, and Hwang, 2002a) used to calculate the mutation rate. Whether the selection methods (the use of antiviral drugs), experimental bias, or other unknown factors, such as the virus stocks and/or host cells used, could lead to the differences require further studies. Perhaps it is important to examine clinical isolates with limited passages in cell cultures, which may avoid the viral adaptation. Nevertheless, the study by Lu et al. (Lu, Hwang, and Hwang, 2002a) demonstrates that HSV-1 *pol* mutants can replicate the *tk* gene with different mutation spectra (see below).

3.1.2 *Lac Z* mutagenesis assay

The *lacZ* mutagenesis assay has also been applied to examine the mutation frequency of the *lacZ* gene when it is inserted into the viral genome (Hwang et al., 2003; Pyles and Thompson, 1994). This assay is based on observing the relative ratio of the number of white/light blue plaques over the total number of plaques examined by plaque assay after X-Gal staining. The advantage of this assay is its simple procedure of X-Gal staining of the plaques formed on cultured monolayers. However, identifying plaques with mutated *lacZ* genes may not be as simple as expected since bias could be derived from cells infected with a mixture of viruses containing wild-type and mutated *lacZ* genes; a similar bias also can be observed in the TK mutagenesis assay. This method may not be sensitive enough to detect all mutations, similar to the sensitivity issue of the TK mutagenesis assay. Therefore, we developed a more sensitive mutagenesis assay, the *supF* mutagenesis assay to study the replication fidelity of HSV.

3.1.3 *SupF* mutagenesis assay

The *supF* mutagenesis assay (Fig. 1) was first introduced by Seidman and colleagues (Seidman et al., 1985) to examine the mutagenic effect of carcinogens in mammalian cells using a shuttle plasmid containing SV40 DNA sequences for its replication in SV40-permissive cells and an *E. coli* amplicon for recovering DNA from *E. coli*. The shuttle plasmid contains the *supF* gene, which is a bacterial suppressor tRNA gene that can serves as a mutagenesis marker. The *supF* gene can suppress the amber codon present in the β-galactosidase (*lacZ*) gene, forming blue colonies in the presence of X-gal and IPTG in *E. coli* host that harbor the amber mutation in the *lacZ* gene. Mutated and inactivated *supF* genes, on the other hand, fail to suppress the amber mutation and are unable to express the β-galactosidase enzyme, and thus, produce white colonies. Measuring the ratio of the number of white/light blue colonies over the total number of colonies reveals the mutation frequency. Furthermore, the short coding sequences (~90 bp) can be easily sequenced to identify the mutation. Other advantages of the *supF* mutagenesis assay include the low spontaneous mutation background and that more than 96% of possible changes in the *supF* gene have been demonstrated to become inactive and fail to express blue colonies. Therefore, it is a very sensitive assay (reviewed in (Canella and Seidman, 2000)).

We have modified and inserted the *supF* amplicon into the *tk* locus, allowing measurement of the *supF* mutation frequency in the context of the viral genome during viral replication (Hwang and Hwang, 2003; Hwang, Liu, and Hwang, 2002; Hwang et al., 2004). Furthermore, the *supF* amplicon can be modified to contain the origin (*ori*) sequences

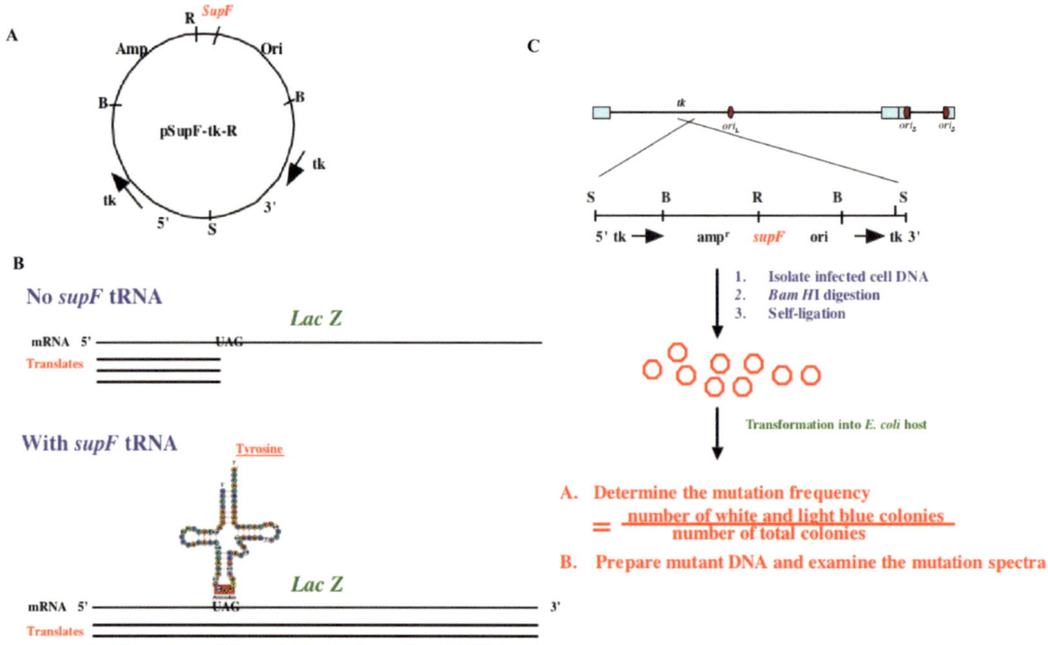

Fig. 1. *SupF* mutagenesis assay used in HSV-1 DNA replication fidelity. (A). Map of the plasmid DNA used for the construction of recombinant virus. (B). The action of *supF* tRNA in suppression of the amber codon in the *lacZ* gene in *E. coli*. In the absence of the *supF* tRNA only the truncated β-galatosidase proteins are translated due to the presence of an amber codon in the *lacZ* gene. In the presence of the *supF* tRNA the amber codon is suppressed by the insertion of a tyrosine residue and leads to the continuous synthesis of the full-length β-galatosidase protein. (C). Experimental procedures of the *supF* mutagenesis assay. The top line denotes the linear DNA of HSV-1. The relative locations of the thymidine kinase (*tk*) locus and origins of DNA replication (*oriL* and *oriS*) are shown. The components of an integrated *supF* amplicon within the *tk* locus are shown. The procedures of the mutagenesis assay are briefly illustrated.

required for HSV-1 DNA replication and applied as a shuttle plasmid for transient DNA replication in HSV-infected cells for the mutagenesis assay (Hwang et al., 1999), an assay similar to that applied by Seidman et al. (Seidman et al., 1985). The assay requires a minimal manipulation of DNA samples, which includes isolation and purification of total infected cell DNA, enzyme digestion, and ligation of the *supF*-containing amplicon. The *supF*-containing amplicon can then be recovered in *E. coli* for the blue/white selection and the measurement of the mutation frequency, again represented as the ratio of the number of white/light blue colonies to total number of colonies recovered. Figure 1 illustrates the *supF* mutagenesis assays used for the study of HSV-1 replication fidelity. Studies of recombinant viruses derived from the HSV-1 KOS strain and the transient replication assay using the modified shuttle plasmid have revealed that the KOS virus replicates the *supF* genes at a mutation frequency (Hwang, Liu, and Hwang, 2002; Hwang et al., 1999), which is consistent with that observed for the *supF* amplicon propagated in mammalian cells (Seidman et al., 1985).

4. Polymerase activity and DNA replication fidelity

4.1 Multiple activities of HSV-1 polymerase

DNA polymerase is the pivotal enzyme involved in DNA replication and fidelity. HSV-1 DNA polymerase is composed of the catalytic subunit encoded by the polymerase gene (*pol*) and the accessory protein processivity factor (or UL42) encoded by the *UL42* gene. The Pol subunit is a 1,235 amino acid polypeptide (Gibbs et al., 1988). It shares sequence homology with α-, δ-, and prokaryotic DNA Pols (Bernad et al., 1989; Brown, 2004) that contribute to the polymerization activity (the polymerase domain) and contains conserved motifs, namely Exo I, II, and III, common to other Pols possessing exonuclease activity (Bernad et al., 1989). Although a structural study reveals that HSV-1 Pol contains separated polymerase and exonuclease domains (Liu et al., 2006), the conserved δ-region C overlaps with the Exo III motif and the conserved region IV with the Exo II motif, suggesting the interdependence of DNA polymerase and its associated 3′-exonuclease proofreading activity (reviewed in (Coen, 1996)). In addition to these two functional components, HSV-1 Pol also contains a C-terminal domain that is required for Pol's interaction with the accessory protein UL42 (Digard and Coen, 1990). Fig. 2 depicts the regions of Pol possessing these functional domains or activities.

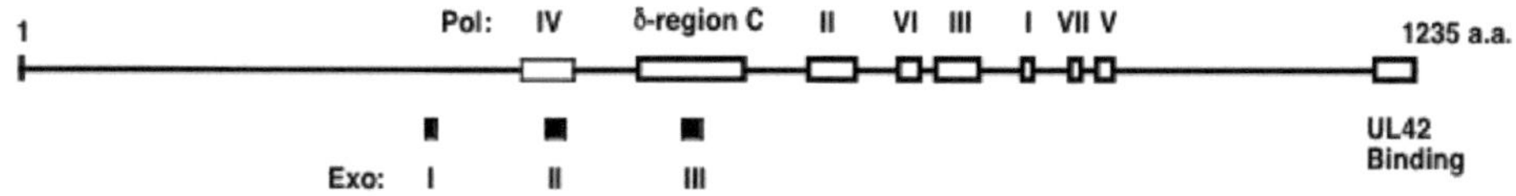

Fig. 2. Map of HSV-1 Pol polypeptide. The Pol protein is composed of 1,235 amino acids (a.a.). The labels above the line depict the relative locations of conserved regions I –VII and δ-region C, which are conserved among the polymerase domains of other Pol proteins. The labels below the line indicate the relative locations of conserved exonuclease motifs (Exo I, II, and III) and the UL42 binding domain located at the C terminus. The overlapping regions between the conserved polymerase and exonuclease sequences argue for the structural and functional interdependence of two activities.

Genetic and biochemical studies of mutations within the conserved regions of the polymerase domains confirm that these sequences are critical for the polymerase activity as mutations within these conserved regions confer altered sensitivity to certain antiviral drugs, which are nucleoside or pyrophosphate analogs (Gibbs et al., 1988; Hall et al., 1984; Hall et al., 1985). Regarding viral DNA replication fidelity, the effect of mutations in conserved regions of the polymerase domain, including those in both the polymerase and exonuclease domains, have been studied and summarized below.

4.2 Polymerase mutation affects the replication fidelity

The TK mutagenesis assay demonstrates that mutations in Pol can result in anti-mutator or mutator phenotypes (Hall et al., 1984; Hall et al., 1985). Such studies have provided the first evidence that HSV-1 Pol can regulate the replication fidelity of viral DNA and that TK mutagenesis is a useful means to measure the mutation frequency of HSV-1. Biochemical study has also demonstrated that mutant Pol can have the anti-mutator phenotype (PAA^{r}5) and that the improved fidelity can be attributed to the improved nucleotide selectivity (Hall et al., 1985). Sequencing has subsequently demonstrated that such a *pol* mutant contains a mutation within the conserved region of the polymerase domain (Gibbs et al., 1988). Examination of several *tk* mutants also demonstrates that the mutant Pol (PAA^{r}5) replicates the *tk* genes with different mutation types compared with those mediated by wild-type Pol (Hwang and Chen, 1995). PAA^{r}5 mutant Pol generates only frameshift changes, whereas the wild-type Pol generates tk mutants of both base substitutions and frameshift mutations at 1:1 ratio. Therefore, HSV-1 Pol is critical for regulating replication fidelity.

Enzymatic studies of wild-type and PAA^{r}5 Pols demonstrate that the mutant PAA^{r}5 Pol has higher K_m of nucleoside triphosphates (dNTPs) relative to wild-type Pol (Hall et al., 1985; Huang et al., 1999), suggesting that the mutant Pol may have the better selectivity of incoming dNTPs. Study of the HSV-1 Pol model, based on the known structure of RB69 Pol, also suggests that arginine residue 842 of HSV-1 Pol is in close proximity to the sugar ring of dNTPs and that the mutation of arginine to serine (R842S; conserved region III; Fig. 2) in PAA^{r}5 Pol may weaken the interaction of Pol with dNTPs.

The *supF* mutagenesis assay further demonstrates that the PAA^{r}5 mutant replicates DNA with an altered fidelity relative to the parental strain KOS virus. This mutant Pol induces differences in the type and distribution of base substitutions relative to those by wild-type Pol (Hwang, Liu, and Hwang, 2002), suggesting that the amino acid change in PAA^{r}5 Pol results in alterations in its replication fidelity. However, this mutant Pol has a modest mutator activity in replicating the *supF* gene (Hwang, Liu, and Hwang, 2002), which is in contrast to the anti-mutator activity observed by the TK mutagenesis assay (Hall et al., 1984; Hall et al., 1985; Hwang and Chen, 1995). Perhaps the sequence contents of the target genes contribute to the differences, similar to those observed for other Pols (reviewed in (Goodman et al., 1993)). Alternatively, the assay method could influence the outcomes of the studies (see below).

The *supF* mutagenesis study also revealed that another Pol mutant (L774F) has an anti-mutator phenotype (Hwang et al., 2004). This mutant contains a mutation in conserved region VI of the polymerase domain and confers altered drug sensitivities, supporting that this conserved region plays a role in forming the structural and functional polymerase active site. Studies of mutations in this conserved region of other Pols, together with the structural information of RB69 and HSV-1 Pols (Wang et al., 1997; Liu et al., 2006), suggest that conserved region VI has a functional role in the HSV-1 Pol interaction with incoming dNTPs. In relation to the thumb, palm and finger subdomains of Pol, the L774F mutation, with a hydrophobic phenylalanine replacing the leucine residue, may induce a local structure change of the finger subdomain and cause the finger subdomain to adapt a different orientation relative to other polymerase subdomains. The slight structural change of L774F may affect the relative position of the finger residues and subsequently lead to an altered catalytic reaction, binding affinity of dNTP and rate of polymerization, which may result in higher DNA replication fidelity (Hwang et al., 2004). Further enzymatic and structural studies of the mutant Pol will be necessary to demonstrate the proposed mechanism leading to the higher replication fidelity.

5. Pol's exonuclease activity and DNA replication fidelity

The 3′-5′ exonucleolytic proofreading activity plays a significant role in maintaining DNA replication fidelity. A Pol lacking the proofreading activity replicates DNA with a 10- to 100-fold less fidelity than that with such activity (reviewed in (Kunkel, 1988)).

5.1 Mutator phenotype of HSV-1 Pol with defective exonuclease activity

HSV-1 Pol has an intrinsic exonuclease activity that is mapped to the N-terminal half of the protein (Weisshart et al., 1994) and contains three conserved Exo motifs found in all Pols with proofreading activity. Mutations of the highly conserved residues within these Exo motifs result in the loss of exonuclease activity accompanied with the altered polymerase activity *in vitro* (Baker and Hall, 1998; Hall et al., 1995; Hwang et al., 1997; Kuhn and Knopf, 1996). However, the degree and extent of the altered polymerase activity due to the mutations within the Exo motifs vary from study to study. For example, the Exo I mutant of D368A was found to retain wild-type levels of polymerase activity and to extend from a mismatched base at the 3′-end of the primer (Kuhn and Knopf, 1996; Song et al., 2004), while another study demonstrated the failure of extension from a mismatched base (Baker and Hall, 1998). It is possible that the differences in assay conditions and the primer-templates used could lead to such differences. Nevertheless, it is evidenced that a Pol with defective exonuclease activity is highly mutagenic (Baker and Hall, 1998).

Studies of Exo III mutant Pols also demonstrate the roles of conserved residues Y577 and D581 on exonuclease activities. Mutants of Y577A, Y577H, D581A, and the double substitutions Y577H/D581A are defective in exonuclease activity and impaired in polymerase activity (Hwang et al., 1997; Kuhn and Knopf, 1996). The TK mutagenesis study demonstrates that Y577H and Y577H/D581A recombinant viruses are highly mutagenic relative to the parental wild-type virus (Hwang et al., 1997). On the other hand, the *supF* mutagenesis assay reveals the modest effects of the exonuclease activity on replication fidelity (Hwang, Liu, and Hwang, 2002). It is possible that different sequence content of the target genes could contribute to the difference of mutation frequency. Alternatively the assay method could play a key factor affecting the detection and measurement of mutations. For example, the TK mutagenesis assay can only identify the mutants among viable viruses, whereas the *supF* mutagenesis assay examines total DNA being replicated regardless of whether the mutations (in essential genes) are lethal. The higher magnitude of the mutation frequencies observed in the *tk* mutagenesis study may be theoretically explained by the fact that the *tk* mutation frequency could be amplified due to the increases of lethal mutations that reduces the total number of progeny viruses been analyzed on cell cultures. Nevertheless, the exonuclease-deficient Pol mutants replicate both target genes with significant difference of mutation spectra compared to those induced by the wild-type Pol (Hwang and Hwang, 2003; Lu, Hwang, and Hwang, 2002b).

5.2 Exonuclease deficient polymerase induces altered mutation spectra

Examining *tk* mutants derived from wild-type strain KOS demonstrates that the majority of drug-resistant *tk* mutants are frameshift mutations (45 out of 66 mutants examined; 67%), containing insertion or deletion of one or two nucleotides in the regions containing homonucleotide runs. In contrast, the Y7 recombinant virus, which contains the Y577H mutation in the Exo III motif, replicates the *tk* gene with significantly less frameshift mutations (21%; $p < 0.005$) relative to wild-type virus (Lu, Hwang, and Hwang, 2002b). Furthermore, although the majority of substitutions are transitional changes in mutants derived from both wild-type and exonuclease-deficient viruses, they distribute differently (Lu, Hwang, and Hwang, 2002b). These findings imply that HSV Pol can incorporate mispaired nucleotides, and most of the misinsertions are corrected by the proofreading activity during DNA synthesis. Furthermore, the Y577H mutation not only loses exonuclease activity but also alters the polymerase activity as it replicates misinsertions at positions distinct from those of wild-type Pol. Only 3 identical base substitutions are found among 15 and 52 *tk* mutations replicated by wild-type and exonuclease negative Pol, respectively (Lu, Hwang, and Hwang, 2002b). Theoretically, one would expect to observe more identical substitutions in both groups if the exonuclease Pol does not have altered polymerase activity. The observation that recombinant Y7 (Y577H) virus also exhibits altered drug sensitivities relative to wild-type virus further supports that the Exo III motif has a role on the polymerization activity (Hwang et al., 1998) and that the polymerase and exonuclease domains of HSV-1 Pol are interdependent structurally and functionally, also as suggested by the overlap between conserved δ-region C and Exo III motif (Fig. 2).

Not surprisingly, *supF* mutagenesis studies of the Exo III mutant demonstrate modest increases of the *supF* mutation frequency (Hwang and Hwang, 2003). This is sharply different from the several hundred fold increases of *tk* mutation frequency replicated by such mutant viruses (Hwang et al., 1997). Presumably the sequence content between two target genes and the assay methods, as discussed above, contribute to these differences. In agreement with these assumptions, the *in vitro* mutagenesis study of an Exo I mutant Pol using the *lacZα* reversion mutagenesis assay demonstrates increases of 3- to 18-fold in the reversion frequencies, depending on the dNTPs concentrations (Baker and Hall, 1998).

5.3 Enzyme kinetics of exonuclease deficient polymerase

Enzymatic studies of steady (and perhaps pre-steady) state kinetics of the Pol protein will provide information to illustrate the affinity of Pol on dNTPs within the context of a matched or mismatched 3′-terminus and the relative catalytic activity of Pol's incorporation of incoming dNTPs. Based on the kinetic data the extension efficiency and misinsertion efficiency of the Pol from a primer-template (p/t) can be obtained to indicate a possible mechanism of how a Pol discriminates between correct and incorrect nucleotide during the polymerization reaction. Although little information of enzyme kinetics is available, Baker and Hall (Baker and Hall, 1998) have demonstrated that both wild-type and the Exo I mutant Pol D368A have high affinity (low K_m) for correct nucleotide incorporation from a matched p/t, and these Pols exhibit extremely high K_m (in the order of 3 magnitudes) for nucleotide incorporation from a mismatched p/t. Furthermore, the kinetic data demonstrate that exonuclease activity is required for removal of the misinserted nucleotides by slowing the primer extension (low V_{max} for nucleotide incorporation at the mispaired 3′-termini) and reinsertion of the correct base to resume the efficient extension. Thus an enzyme lacking the ability to remove the mispaired base significantly reduces the extension efficiency from the mispaired 3′-termini. Consistent with the results discussed above, we observed that both Y577H and Y577H/D581A mutant Pols had altered K_m, V_{max}, and extension efficiency from mispaired 3′-termini dependent on the mismatched 3′-base. Furthermore, both mutant Pols exhibited increases in infidelity (f_{inc}), determined as the ratio of $(K_m/V_{max})_{incorrect}/(K_m/V_{max})_{correct}$ (unpublished data). Additional information of the kinetic approach addressing the mechanism affecting the fidelity of HSV-1 Pol can be found in a recent review (Zhu et al., 2010).

6. Processivity factor and DNA replication fidelity

6.1 UL42 functions as a processivity factor

The UL42 protein was originally identified as a non-specific double-stranded DNA (dsDNA) binding protein (Marsden et al., 1987; Powell and Purifoy, 1976) and was defined as a processivity factor for Pol (Gottlieb et al., 1990). Unlike other known processivity factors, UL42 binds DNA directly. It also directly interacts with the Pol subunit to form the Pol/UL42 heterodimer, which binds more tightly to the p/t-DNA than to single-stranded DNA (ssDNA). On the other hand, Pol alone binds more tightly to ssDNA than to p/t-DNA (Weisshart, Chow, and Coen, 1999). Therefore, the Pol/UL42 heterodimer exhibits a ~2-fold faster association rate and a ~10-fold slower dissociation rate to p/t-DNA than does Pol alone. However, the increased affinity and stability of the Pol/UL42 complex to p/t-DNA does not alter the elongation rate relative to Pol alone (Weisshart, Chow, and Coen, 1999). The increased half-life, but not the elongation rate, of UL42/Pol on p/t-DNA compared with the Pol subunit alone could afford a greater ability for the excision of a misincorporated base by the exonuclease activity intrinsic to wild-type Pol (Chaudhuri, Song, and Parris, 2003). This suggests that, in addition to its processivity, UL42 may enhance the fidelity of wild-type Pol in viral DNA replication via the exonuclease activity.

6.2 Processivity factor and replication fidelity

Although the effect of UL42 on DNA replication fidelity at the nucleotide level has not been examined, studies from other systems demonstrate that the processivity factor can influence replication fidelity. For example, the T7 Pol processivity factor thioredoxin can increase the fidelity of single-nucleotide insertions by an exonuclease-deficient T7 Pol. It can also increase the frequencies of certain base substitutions and deletions (Kunkel, Patel., and Johnson, 1994). These findings imply that slippage may occur during enzyme dissociation or reassociation and that thioredoxin enhances the processivity of Pol by preventing it from dissociating from the p/t, thereby reducing the slippage-mediated insertion mutations. Paradoxically, the reduced accuracy of certain base substitutions synthesized by T7 Pol in the presence of thioredoxin also implies that it promotes the extension of mismatches and misalignments. Therefore, the processivity factor can act as an anti-mutator factor in the slippage-mediated insertion mutations and as a mutator factor in base substitutions and deletions. Recent studies also demonstrate that the accessory protein gp45 of bacteriophage BR69 Pol can modulate site-specific mutation rates in the target gene compared to those by the Pol alone, although the overall mutation rate increases only modestly (Bebenek et al., 2002; Bebenek et al., 2005). The sliding clamp protein PCNA that enhances the processivity of replicative DNA Pol in eukaryotes can promote the bypass of DNA lesions (Mozzherin et al., 1997; O'Day, Burgers, and Taylor, 1992) and acts as a mutator factor. Studies have also demonstrated that mutations in genes encoding PCNA or subunits of replication factor C

(RFC) increase mutation frequency *in vivo* (Chen et al., 1999; Johnson et al., 1996; McAlear et al., 1994; McAlear, Tuffo, and Holm, 1996; Umar et al., 1996).

Several UL42 mutations that increase or decrease DNA binding without affecting its interaction with Pol have been constructed (Komazin-Meredith et al., 2008; Randell et al., 2005). These studies suggest that UL42 interacts with DNA via interaction between the basic charged residues located on the surface of the molecule and the negatively charged DNA. Recombinant viruses expressing UL42 with increased DNA binding exhibits impaired phenotypes, including the formation of smaller plaques, decrease replication of progeny and synthesis of DNA with higher ratio of DNA copies per plaque forming unit (PFU) (Jiang et al., 2009). As expected the mutants are more mutagenic than the control virus expressing wild type UL42 (Jiang et al., 2009). Similarly mutants with decreased DNA binding also have defective phenotypes and are highly mutagenic (Jiang et al., 2007a), and that mutants with no detectable DNA binding are deleterious in viral growth and DNA synthesis (Jiang et al., 2007b). These studies provide information that UL42 cannot bind DNA too tightly or too weakly and that any perturbation of DNA binding can impact virus production and replication fidelity. Future studies of the effects of mutation on the enzyme kinetics and on the mutation spectra at the nucleotide level will be invaluable for understanding the mechanisms attributed to UL42 in regulating DNA replication fidelity.

7. Nucleotide metabolism enzymes and DNA replication fidelity

In addition to the TK enzyme, HSV-1 also encodes several genes expressing nucleotide metabolism enzymes, including deoxyuridine triphosphatease (dUTPase), uracil-N-glycosidase (UNG), and ribonucleotide redutase (RR). The dUTPase can convert dUTP to dUMP, which can subsequently lead to an increased dTTP pool and a decreased dUTP pool. The UNG enzyme can remove uracil bases, which are resulted from deamination of cytosines, on DNA. The activity of RR is to convert ribonucleoside diphosphates to the corresponding deoxyribonucleoside diphosphates. Theoretically, these enzymes may act to maintain an optimal condition favoring HSV-1 DNA replication. The study of Pyles and Thompson (Pyles and Thompson, 1994), however, demonstrates intriguing results of how viruses lacking the expression of these enzymes affect the replication fidelity in infected cells. Using recombinant viruses containing a deletion of tested genes and the *lacZ* reporter system the viral dUTPase is shown to have an antimutator activity, whereas the viral TK has the mutator activity. While the UNG^- viruses replicated the *lacZ* gene with no significant difference of the mutation frequency relative to that of UNG^+ recombinants, continuous passage of UNG^- viruses lead an increased mutation frequency, suggesting its antimutator activity. Furthermore, the interaction between UNG and Pol and the association of UNG with viral replisome also suggest a role UNG in regulating DNA replication fidelity (Bogani et al., 2010). There is no information whether HSV-1 encoded ribonucleotide redutase plays a role on replication fidelity.

In contrast to the observed mutator activity of the TK enzyme (Pyles and Thompson, 1994), we demonstrated that the TK enzyme of strain KOS does not possess the mutator activity; recombinant viruses harboring either the *lacZ* or *supF* gene replicate both genes with equal fidelity in HSV-1 TK expressing or non-expressing cells (Hwang et al., 2003). Although it is not clear what the factor leads to the difference, one may wonder why the virus were encoding a mutagenic gene. However, it is also important to note that each recombinant virus, including those used to establish the baseline relative mutation frequency, constructed by Pyles and Thompson (Pyles and Thompson, 1994) harbors the integrated *lacZ* gene at different location in the viral genome, which may affect the replication fidelity (see section 8.2). Further studies using recombinant viruses containing the reporter gene integrated at the defined location and with or without the expression of gene to be examined are necessary to demonstrate the effects of these nucleotide metabolism enzymes on replication fidelity.

8. Other factors may affect the replication fidelity

8.1 Single-stranded DNA binding protein and replication fidelity

Little information is available regarding the contribution of other accessory proteins in DNA replication fidelity. However, a recent *in vitro* study of DNA replication fidelity using RB69 Pol with and without accessory proteins, including single-stranded DNA binding protein (SSB), the processivity clamp, and the clamp-loading proteins, demonstrated that these proteins induced altered mutation rates in a site-specific manner, although the overall mutation rate of the target gene did not differ significantly relative to that by Pol alone (Bebenek et al., 2002; Bebenek et al., 2005). Thus, SSB protein and the other accessory proteins also play a role on replication fidelity.

Our previous study examining the effect of an exonuclease-deficient Pol mutant, Y7(Y577H), on replication fidelity suggests the possibility that other DNA replicative proteins may have effects on regulating the replication fidelity (Hwang and Hwang, 2003). The mutagenic ability of the exonuclease-deficient Y7 Pol is expected to generate various mutations in the entire genome, including genes coding for Pol and other replicative proteins, and result in heterogeneous populations in viral stocks. Examining the *pol* gene sequences confirms the presence of heterogeneous *pol* sequences in a single viral stock. Marker rescue experiments in which the mutated *pol* is rescued to the wild-type sequences demonstrate that several rescued recombinants exhibit higher fidelity than those with wild-type Pol. These allow one to test the hypotheses that there are mutations in other replicative genes, which may contribute to the higher replication fidelity of the *supF* gene. It is also important to explore the mechanisms by which SSB may regulate replication fidelity in infected cells since this protein associates and colocalizes with cellular DNA repair and recombination proteins (Taylor and Knipe, 2004; Wilkinson and Weller, 2004) and the SSB protein is able to promote recombination *in vitro* (Nimonkar and Boehmer, 2002; Nimonkar and Boehmer, 2003; Nimonkar and Boehmer, 2004; Reuven et al., 2004). Along this line the contributions of other cellular replicative proteins in HSV DNA replication warrant for future studies.

8.2 Can the position of target gene influence replication fidelity?

The genomes of all alpha-herpesviruses, including HSV-1, are composed of unique long (UL) and short (US) sequences and repeated sequences that segment the unique regions. Study of proteins conserved among six alpha-herpesviruses reveals that US proteins are more divergent than those encoded by UL sequences (Brown, 2004). The study further indicates that proteins encoded by sequences at the repeat regions, UL1, UL56, US1, and US12, are highly divergent than those of other regions (Brown, 2004). This observation suggests that selective sequences within the viral genome have a comparatively rapid evolutionary rate or high mutation rate. It is possible that the virus has evolved to arrange the sequences in clusters that can be the targets of different mutation rates. If this is the case, then one may speculate that HSV may have position-dependent DNA replication fidelity, which we have described as the position effect (Hwang et al., 2003). This may also explain that the proteins clustered in the middle of the UL regions (between UL27 and UL33) are highly conserved as they are essential for viral replication. However, two proteins required for viral DNA replication, UL42 and UL8, that encode a helicase/primase subunit are highly divergent. Perhaps, these essential proteins quickly evolved to have multiple functions to include differential activity critical for each virus's life cycle.

8.3 Sequence context, replication mode and replication fidelity

Consistent with other studies (reviewed in (Goodman et al., 1993), *tk* and *supF* mutagenesis assays also demonstrate that the sequence content affects HSV-1 replication fidelity. We demonstrate that the *supF* mutation spectra observed in the plasmid-borne replication assay differ from those replicated as a part of viral genome (Hwang, Liu, and Hwang, 2002; Hwang et al., 1999). The differences could be related to the mechanism of how DNA is replicated in infected cells. For example, viral genome replication involves the formation of head to tail arranged DNA concatemers and branched structure, presumably mediated by a recombination mechanism; the processing and cleavage of complex DNA molecules are required for DNA packaging and maturation of viral particles (Bataille and Epstein, 1997; Slobedman, Zhang, and Simmons, 1999). On the other hand, the *ori*-based plasmid may not replicate by the same mechanisms. It is reasonable to hypothesize that the lack of viral repeat sequences in the *ori*-containing plasmid DNA may not form isomers similar to those observed in genomic DNA replication, and that the mechanisms involved in branch DNA formation may not be obvious. Further studies are required to determine whether the plasmid-borne DNA is replicated with a different mechanism relative to viral genomic DNA replication.

9. Conclusions

A large body of literature discusses DNA replication fidelity in both prokaryotic and eukaryotic cells, yet limited information is available regarding how HSV DNA replication is regulated to maintain a certain degree of fidelity. Understanding the mechanisms regulating HSV DNA replication fidelity may lead to comprehension of how drug resistant mutants develop. The proteins that regulate replication fidelity definitely play roles in HSV DNA replication. In the aspect of antiviral therapy, the knowledge gained from such studies may lead to the design of new strategies to combat HSV diseases.

10. Acknowledgement

I thank C. W. Knopf, J. W. Drake, D. M. Coen and L. B. Crawford for valuable comments on this article. The study was supported by NIH grant AI056359.

11. References

Baker, R. O., and Hall, J. D. (1998). Impaired Mismatch Extension by a Herpes Simplex DNA Polymerase Mutant with an Editing Nuclease Defect. *Journal of Biological Chemistry* Vol.273, No.37, pp. 24075-24082.

Bataille, D., and Epstein, A. L. (1997). Equimolar generation of the four possible arrangements of adjacent L components in herpes simplex virus type 1 replicative intermediates. *Journal of Virology* Vol.71, No.10, pp. 7736-7743.

Bebenek, A., Carver, G. T., Dressman, H. K., Kadyrov, F. A., Haseman, J. K., Petrov, V., Konigsberg, W. H., Karam, J. D., and Drake, J. W. (2002). Dissecting the fidelity of bacteriophage RB69 DNA polymerase: site-specific modulation of fidelity by polymerase accessory proteins. *Genetics* Vol.162, No.3, pp. 1003-1018.

Bebenek, A., Carver, G. T., Kadyrov, F. A., Kissking, G. E., and Drake, J. W. (2005). Processivity clamp gp45 and ssDNA-binding-protein gp32 modulate the fidelity of bacteriophage RB69 polymerase in a sequence-specific manner, sometime enhancing and sometimes compromising accuracy. *Genetics* Vol,169, No.4, pp. 1815-1824.

Bernad, A., Blanco, L., Lazaro, J. M., Martin, G., and Salas, M. (1989). A conserved 3'- 5' exonuclease active site in prokaryotic and eukaryotic DNA polymerases. *Cell* 59, Vol.59, No.1, pp. 219-228.

Bogani, F., Corredeira, I., Fernandez, V., Sattler, U., Rutvisuttinunt, W., Defais, M., and Boehmer, P. E. (2010). Association between the herpes simplex virus-1 DNA polymerase and uracil DNA glycosylase. *Journal of Biological Chemistry* Vol.285, No.36, pp. 27664-27672.

Brown, J. (2004). Effect of gene location on the evolutionay rate of amino acid substitutions in herpes simplex virus proteins. *Virology* Vol.330, No.1, pp. 209-220.

Canella, K. A., and Seidman, M. M. (2000). Mutation spectra in *SupF*: Approaches to elucidating sequence context effects. *.Mutation Research* Vol.450, No.1, pp. 61-73.

Chaudhuri, M., Song, L., and Parris, D. S. (2003). The Herpes Simplex Virus Type 1 DNA Polymerase Processivity Factor Increases Fidelity without Altering Pre-steady-state Rate Constants for Polymerization or Excision. *Journal of Biological Chemistry* Vol.278, No.11, pp. 8996-9004.

Chen, C., Merrill, B., Lau, P., Holm, C., and Kolodner, R. D. (1999). Saccharomyces cerevisiae pol30 (Proliferating Cell Nuclear Antigen) mutations impair replication fidelity and mismatch repair. *Molecular and Cellular Biology* Vo.19, No.11, pp. 7801-7815.

Coen, D. M. (1996). Viral DNA polymerases. In: DNA replication in eukaryotic cells. Monograph 31. (Ed. Depamphilis, M. L.) Cold Spring harbor, N. Y. pp. 495-523.

Digard, P., and Coen, D. M. (1990). A novel functional domain of an alpha-like DNA polymerase. The binding site on the herpes simplex virus polymerase for the viral UL42 protein. *Journal of Biological Chemistry* Vol.265, No.29, pp. 17393-17396.

Drake, J. W., and Hwang, C. B. C. (2005). On the mutation rate of herpes simplex virus type 1. *Genetics* Vol.170, No.2, pp. 969-970.

Furman, P. A., St. Clair, M. H., Fyte, J. A., Rideout, J. L., Keller, P. M., and Elion, G. B. (1979). Inhibition of herpes simplex virus induced DNA polymerase activity and viral DNA replication of 9-(2-hydroxyethoxymethyl)guanine and its triphosphate. *Journal of Viorlogy* Vol.32, No.1, pp. 72-77.

Gibbs, J. S., Chiou, H. C., Bastow, K. F., Cheng, Y. C., and Coen, D. M. (1988). Identification of amino acids in herpes simplex virus DNA polymerase involved in substrate and drug recognition. *Proceedings of the National Academy of Sciences of the United States of America* Vol.85, No.18, pp. 6672-6676.

Gibbs, J. S., Weisshart, K., Digard, P., deBruynKops, A., Knipe, D. M., and Coen, D. M. (1991). Polymerization activity of an α-like DNA polymerase requires a conserved 3' - 5' exonuclease active site. *Molecular and Cellular Biology* Vol.11, No.9, pp. 4786-4795.

Goodman, M. F., Creighton, S., Bloom, L. B., and Petruska, J. (1993). Biochemical basis of DNA replication fidelity. *Critical Reviews of Biochemistry and Molecular Biology* Vol.28, No.2, pp. 83-126.

Gottlieb, J., Marcy, A. I., Coen, D. M., and Challberg, M. D. (1990). The herpes simplex virus type 1 UL42 gene product: a subunit of DNA polymerase that functions to increase processivity. *Journal of Virology* Vol.64, No.12, pp. 5976-5987.

Hall, J. D., Coen, D. M., Fisher, B. L., Weisslitz, M., Randall, S., Almy, R. E., Gelep, P. T., and Schaffer, P. A. (1984). Generation of genetic diversity in herpes simplex virus: an antimutator phenotype maps to the DNA polymerase locus. *Virology* Vol.132, No.1, pp. 26-37.

Hall, J. D., Furman, P. A., St. Clair, M. H., and Knopf, C. W. (1985). Reduced *in vivo* mutagenesis by mutant herpes simplex DNA polymerase involves improved nucleotide selection. *Proceedings of the National Academy of Sciences of the United States of America* Vol.82, No.11, pp. 3889-3893.

Hall, J. D., Orth, K. L., Sander, K. L., Swihart, B. M., and Senese, R. A. (1995). Mutations within conserved motifs in the 3'-5' exonuclease domain of herpes simplex virus DNA polymerase. *Journal of General Virology* Vol.76, No.12, pp. 2999-3008.

Huang, L., Ishii, K. K., Zuccola, H., Gehring, A. M., Hwang, C. B., Hogle, J., and Coen, D. M. (1999). The enzymological basis for resistance of herpesvirus DNA polymerase mutants to acyclovir: relationship to the structure of alpha-like DNA polymerases. *Proceedings of the National Academy of Sciences of the United States of America* Vol.96, No.2, pp. 447-52.

Hwang, C. B. C., and Chen, H. J.-H. (1995). An altered spectrum of herpes simplex virus mutations mediated by an antimutator DNA polymerase. *Gene* Vol.152, pp. 191-193.

Hwang, Y. T., and Hwang, C. B. C. (2003). Exonuclease-deficient polymerase mutant of herpes simplex virus type 1 induces altered spectra of mutations. *Journal of Virology* Vol.77, No.5, pp. 2946-2955.

Hwang, Y. T., Liu, B.-Y., and Hwang, C. B. C. (2002). Replication fidelity of the SupF gene integrated in the thymidine kinase locus of herpes simplex virus type 1. *Journal of Virology* Vol.76, No8, pp.3605-3614.

Hwang, Y. T., Liu, B. Y., Coen, D. M., and Hwang, C. B. (1997). Effects of mutations in the Exo III motif of the herpes simplex virus DNA polymerase gene on enzyme activities, viral replication, and replication fidelity. *Journal of Virology* Vol.71, No.10, pp.7791-7798.

Hwang, Y. T., Liu, B. Y., Hong, C. Y., Shillitoe, E. J., and Hwang, C. B. C. (1999). Effects of exonuclease activity and nucleotide selectivity of the herpes simplex virus DNA polymerase on the fidelity of DNA replication in vivo. *Journal of Virology* Vol.73, No.7, pp. 5326-5332.

Hwang, Y. T., Smith, J. F., Gao, L., and Hwang, C. B. (1998). Mutations in the Exo III motif of the herpes simplex virus DNA polymerase gene can confer altered drug sensitivities. *Virology* Vol.246, pp. 298-305.

Hwang, Y. T., Wang, Y.-A., Lu, Q., and Hwang, C. B. C. (2003). Thymidine kinase of herpes simplex virus type 1 strain KOS lacks mutator activity. *Virology* Vol.305, pp. 388-396.

Hwang, Y. T., Zuccola, H. J., Lu, Q., and Hwang, C. B. C. (2004). A Point Mutation within Conserved Region VI of Herpes Simplex Virus Type 1 DNA Polymerase Confers Altered Drug Sensitivity and Enhances Replication Fidelity. *Journal of Virology* Vol.78, No.2, pp. 650-657.

Jiang, C., Hwang, Y. T., Randell, J. C., Coen, D. M., and Hwang, C. B. (2007a). Mutations that decrease DNA binding of the processivity factor of the herpes simplex virus DNA polymerase reduce viral yield, alter the kinetics of viral DNA replication, and decrease the fidelity of DNA replication. *Journal of Virology* Vol.81, No.7, pp. 3495-3502.

Jiang, C., Hwang, Y. T., Wang, G., Randell, J. C., Coen, D. M., and Hwang, C. B. (2007b). Herpes simplex virus mutants with multiple substitutions affecting DNA binding of UL42 are impaired for viral replication and DNA synthesis. *Journal of Virology* Vol.81, No.21, pp. 12077-12079.

Jiang, C., Komazin-Meredith, G., Tian, W., Coen, D. M., and Hwang, C. B. C. (2009). Mutations That Increase DNA Binding by the Processivity Factor of Herpes Simplex Virus Affect Virus Production and DNA Replication Fidelity. *Journal of Virology* Vol.83, No.15, pp. 7573-7580.

Johnson, R. E., Kovvali, G. K., Guzder, S. N., Amin, N. S., Holm, C., Habraken, Y., Sung, P., Prakash, L., and Prakash, S. (1996). Evidence for the involvement of proliferating cell nuclear antigene in DNA mismatch repair. *Journal of Biological Chemistry* Vol.271, No.45, pp. 27987-27990.

Kimberlin, D. W., and Whitley, R. J. (1996). Antiviral resistance: mechanisms, clinical significance, and future implications. *Journal of Antimicrobial and Chemotherapy* Vol.37, No.37, pp. 403-421.

Komazin-Meredith, G., Santos, W. L., Filman, D. J., Hogle, J. M., Verdine, G. L., and Coen, D. M. (2008). The positively charged surface of herpes simplex virus UL42 mediates DNA binding. *Journal of Biological Chemistry* Vol.283, No.10, pp. 6154-61.

Kuhn, F. J. P., and Knopf, C. W. (1996). Herpes Simplex Virus Type 1DNA Polymerase. Mutational analysis of the 3' - 5' exonuclease domain. *Journal of Biological Chemistry* Vol.271, No.46, pp. 29245-29254.

Kunkel, T. A. (1988). Exonucleolytic proofreading. *Cell* Vol.53, No.6, pp. 837-840.

Kunkel, T. A., Patel., S. S., and Johnson, K. A. (1994). Error-Prone Replication of Repeated DNA Sequences by T7 DNA Polymerase in the Absence of its Processivity Subunit.

Proceedings of the National Academy of Sciences of the United States of America Vol.91, No.15, pp. 6830-6834.

Liu, S., Knafels, J. D., Chang, J. S., Waszak, G. A., Baldwin, E. T., Deibel, M. R., Jr., Thomsen, D. R., Homa, F. L., Wells, P. A., Tory, M. C., Poorman, R. A., Gao, H., Qiu, X., and Seddon, A. P. (2006). Crystal structure of the herpes simplex virus 1 DNA polymerase. Journal of Biological Chemistry Vol.281, No.26, pp. 18193-18200.

Lu, Q., Hwang, Y. T., and Hwang, C. B. (2002a). Detection of mutations within the thymidine kinase gene of herpes simplex virus type 1 by denaturing gradient gel electrophoresis. *Journal of Virological Methods* Vol.99, No.1-2, pp. 1-7.

Lu, Q., Hwang, Y. T., and Hwang, C. B. C. (2002b). Mutation Spectra of Herpes Simplex Virus Type 1 Thymidine Kinase Mutants. *Journal of Virology* Vol.76, No.11, pp. 5822-5828.

Marcy, A. I., Yager, D. R., and Coen, D. M. (1990). Isolation and characterization of herpes simplex virus mutants containing enigneered mutations at the DNA polymerase locus. *Journal of Viorlogy* Vol.64, No.5, pp. 2208-2216.

Marsden, H. S., Campbell, M. E. M., Haarr, L., Frame, M. C., Parris, D. S., Murphy, M., Hope, R. G., Muller, M. T., and Preston, C. M. (1987). The 65,000-M_r DNA-binding and virion *trans*-inducing proteins of herpes simplex virus type 1. *Journal of Virology* Vol.61, No.8, pp. 2428-2437.

McAlear, M. A., Howell, E. A., Espenshade, K. K., and Holm, C. (1994). McAlear, M. A., Howell, E. A., Espenshade, K. K., and Holm, C. (1994). Proliferating cell nuclear antigen (pol30) mutations suppress cdc44 mutations and identify potential regions of interaction between the two encoded proteins. *Molecular and Cellular Biology* Vol.14, No.7, pp. 4390-4397.

McAlear, M. A., Tuffo, K. M., and Holm, C. (1996). The large subunit of replication factor C (Rfc1p/Cdc44p) is required for DNA replication and DNA repair in Saccharomyces cerevisiae. *Genetics*
Vo1.42, No.1, pp. 65-78.

Mozzherin, D. J., Shibutani, S., Tan, C. K., Downey, K. M., and A., F. P. (1997). Proliferating cell nuclear antigen promotes DNA synthesis past template lesions by mammalian DNA polymerase delta. *Proceedings of the National Academy of Sciences of the United States of America* Vol.94, No.12, pp. 6126-6131.

Nimonkar, A. V., and Boehmer, P. E. (2002). In Vitro Strand Exchange Promoted by the Herpes Simplex Virus Type-1 Single Strand DNA-binding Protein (ICP8) and DNA Helicase-Primase. *Journal of Biological Chemistry* Vol.277, No.17, pp. 15182-15189.

Nimonkar, A. V., and Boehmer, P. E. (2003). Reconstitution of recombination-dependent DNA synthesis in herpes simplex virus 1. *Proceedings of the National Academy of Sciences of the United States of America* Vol.100, No.18, pp. 10201-10206.

Nimonkar, A. V., and Boehmer, P. E. (2004). Role of Protein-Protein Interactions during Herpes Simplex Virus Type 1 Recombination-dependent Replication. *J. Biol. Chem.* 279, 21957-21965.

O'Day, C. L., Burgers, P. M., and Taylor, J. S. (1992). PCNA-induced DNA synthesis past cis-syn and trans-syn-I thymine dimers by calf thymus DNA polymerase delta in vitro. *Nucleic Acids Research* Vol.20, No.20, pp. 5403-5406.

Parris, D. S., and Harrington, J. E. (1982). Herpes simplex virus variants resistant to high concentrations of acyclovir exist in clincal isolates. *Antimicrobial Agents and Chemotherapy* Vol.22, No.1, 71-77.

Powell, K. L., and Purifoy, D. J. M. (1976). DNA-binding proteins of cells infected with herpes simplex virus type 1 and type 2. *Intervirology* Vol.7, No.4-5, pp. 225-239.

Pyles, R. B., and Thompson, R. L. (1994). Mutations in accessory DNA replicating functions alter the relative mutation frequency of herpes simplex virus type 1 strains in cultured murine cells. *Journal of Virology* Vol.68, No.7, pp. 4514-4524.

Randell, J. C., Komazin, G., Jiang, C., Hwang, C. B., and Coen, D. M. (2005). Effects of substitutions of arginine residues on the basic surface of herpes simplex virus UL42 support a role for DNA binding in processive DNA synthesis. *Journal of Virology* Vol.79, No.18, pp. 12025-34.

Reardon, J. E., and Spector, T. (1989). Herpes simplex virus type 1 DNA polymerase. Mechanism of inhibition by acyclovir triphosphate. *Journal of Biological Chemistry* Vol.264, No.32, pp. 7405-7411.

Reuven, N. B., Willcox, S., Griffith, J. D., and Weller, S. K. (2004). Catalysis of strand exchange by the HSV-1 UL12 and ICP8 proteins: potent ICP8 recombinase activity is revealed upon resection of dsDNA substrate by nuclease. *Journal of Molecular Biology* Vol.342, No.1, pp. 57-71.

Seidman, M. M., Dixon, K., Razzaque, A., Zagursky, R. J., and Berman, M. L. (1985). A shuttle vector plasmid for studying carcinogen-induced point mutations in mammalian cells Gene. *Gene* Vol.38, 233-237.

Slobedman, B., Zhang, X., and Simmons, A. (1999). Herpes Simplex Virus Genome Isomerization: Origins of Adjacent Long Segments in Concatemeric Viral DNA. *Journal of Virology* Vol.73, No.1, pp. 810-813.

Song, L., Chaudhuri, M., Knopf, C. W., and Parris, D. S. (2004). Contribution of the 3'- to 5'-Exonuclease Activity of Herpes Simplex Virus Type 1 DNA Polymerase to the Fidelity of DNA Synthesis. *Journal of Biological Chemistry* Vol.279, No.18, pp. 18535-18543.

Taylor, T. J., and Knipe, D. M. (2004). Proteomics of herpes simplex virus replication compartments: association of cellular DNA replication, repair, recombination, and chromatin remodeling proteins with ICP8. *Journal of Virology* Vol.78, No.11, pp. 5856-5866.

Umar, A., Buermeyer, A. B., Simon, J. A., Thomas, D. C., Clark, A. B., Liskay, R. M., and Kunkel, T. A. (1996). Requirement for PCNA in DNA mismatch repair at a step preceding DNA resynthesis. *Cell* Vol.87, No.1, pp. 65-73.

Wang, J., Sattar, A. K., Wang, C. C., Karam, J. D., Konigsberg, W. H., and Steitz, T. A. (1997). Crystal structure of a pol α family replication DNA polymerase from bacteriophage RB69. *Cell* Vol.89, No.7, pp. 1087-1099.

Weisshart, K., Chow, C. S., and Coen, D. M. (1999). Herpes simplex virus processivity factor UL42 imparts increased DNA-binding specificity to the viral DNA polymerase and decreased dissociation from primer-template without reducing the elongation rate. *Journal of Virology* Vol.73, No.1, pp. 55-66.

Weisshart, K., Kuo, A. A., Hwang, C. B., Kumura, K., and Coen, D. M. (1994). Structural and functional organization of herpes simplex virus DNA polymerase investigated by limited proteolysis. *Journal of Biological Chemistry* Vol.269, No.36, pp. 22788-22796.

Wilkinson, D. E., and Weller, S. K. (2004). Recruitment of cellular recombination and repair proteins to sites of herpes simplex virus type 1 DNA replication is dependent on the composition of viral proteins within prereplicative sites and correlates with the induction of the DNA damage response. *Journal of Virology* Vol.78, No.9, pp. 4783-4796.

Zhu, Y;., Stroud, J., Somg, L., and Parris D. S. (2010). Kinetic approaches to understanding the mechanisms of fidelity of the herpes simplex virus type 1 DNA polymerase. *Journal of Nucleic Acids* Vol.2010, ID 631595. Doi:10,4061/631595

8

DNA Polymerase Processivity Factor of Human Cytomegalovirus May Be a Key Molecule for Molecular Coupling of Viral DNA Replication to Transcription

Hiroki Isomura
Division of Virology, Aichi Cancer Center Research Institute
Japan

1. Introduction

Human cytomegalovirus (HCMV) is a member of the betaherpesvirus family. Like all herpesviruses, HCMV is an enveloped, double-stranded DNA virus. The genome of HCMV is 240,000 bp in size with at least 150 known open reading frames (ORFs) (Dunn, Chou et al. 2003). A majority of the ORFs are nonessential for viral replication in cell culture. These nonessential ORFs likely encode proteins with redundant functions or proteins that may be required for replication in the human host. In addition, several ORFs are beneficial but not required for replication. However, approximately one-quarter, or 41 ORFs, are absolutely required for viral replication (Yu, Silva et al. 2003). The UL44 gene is essential.

During productive infection, HCMV genes are expressed in a temporal cascade, designated immediate early (IE), delayed early, and late. The major IE genes (MIE) UL123/122 (IE1/IE2) play a critical role in subsequent viral gene expression and the efficiency of viral replication (Meier and Stinski 1997; Meier and Pruessner 2000; Meier, Keller et al. 2002; Isomura and Stinski 2003; Isomura, Tsurumi et al. 2004; Isomura, Stinski et al. 2005). The IE72 protein, the predominant product of the IE1 transcript, is encoded by exons 2 and 3 spliced to exon 4. The IE86 protein, the predominant product of the IE2 transcript, is encoded by exons 2 and 3 spliced to exon 5. Translation of the IE1 and IE2 transcripts begins in exon 2. The IE72 protein is not essential for viral replication at high MOI, but the IE86 protein is essential (Marchini, Liu et al. 2001). The early viral genes encode proteins necessary for viral DNA replication (Pari and Anders 1993). Following viral DNA replication, delayed early and late viral genes are expressed which encode structural proteins for virion production.

The UL 44 protein (pUL44), which binds double-stranded DNA, is an essential accessory protein for viral DNA replication and interacts specifically with the viral DNA polymerase encoded by UL54 (Pari, Kacica et al. 1993; Ripalti, Boccuni et al. 1995). pUL44 increases processivity of the polymerase along the viral DNA template (Ertl and Powell 1992; Weiland, Oien et al. 1994; Zuccola, Filman et al. 2000). The accumulation of the pUL44 is to strikingly high levels at late times after infection (Stinski 1978; Geballe, Leach et al. 1986). Its late kinetics of transcription and the high level of expression suggest an additional important role for viral replication. pUL44 is phosphorylated by the viral UL97 protein kinase (pUL97) in infected cells (Krosky, Baek et al. 2003). Phosphorylation by pUL97 is not required for pUL44 to interact with the catalytic subunit of the viral DNA polymerase (Ertl and Powell 1992; Weiland, Oien et al. 1994).

The HCMV UL44 transcription unit initiates at three distinct sites, which are separated by approximately 50 nucleotides and are differentially regulated during productive infection. Two of these start sites, the distal and the proximal, are active at early times, whereas the middle start site is inactive until late times (Leach and Mocarski 1989). Expression from the late start site is dependent upon viral DNA replication.

We investigated whether the late start site is necessary for efficient viral DNA replication in human fibroblast cells.

2. Distinct regulation of HCMV DNA polymerase prosessivity factor

Transcriptional regulation of UL44 gene expression occurs at two levels. The two transcription start sites that are activated early in infection presumably respond to IE proteins. Each contains a conventional TATA element, which is the only region of significant homology between start sites 1 and 3. Late in infection, sequences that are dependent on DNA replication result in transcriptional activation at start site 2 (Leach and Mocarski 1989). This is referred to as a late viral promoter.

2.1.1 Effect of the TATA elements on UL44 transcription

To determine the role of the late UL44 promoter, we constructed recombinant viruses with the distal-early or the middle-late UL44 TATA elements mutated (dlTATA1, or dlTATA2, respectively) (Fig. 1).

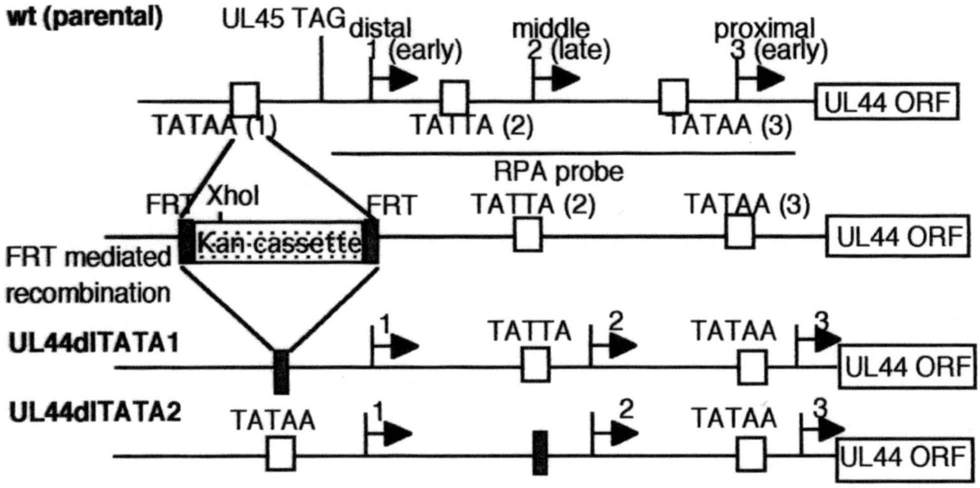

Fig. 1. Structure of recombinant HCMV BAC DNAs. Recombinant viruses with TATA element mutations. UL44 transcription initiates at three distinct sites (labeled as start site 1, 2, and 3), which are separated by approximately 50 nucleotides. Two of these start sites, the distal and proximal, were active at early times after infection, whereas the middle start site was inactive until late times. The distal or middle TATA element was replaced by KanR with FRT sequence flanking. KanR was excised by FLP-mediated recombination.

To detect all the transcripts derived from the different start sites, RNase protection assay was employed. Three major transcripts initiating at the spatially distinct start sites were detected 2 and 3 days after infection with wild type virus (wt) (Fig. 2). Consistent with a previous report (Leach and Mocarski 1989), the middle transcript was not detected with wt and dlTATA1 in infected cells maintained in the presence of phosphonoacetic acid (PAA), which is an inhibitor of HCMV DNA synthesis for 48 h (Fig. 2, lanes: 12 and 13), indicating that the TATA2 element was activated upon viral DNA replication. Substitution of the TATA2 element caused loss of the late transcript initiating at start site 2. (Fig. 2, lanes: 6 to 11). The levels of the middle and the proximal transcripts derived from dlTATA1 were slightly lower than those of wt at 2 d.p.i. (Fig. 2, lanes: 6 and 7). Since levels of the proximal transcripts were similar between wt and dlTATA1 in the presence of PAA for 48 h. (Fig. 2, lanes: 12 and 13), substitution of the TATA1 element affects the transcription initiating at

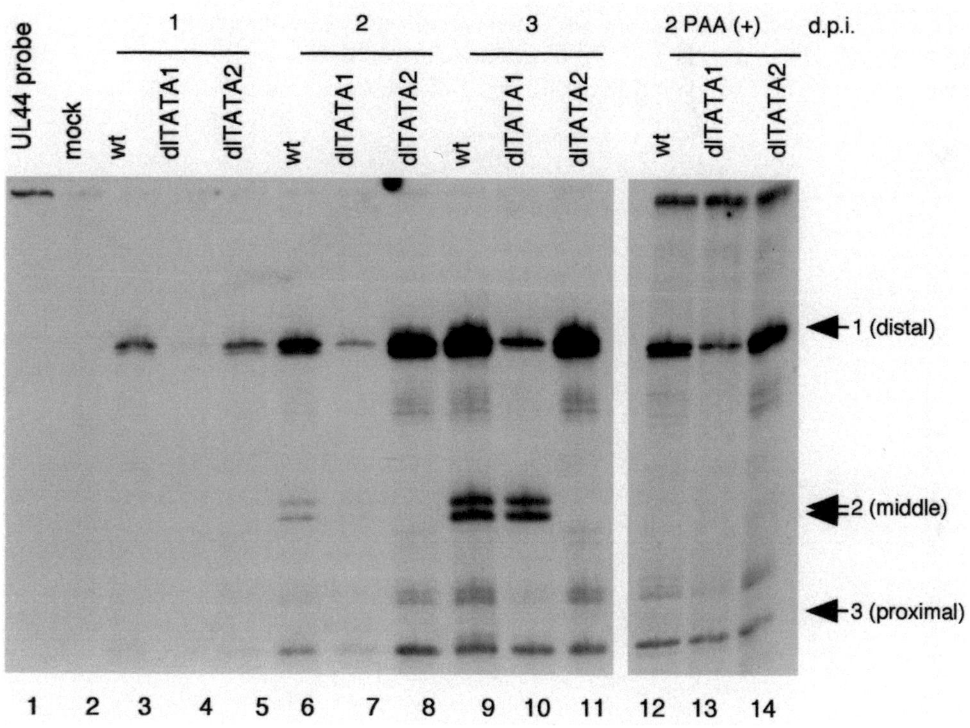

Fig. 2. Effect of substitution for each TATA element on the UL44 transcription in cells infected with wt and recombinant viruses. Cytoplasmic RNAs were harvested at 1, 2, and 3 days after infection with an MOI of approximately 1. Twenty micrograms of RNA was hybridized to ^{32}P-labeled antisense UL44 promoter probe at 37 ^{o}C overnight before digestion with RNase T1. Antisense UL44 probe contains sequence upstream of the transcription start site of all the UL44 transcripts. The protected RNA fragments were subjected to electrophoresis in denaturing 6% polyacrylamide gels. Lanes: 1, Probe lacked RNase T1; 2, mock; 3, 6, 9, and 12 wt; 4, 7, 10, and 13 dlTATA1; 5, 8, 11, and 14 dlTATA2; 3 to 5, 1 d.p.i.; 6 to 8 2 d.p.i.; 9 to 11, and 12 to 14, 3 d.p.i.; 12 to 14 in the presence of phosphonoacetic acid (PAA). Arrow1, 2, or 3 indicates the transcript initiating at start site 1, 2, or 3, respectively.

start site 2 and 3 in a viral DNA replication dependent manner. Since pUL44 is an essential viral protein that acts as a processivity factor for the catalytic subunit of the viral DNA polymerase (pUL54) (Ertl and Powell 1992; Pari, Kacica et al. 1993; Weiland, Oien et al. 1994; Ripalti, Boccuni et al. 1995; Zuccola, Filman et al. 2000), loss of transcription start site 1 was responsible for the lower level of viral DNA replication of recombinant virus dlTATA1. Taken together, mutation of the distal or middle TATA element reduced the transcription from the corresponding start sites.

2.1.2 The middle element had no effect on viral DNA synthesis

We compared viral DNA replication of the recombinant viruses with wt at high or low MOI. While the relative input of viral genomes for an MOI equivalent to approximately 1 differed between 0.001 and 0.0007 for wt, dlTATA1, and dlTATA2 (Fig. 3a), viral DNA of dlTATA1 was 5 to 10 times lower compared to wt after infection at an MOI of approximately 1 or 0.01 (Fig. 3a and b, respectively) and dlTATA2 was similar to wt in relative amount (Fig. 3a and b, respectively). These results indicate that the reduction of late gene expression in the cells infected with dlTATA2 was not due to reduced DNA template for transcription.

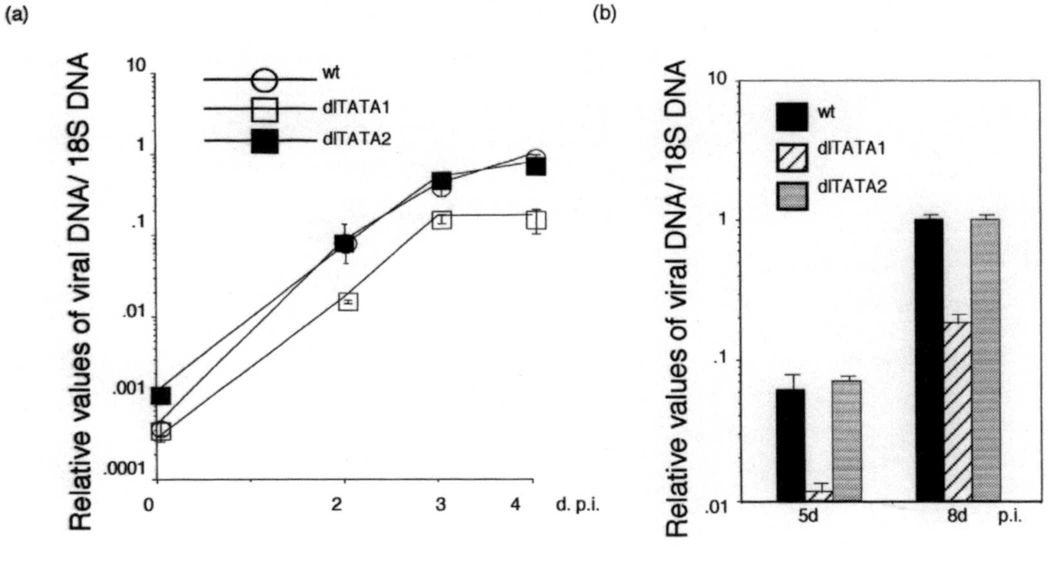

Fig. 3. Analysis of viral DNA replication after high or low MOI infection with wt and recombinant viruses. HFF cells were infected with wt or recombinant viruses at an MOI of approximately 1 or 0.01 and analyzed for viral DNA replication. Viral DNA was quantified by real-time PCR with gB primers and probe as described in the Materials and Methods. Real-time PCR with 18S primers and probe were also performed to serve as an internal control. Data are averages of three independent experiments. (a) HFF cells were infected with wt, dlTATA1, or dlTATA2 at an MOI of approximately 1 and harvested at 2, 3, and 4 d.p.i. Each value, relative to the level of the wt DNA at 4 d.p.i., was calculated and plotted. (b) HFF cells were infected with wt, dlTATA1, or dlTATA2 at an MOI of approximately 0.01 and harvested at 5, and 8 d.p.i. Each value, relative to the level of the wt DNA at 8 d.p.i., was calculated and plotted.

2.1.3 The distal and middle TATA element had an impact on the viral delayed early and late gene transcription

To compare the overall viral delayed early and late transcription of the recombinant viruses with wt, cells were assayed for immediate early, early, delayed early and late gene transcripts by Northern blotting at 1, 2, and 3 d.p.i. RNA from infected cells maintained in the presence of PAA for 2 d was also assayed. RNA analysis after PAA treatment for 48 h did not show a significant difference of IE1 RNAs between wt, dlTATA1, and dlTATA2 (Fig. 4a, lanes: 7 to 9, and Fig. 4e). In contrast, the level of IE RNAs from dlTATA1 was approximately two-fold lower than that of wt and dlTATA2 2 and 3 d. p.i (Fig. 4a. lanes: 5 and 6, and 10 and 11, and Fig. 4e). This might suggest that viral DNA replication modulated the IE transcription from the MIE promoter. In the absence of PAA, the amount of UL44 RNA from dlTATA1 was more than two-fold lower than that from wt at 1, 2, and 3 d.p.i. (Fig. 4b, lanes: 1 and 2, 4 and 5, and 10 and 11, and Fig. 5e). There was no significant difference in the amount of UL44 RNA between wt and dlTATA2 at 1 and 2 d. p.i. (Fig. 4, lanes: 1 and 3, and 4 and 6, and Fig. 5e). In contrast, the level of UL44 transcript from dlTATA2 was approximately 2-fold lower than that of wt at 3 d p.i. (Fig. 4b, lanes: 10 and 12, and Fig. 5e). The reduction of the UL44 transcript in the cells infected with dlTATA1 or dlTATA2 correlates with the loss of the corresponding early or late transcript initiating at start site 1 or 2, respectively (see figure 2).

The UL99 ORF, which encodes a tegument protein of HCMV, is located in a complex region of HCMV with a series of 3′-coterminal transcripts (Wing and Huang 1995). All the transcripts utilize a common polyadenylation site downstream of ORF UL99 (Wing and Huang 1995). Thus, real-time PCR analysis using the UL99 primers and probe detects the total amount of the UL92 to 99 transcripts. The pp28 tegument protein is translated from two mRNAs of 1.6 and 1.3 kb. The 1.3 kb mRNA is of relatively low abundance (Adam, Jervey et al. 1995). Northern blot analysis using the UL99 probe showed that in the presence of PAA, the 1.6 kb mRNA from the UL99 promoter was not detectable, thus UL99 is a true late gene (Fig. 4c, lanes: 7 to 9) as reported previously (Adam, Jervey et al. 1995). Consistent with the previous report (Wing and Huang 1995), analysis of PAA-treated RNA also showed that mRNAs initiating upstream of each of the potential ORFs in this region contained late transcripts (Fig. 4c lanes: 7 to 9). We did not detect differences in the level of steady-state mRNAs between wt and dlTATA2 at 1 and 2 d.p.i. but we did detect it at 3 d.p.i. (Fig. 4c, lanes: 1 and 3, 4 and 6, and 10 and 12). From a quantitative analysis using real-time RT-PCR analysis, the amount of the UL92 to 99 transcripts for dlTATA1 and dlTATA2 was more than two-fold lower at 2 and 3 d.p.i, respectively (Fig. 4e). These results indicate that the early or late transcripts initiating at start site 1 or 2 of the UL44 gene facilitated delayed early and late transcription.

To determine whether the product from the UL44 late transcript initiating at start site 2 affected other late gene expression, Northern blot analysis using the UL75, which encodes a glycoprotein of HCMV, probe was also performed. Three mRNAs were detected (Fig. 4d). Two transcripts, 4.5 and 5.5 kbp, corresponding to the UL76, and UL77 and UL78 genes, respectively, which utilize different transcription start sites as reported previously (Wang, Duh et al. 2004). An analysis of the transcripts of the recombinant virus with an UL76 ORF deletion determined the transcript from the UL76 promoter in the three mRNAs. The direction of transcription of the UL75 ORF is opposite to that the UL76, 77, or 78 ORFs. Thus, real-time RT-PCR analysis using the UL75 primers and probes detects only the UL75 transcript. The initiation site of UL75 transcript was determined by primer extension as

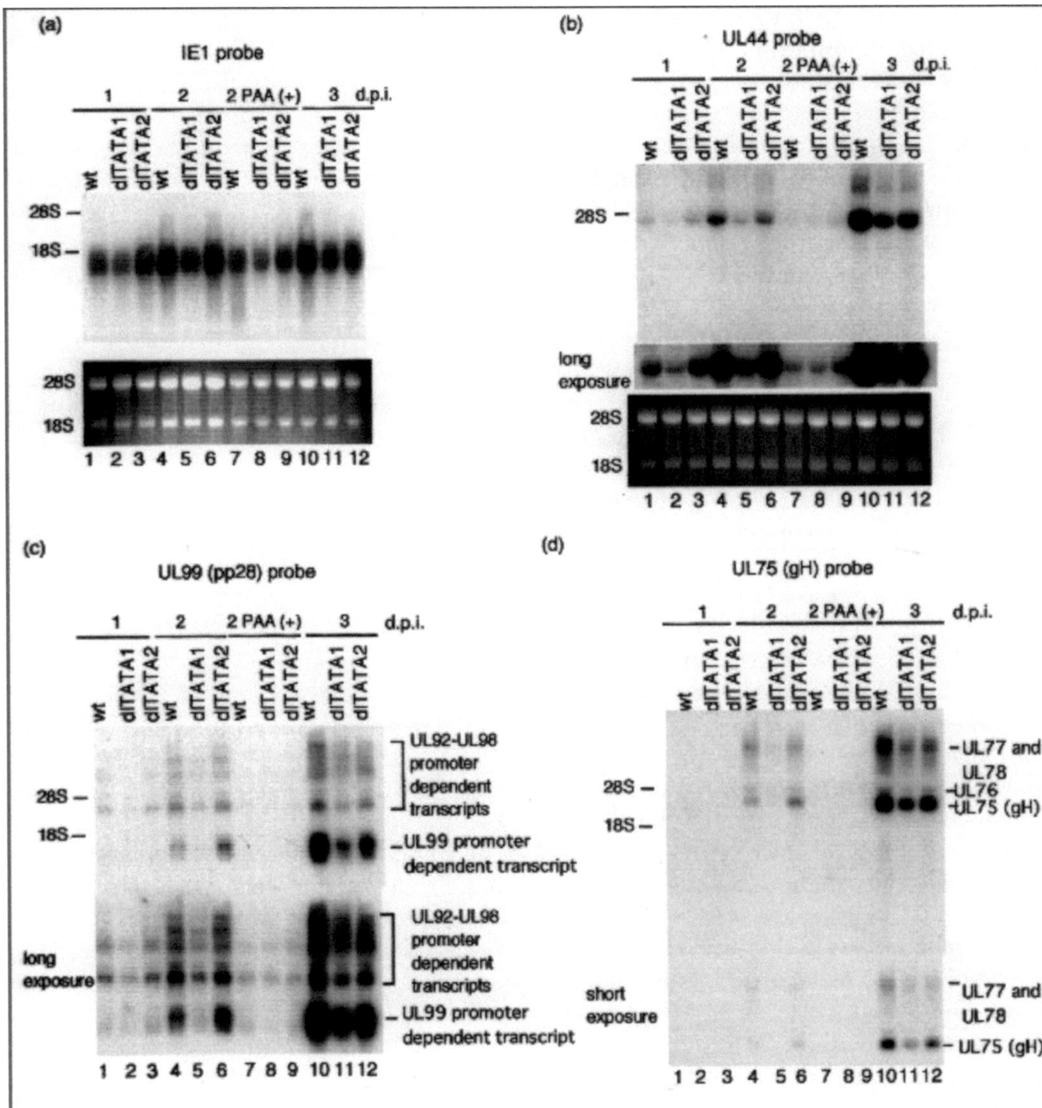
(a)
IE1 probe
1
2
2 PAA (+)
3 d.p.i.
wt
dlTATA1
dlTATA2
28S
18S
1 2 3 4 5 6 7 8 9 10 11 12
(b)
UL44 probe
long exposure
(c)
UL99 (pp28) probe
UL92-UL98 promoter dependent transcripts
UL99 promoter dependent transcript
long exposure
(d)
UL75 (gH) probe
UL77 and UL78
UL76
UL75 (gH)
short exposure

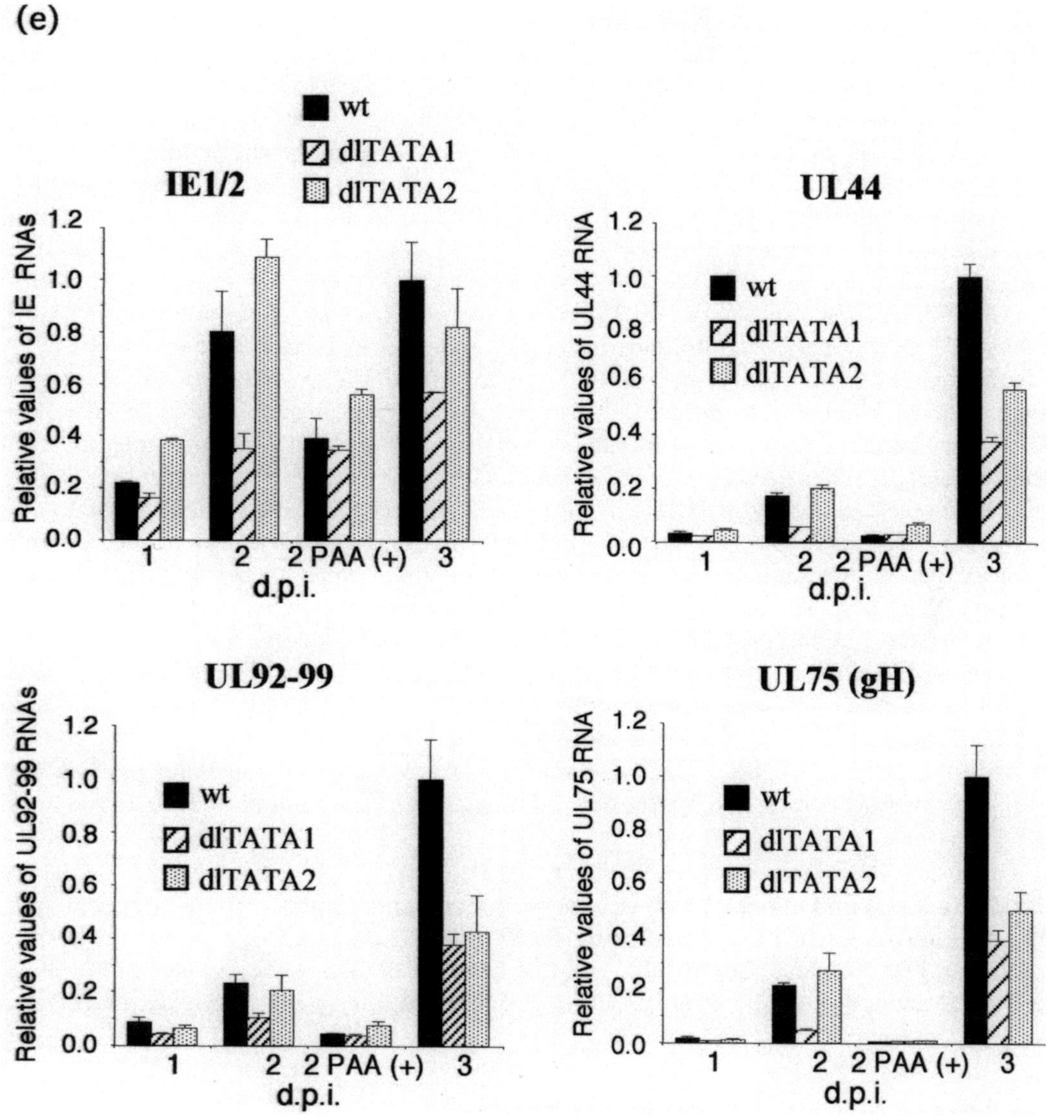

Fig. 4. Analysis of UL44 and the subsequent gene transcription after infection with wt and recombinant viruses. HFF cells were infected with an MOI (multiplicity of infection) of approximately 1 and cytoplasmic RNA was harvested at 1, 2, and 3 d.p.i. as described in Materials and Methods. (a-d) Northern blotting for IE1, UL44, UL99 (pp28), or UL75 (gH). 28S and 18S ribosomal RNA served as controls for an equal amount of RNA loading. Lanes: 1, 4, 7, and 10, wt: 2, 5, 8, and 11, dlTATA1; 3, 6, 9, and 12, dlTATA2; 1 to 3, 1 d.p.i.; 4 to 6, 2 d.p.i..; 7 to 9, 2 d.p.i.. in the presence of PAA; 10 to 12, 3 d.p.i. (a) Analysis with IE1 probe; (b) Analysis with UL44 probe; (c) Analysis with UL99 (pp28) probe; (d) Analysis with UL75 (gH) probe. (e) Real-time RT-PCR for analysis for IE1/2, UL44, UL92-99 and UL75 (gH) gene transcripts.

described previously (McWatters, Stenberg et al. 2002). RNA analysis from PAA-treated cells for 48 h suggested that the UL75 is a true late viral gene (Fig. 4d, lanes 7 to 9 and long exposure: data not shown). Since a small amount of the transcripts from the UL76, UL77 and UL78 promoters were detected in PAA-treated cells after long exposure (data not shown), UL76, 77, and 78 were delayed early viral genes. Similar to the result using the probe for UL99, the level of steady-state mRNAs from the UL76, and the UL77 and UL78 promoters in the cells infected with dlTATA2 was lower compared to wt at 3 d.p.i. (Fig. 4d, lanes 10 and 12). Likewise, the transcript from the UL75 promoter was also approximately 2-fold lower for dlTATA2 at 3 d. p.i. (Fig. 4d, lanes: 10 and 12, and Fig. 4e). The steady-state mRNAs from UL75, UL76, and UL77 and UL78 promoters in the cells infected with dlTATA1 were lower at 2, and 3 d.p.i. (Fig. 4d, lanes: 5 and 6, and 10 and 11, and Fig. 4e). Since DNA replication of recombinant virus dlTATA2 was similar to wt, reduction in viral gene expression was not due to reduced DNA template for transcription. Taken together, the UL44 gene product from the late transcript initiating at start sites 2 has an impact on viral delayed early and late gene transcription independently of viral DNA replication.

pUL44 is detected at sites of HCMV DNA replication centers in the nucleus (Penfold and Mocarski 1997; Park, Kim et al. 2006). Viral replication centers also serve as foci for viral gene expression, presumably in part by concentrating templates for transcription with the proteins that carry out or regulate this process. The herpes simplex virus (HSV) single-stranded DNA-binding protein, ICP8 is also located at viral DNA replication centers in the nucleus and stimulates multiple late viral gene promoters (Gao and Knipe 1991). A recent report shows that ICP8 co-precipitates with chromatin remodeling factors (Taylor and Knipe 2004). Whether or not pUL44 is also associated with ATP-dependent nucleosome remodeling proteins on the HCMV genome is not known, but it might be possible that pUL44 recruits activating chromatin remodeling factors to late viral promoters at late times after infection.

2.1.4 The distal and middle TATA element reduced accumulation of late viral protein

We determined whether the reduction of these viral gene transcriptions affected expression of the viral late proteins. Compared to wt, the levels of the late viral protein pp28 (pUL99) were 16.7 and 7.4 -fold lower for dlTATA1 and dlTATA2, respectively (Fig. 5, lanes: 8 and 9).

2.1.5 Growth kinetics of the recombinant viruses

Since accumulation of late viral protein for the recombinant viruses was reduced, we compared the growth of the recombinant viruses with wt at low or high MOI. HFF cells were infected with wt or recombinant virus at an MOI of approximately 0.01 or 1. Virus from infected cultures at 1,5, 8, 11 and 14 d.p.i. or 1, 4, 5, 7, and 9 d.p.i., respectively, were assayed as described in the Materials and Methods. Viral growth of dlTATA1 or dlTATA2 was slightly delayed compared to the wt at low and high MOI infection (Fig. 6a and b). We detected approximately a 5 to 10-fold difference in viral replication at low MOI infection between wt and dlTATA2 at 5 and 8 d.p.i. (Fig. 6a), while DNA replication of dlTATA2 was similar at the same time (see figure 3a and b). Likewise, at high MOI infection, the viral titer of dlTATA2 was approximately 10-fold lower than that of wt at 4 and 5 d.p.i.. (Fig. 6b), while viral DNA replication of dlTATA2 was similar to wt (see figure 3a and b). Therefore, insufficient expression of the late gene product of UL44 was linked to delayed viral growth.

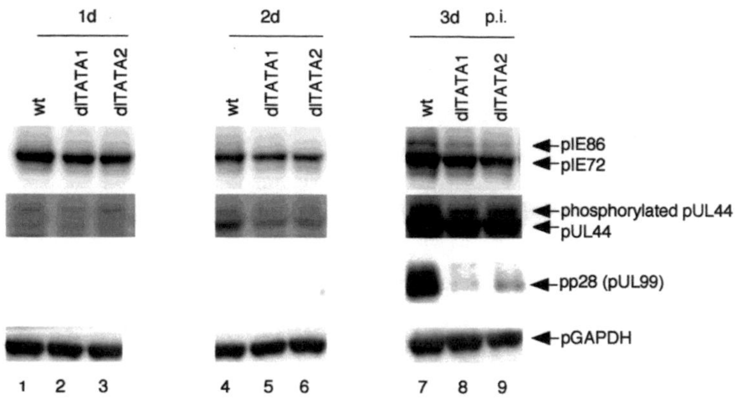

Fig. 5. Analysis of viral protein expression after infection with wt and recombinant viruses. HFF cells were infected with the wt and the recombinant viruses at an MOI of 1 and analyzed for viral proteins. Immediate early pIE72 (UL123), pIE86 (UL122), early ppUL44, and late pp28 proteins were analyzed 1, 2, and 3 d p.i. Anti-pGAPDH (p36) antibody was used to show equal protein loading. Lanes: 1, 4, and 7, wt; Lanes: 2, 5, and 8, dlTATA1; 3, 6, and 9, dlTATA2. Lanes 1-3, 1 d p.i.; 4-6, 2 d p.i.; 7-6, 3 d p.i.

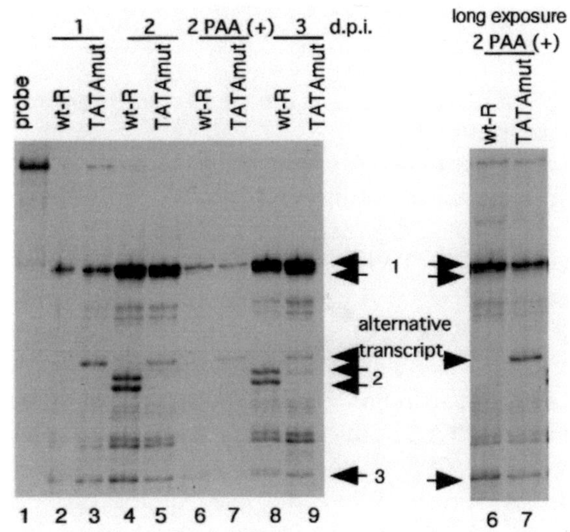

Fig. 6. Analysis of viral DNA replication after high or low MOI infection with wt and recombinant viruses. HFF cells were infected with wt or recombinant viruses at an MOI of approximately 1 or 0.01 and analyzed for viral DNA replication. Viral DNA was quantified by real-time PCR with gB primers and probe as described in the Materials and Methods. Real-time PCR with 18S primers and probe were also performed to serve as an internal control. Data are averages of three independent experiments. (a) HFF cells were infected with wt, dlTATA1, or dlTATA2 at an MOI of approximately 1 and harvested at 2, 3, and 4 d.p.i. Each value, relative to the level of the wt DNA at 4 d.p.i., was calculated and plotted. (b) HFF cells were infected with wt, dlTATA1, or dlTATA2 at an MOI of approximately 0.01 and harvested at 5, and 8 d.p.i. Each value, relative to the level of the wt DNA at 8 d.p.i., was calculated and plotted.

2.2.1 Effect of the TATA sequence in the UL44 middle promoter on the kinetics of transcription and the start site selection

What determines the kinetics of the UL44 late transcript start site is unclear. An important parameter governing transcription initiation is the relative concentration of the viral DNA template and the promoter sequence. As discussed previously (Leach and Mocarski 1989), The UL44 early promoters have a canonical TATA sequence of "TATAA". In contrast, the viral late or middle TATA element is a noncanonical sequence of "TATTATTA" (Fig. 1). To determine the significance of the noncanonical TATA sequence on UL44 late gene expression from the middle promoter, we constructed recombinant viruses with the UL44 middle TATA sequence of "TATTATTA" mutated to "TATataaA", to contain a canonical TATA sequence, "TATAA" and the revertant (wt-R) (Fig. 1). The lower case letters indicate the mutated bases. The proximal and distal transcripts were similar between wt-R and TATAmut at 1, 2, and 3 d.p.i. (Fig. 7). In contrast, an alternative transcript initiating upstream of start site 2 was detected with TATAmut in infected cells 1, 2, and 3 d p.i. (Fig. 7, lanes 3, 5, and 9). The alternative transcript was not detected with wt-R in the presence of PAA at 48 h but it was detected with TATAmut (Fig. 7, compare lanes 6 and 7). The transcript initiating at start site 2 was also detected with TATAmut, but it was at very low levels at 2 and 3 d p.i. (Fig. 7, lanes 5 and 9). The sequence of the UL44 middle TATA nucleotides affects the kinetics and the TSS selection of the UL44 late transcript.

2.2.2 The noncanonical TATA sequence in the UL44 middle promoter is required for the accumulation of late transcripts

To confirm that the noncanonical TATA sequence is required for the accumulation of late transcripts, we made adenine and thymidine substitutions to generate recombinant viruses TATAmut2 and TATAmut3 (Fig. 8a). As shown in Fig. 3b, when the TATA sequence is mutated to contain a canonical TATA sequence "TATAA", the accumulation of late transcripts was decreased at 2 and 3 d p.i. (compare lanes 9 with 1 to 8). An alternative transcript was detected with TATAmut3 as well as the middle transcripts from the start site 2 at 2 and 3 d p.i. (Fig. 8b, lanes 5 and 8). These transcripts were not detected in the presence of PAA at 2 d p.i. (Fig. 8b, lanes 4 and 6). Since TATAmut contains a repeat of thymine and adenine nucleotides in front of TAA in the UL44 middle promoter (see figure 1), the number of the TA repeats in front of TAA nucleotides may determine the strength of the UL44 middle promoter with TATAmut3. While the level of the distal transcript was similar between TATAmut2 and TATAmut3, the transcripts derived from the UL44 middle promoter with mut2 was lower than those with mut3 at 2 and 3 d p.i. (Fig. 8b: lanes 3, 5, 7, and 8). The noncanonical TATA sequence in the UL44 middle promoter influences the accumulation of late transcripts.

The transcriptional strategies of DNA viruses exhibit a number of common features. Prior to initiation of viral DNA synthesis, during IE and early phases, infected cells are devoted to the production of viral proteins necessary for viral DNA synthesis, efficient expression of viral genes, or the other regulatory functions. Transcription of the late genes requires viral DNA synthesis. However, the molecular coupling of replication to transcription of late genes remains unclear. A part of the newly replicated DNA could serve as templates for transcription. Therefore, one hypothesis is that the increased concentration of transcriptional templates is necessary for initiation of the late UL44 transcription. The relative weak binding

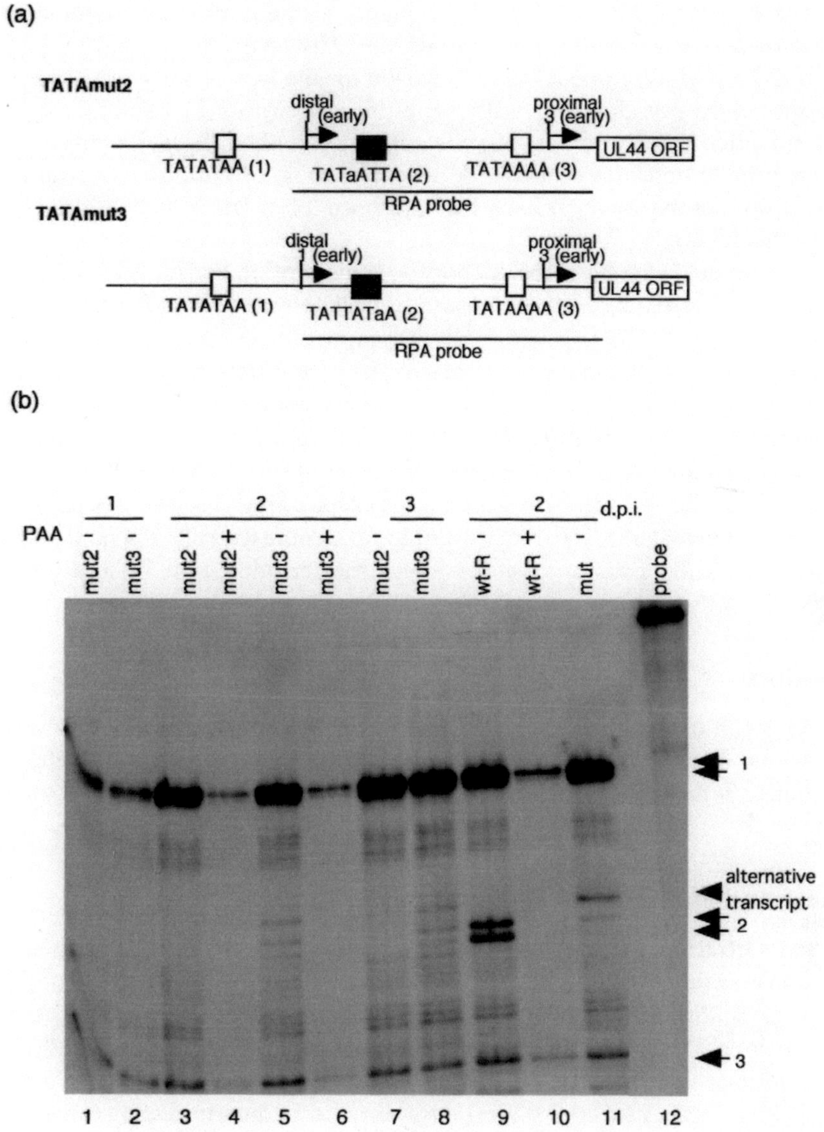

Fig. 7. Effect of the UL44 middle TATA nucleotides on the UL44 transcription in cells infected with wt-R and the recombinant virus. Cytoplasmic RNAs were harvested at 1, 2, and 3 days after infection with an MOI of approximately 3. Twenty micrograms of RNA was hybridized to ^{32}P-labeled antisense UL44 RNA probe at 37 ^{o}C overnight before digestion with RNase T1. Antisense UL44 RNA probe contains sequence upstream of the transcription start site of all the UL44 transcripts. The protected RNA fragments were subjected to electrophoresis in denaturing 6% polyacrylamide gels. Lanes: 1, lacking RNase T1; 2, 4, 6, and 8, wt-R; 3, 5, 7, and 9, TATAmut; 2 and 3, 1 d.p.i.; 4 to 7, 2 d.p.i.; 8 and 9, 3 d.p.i.; 6 and 7, in the presence of phosphonoacetic acid (PAA). Arrow1, 2, or 3 indicates the transcript initiating at start site 1, 2, or 3, respectively. Allowhead indicates the alternative transcript due to the substitution for the UL44 middle TATA nucleotides.

affinity of TBP to the noncanonical TATA sequence at the middle promoter may explain a lack of transcription at early times after infection. However, the weak binding affinity of TBP to the middle promoter is not the only reason for the lack of early transcription because late transcripts were not detected with recombinant viruses TATAmut2 or TATAmut3, while an alternative transcript was significantly detected with TATAmut3. Late specific transcription from a noncanonical TATA sequence may be simply a concentration effect after viral DNA synthesis or reflect the presence of a viral transcription factor that specifically activates a late promoter.

The main function of TATA box is to anchor the transcription preinitiation complex guiding RNA polymerase upstream of the transcription start site (TSS). Therefore, the spacing between TATA box and TSS is functionally important for efficient transcription (Ponjavic, Lenhard et al. 2006), but the underlying mechanisms that determine the start site selection are not understood. As previously shown (Carninci, Sandelin et al. 2006), the preferred canonical sequence for the initiation site is a pyrimidine-purine (PyPu) dinucleotide situated at position -1, +1 relative to TSS. When the UL44 middle TATA element was replaced by a canonical sequence, the distance between the TATA box and TSS was shorten from 32 or 37 to 22 nucleotides. Further studies are required to determine the role of a noncanonical TATA sequence at the middle promoter of the UL44 transcription unit on the viral late gene transcription.

3. Conclusion

While pUL44 accumulates to strikingly high levels at late times after HCMV infection, viral DNA polymerase does not accumulate. The late accumulation of pUL44 depends on the late UL44 promoter, which is required for efficient HCMV delayed early and late gene expression.

4. Materials and methods

Cells and virus titration. Primary human foreskin fibroblast (HFF) cells were maintained in Eagle's minimal essential medium supplemented with 10% fetal calf serum (Sigma, St. Louis, Mo.), penicillin (100 U/ml), and streptomycin (100 μg/ml) at 37°C in 5% CO_2 as described previously (Stinski 1978). The virus titers of wild type (wt) HCMV Towne and recombinant viruses were determined by standard plaque assays on HFF cells as described previously (Meier and Stinski 1997). Viral DNA input was determined by infecting HFF cells in 35 or 60 mm plates in triplicate, and harvesting the cells at 4 h post infection (p.i.) in PCR lysis buffer (10mM Tris-HCl, pH 8.0, 1mM EDTA, 0.001% TritonX-100, and 0.001% SDS) containing 50 μg/ml proteinase K. After 55°C for 100 min, the proteinase K was inactivated at 95°C for 10 min. The relative amount of input viral DNA was estimated by real-time PCR using HCMV gB primers and probes as described previously (Isomura, Tsurumi et al. 2004). For analysis of virus growth kinetics, cells were infected at a multiplicity of 0.01 or 1 plaque-forming unit (PFU)/cell with the wt and the recombinant viruses. At various times after infection, whole cells and supernatant including free virus was collected from infected cultures and three freeze-thaw cycles were performed before titration. Virus titers were determined by the 50% tissue culture infectious dose ($TCID_{50}$) assay on HFF cells as described previously (Nevels, Brune et al. 2004; Nevels, Paulus et al. 2004; Wang and Shenk

2005) except GFP foci rather than CPE were counted. We used Reed-Muench method to calculate $TCID_{50}$. Wt and the recombinant viruses contain the GFP gene substituted for the dispensable, 10-kb US1–US12 region (US, unique short).

RNase protection (RPA) assay. For construction of the antisense UL44 probe, DNA fragment including 5′ upstream of the transcription start site of all the UL44 transcript was amplified by PCR using primer pairs of UL44 F2 RPA primer (5′-CCGCTGGCTCGGCGCGGCTG-3′) and UL44 inner primer as described above, and cloned into TA cloning vector pCRII (Invitrogen). The resulting clone, pUL44 pro-5 was linearized with EcoRV and used as a template for SP6 RNA polymerase. Synthesis by SP6 RNA polymerase on linear pUL44 pro-5 DNA produced a ^{32}P-labeled antisense RNA probe in agreement with the predicted size. Cytoplasmic RNAs from mock-infected or HCMV-infected HFFs were isolated at the indicated times after infection as described previously (Hermiston, Malone et al. 1987; Chang, Malone et al. 1989). DNA replication was inhibited with 200 μg/ml phosphonoacetic acid (PAA) (Sigma, St. Louis, MO.) added to the medium at the time of infection and maintained throughout infection. Twenty micrograms of RNA was hybridized to ^{32}P-labeled antisense UL44 promoter probe at 37 $^{\circ}C$ overnight before digestion with RNase T1 (100U) as described previously (Lashmit, Stinski et al. 1998; Isomura and Stinski 2003). The protected RNA fragments were subjected to electrophoresis in denaturing 6% polyacrylamide gels followed by autoradiography on Hyperfilm MP (Amersham).

Northern blot analysis. Twenty micrograms of cytoplasmic RNA was subjected to electrophoresis in a 1% agarose gel containing 2.2 M formaldehyde and transferred to maximum strength Hybond N+ (Amersham). Northern blot analysis with IE1 probe was performed as described previously (14, 15). UL44, UL99 or UL75 DNA was amplified by PCR using the primer pairs of UL44 ORFF (5′-TGCAGGACATCTCGGACCTGTCGG-3′) and UL44ORFR (5′-CCAGACGCTGCTCAATTGCGCCG-3′), UL99F (5′-TGTGAGTTCGGTACCACGCCCGG-3′) and UL99R (5′-CGTCTAGGTCGTCCGTCTCCTGC-3′), or UL75F (5′-CTGCGAAAAAGATCGGTAGCTGGCC-3′) and UL75R (5′-CGCTGGACCCTCACGCATTTCACCTA-3′), respectively. A radioactive probe was generated by labeling with ^{32}P-dCTP as described above.

Real-time RT-PCR analysis. Reverse transcriptase (RT) (Roche Applied Science, Penzberg, Germany) was used according to the manufacturer's directions to generate first strand cDNA from 2 μg of RNA and 250 ng of oligo-dT primer (Roche) in a final volume of 40 μl. Samples were heat-inactivated at 80°C for 5 min. Amplifications were performed in a final volume of 10 μl containing PLATINUM Quantitative PCR SUPERMIX-UDG cocktail (Invitrogen). Each reaction mixture contained 1 μg of the first-strand cDNA, 5 mM $MgCl_2$, and 500 nM each primer, 250 nM each probe. MIE primers and MIE reporter probe were designed as described previously (Meier, Keller et al. 2002). HCMV UL44, UL92-99, and UL75 forward and reverse primers and reporter probe were designed using Primer Express^{R} (Applied Biosystems) as follows. UL44F: 5′-TTTTCTCACCGAGGAACCTTTC-3′; UL44R: 5′-CCGCTGTTCCCGACGTAAT-3′; UL44 probe: 5′-6-FAM-AGCGTGGCGATCCCTTCGACAA-tetramethyl rhodamine (TAMRA)-3′; UL99-255F: 5′-CCACGACGGCTCCAAGAA-3′; UL99-319R: 5′-TCGGTTTCGGAGCCTTGTC-3′; UL99-275Tprobe: 5′-6-FAM-ACGCGGTGCGCTCGACGTT-TAMRA-3′; UL75-272F:

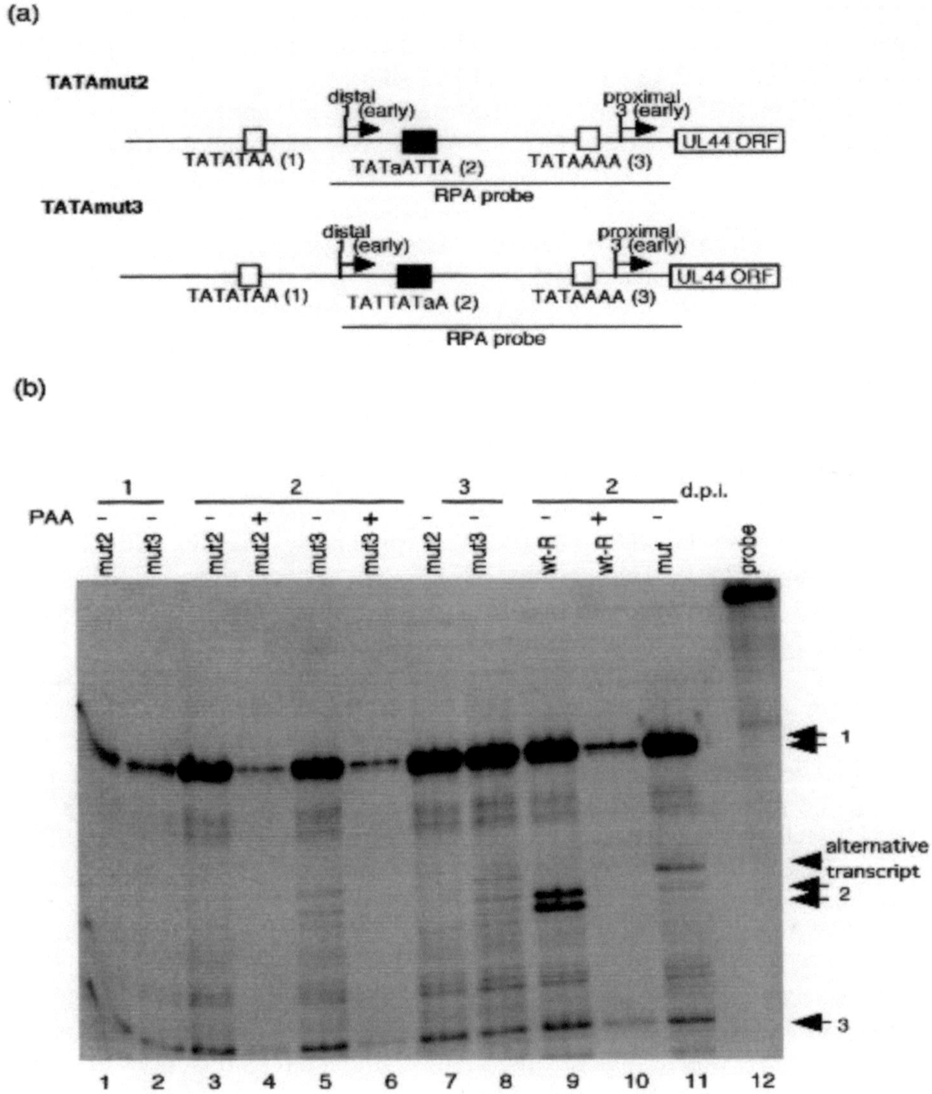

Fig. 8. Effect of a canonical TATA sequence in the UL44 middle promoter on the accumulation of late transcripts. (a) Shematic representation of the recombinant viruses substituted with a canonical TATA sequence. (b) RNAs were harvested at 1, 2, and 3 days after infection with an MOI of approximately 3. RNase protection assay was performed with ^{32}P-labeled antisense UL44 RNA probe at 37 ^{o}C overnight before digestion with RNase T1. The protected RNA fragments were subjected to electrophoresis in denaturing 6% polyacrylamide gels. Lanes: 1, 3, 4, and 7 mut2; 2, 5, 6, and 8 mut3; 9 and 10, wt-R; 11, mut; 12, lacking RNase T1; 1 and 2, 1 d.p.i.; 3 to 6 and 9 to 11, 2 d.p.i.; 7, and 8, 3 d.p.i.; 4, 6, and 10, in the presence of phosphonoacetic acid (PAA); Arrow 1, 2, or 3 indicates the transcript initiating at start site 1, 2, or 3, respectively. Allowhead indicates the alternative transcript due to the substitution for the UL44 middle TATA nucleotides.

5′-TCCATATGCCTCGATGTCTTTT-3′; UL75-339R: 5′-GGTCAGATCTACCTGGTTCAGAAAC-3′; UL75-296Tprobe: 5′-6-FAM-TTGGGCAACCACCGCACTGAGG-TAMRA-3′ (Nihon Gene Research Laboratories Inc., Sendai, Japan). Thermal cycling conditions were an initial 50°C for 2 min and 95°C for 2 min, followed by 40 cycles of 95°C for 15 sec and 60°C for 1 min. Quantitation of relative RNA was accomplished according to a standard curve analysis as described previously (Meier, Keller et al. 2002). Real-time PCR with G6PD primers and probe as described previously (White, Clark et al. 2004) were also performed to serve as an internal control for input RNA. Each real-time RT-PCR assays was performed in triplicate and standardized to threshold cycle values for each viral RNA from HFF cells infected with Rwt crs at 4 d.p.i.

Viral DNA replication assay. After infection with an MOI of 1 or 0.01, cells were collected at 2, 3, and 4 d.p.i. or 5 and 8 d.p.i.., respectively. Cells in 35 mm plates in triplicate were suspended in lysis buffer (50mM Tris-HCl, pH 8.0, 10mM EDTA, 1% SDS and 20μg/ml RNase A) containing 50 μg/ml proteinase K. The replicated viral DNA was quantitated by real-time PCR using HCMV gB primers and probes as described previously (Isomura, Tsurumi et al. 2004; Isomura, Stinski et al. 2005). Real-time PCR with 18S primers and probe purchased from Applied Biosystems (Foster City, CA.) were also performed to serve as an internal control for input DNA. Data are averages of three independent experiments.

5. Acknowlegement

I wish to thank Drs Mark Stinski and Tatsuya Tsurumi for their engagement, advice, and review of various materials.

6. References

Adam, B. L., T. Y. Jervey, et al. (1995). "The human cytomegalovirus UL98 gene transcription unit overlaps with the pp28 true late gene (UL99) and encodes a 58-kilodalton early protein." J. Virol. 69(9): 5304-5310.

Carninci, P., A. Sandelin, et al. (2006). "Genome-wide analysis of mammalian promoter architecture and evolution." Nat Genet 38(6): 626-35.

Chang, C.-P., C. L. Malone, et al. (1989). "A human cytomegalovirus early gene has three inducible promoters that are regulated differentially at various times after infection." J. Virol. 63: 281-290.

Dunn, W., C. Chou, et al. (2003). "Functional profiling of a human cytomegalovirus genome." Proc. Natl. Acad. Sci. U. S. A. 100(24): 14223-14228.

Ertl, P. R. and K. L. Powell (1992). "Physical and functional interaction of human cytomegalovirus DNA polymerase and its accessory protein (ICP36) expressed in insect cells." J. Virol. 66: 4126-4133.

Gao, M. and D. M. Knipe (1991). "Potential role for herpes simplex virus ICP8 DNA replication protein in stimulation of late gene expression." J. Virol. 65(5): 2666-2675.

Geballe, A. P., F. S. Leach, et al. (1986). "Regulation of cytomegalovirus late gene expression: gamma genes are controlled by posttranscriptional events." J. Virol. 57(3): 864-874.

Hermiston, T. W., C. L. Malone, et al. (1987). "Identification and characterization of the human cytomegalovirus immediate-early region 2 gene that stimulates gene expression from an inducible promoter." J. Virol. 61: 3214-3221.

Isomura, H. and M. F. Stinski (2003). "The human cytomegalovirus major immediate-early enhancer determines the efficiency of immediate-early gene transcription and viral replication in permissive cells at low multiplicity of infection." J. Virol. 77(6): 3602-3614.

Isomura, H., M. F. Stinski, et al. (2005). "Two Sp1/Sp3 binding sites in the major immediate-early proximal enhancer of human cytomegalovirus have a significant role in viral replication." J. Virol. 79(15): 9597-9607.

Isomura, H., T. Tsurumi, et al. (2004). "Role of the proximal enhancer of the major immediate-early promoter in human cytomegalovirus replication." J. Virol. 78(23): 12788-12799.

Krosky, P. M., M. C. Baek, et al. (2003). "The human cytomegalovirus UL44 protein is a substrate for the UL97 protein kinase." J. Virol. 77(14): 7720-7727.

Lashmit, P. E., M. F. Stinski, et al. (1998). "A cis-repression sequence adjacent to the transcription start site of the human cytomegalovirus US3 gene is required to down regulate gene expression at early and late times after infection." J. Virol. 72: 9575-9584.

Leach, F. S. and E. S. Mocarski (1989). "Regulation of cytomegalovirus late-gene expression: differential use of three start sites in the transcriptional activation of ICP36 gene expression." J. Virol. 63: 1783-1791.

Marchini, A., H. Liu, et al. (2001). "Human cytomegalovirus with IE-2 (UL122) deleted fails to express early lytic genes." J. Virol. 75(4): 1870-1878.

McWatters, B. J., R. M. Stenberg, et al. (2002). "Characterization of the human cytomegalovirus UL75 (glycoprotein H) late gene promoter." Virology. 303(2): 309-316.

Meier, J. L., M. J. Keller, et al. (2002). "Requirement of multiple cis-acting elements in the human cytomegalovirus major immediate-early distal enhancer for viral gene expression and replication." J. Virol. 76(1): 313-326.

Meier, J. L. and J. A. Pruessner (2000). "The human cytomegalovirus major immediate-early distal enhancer region is required for efficient viral replication and immediate-early gene expression." J. Virol. 74(4): 1602-1613.

Meier, J. L. and M. F. Stinski (1997). "Effect of a modulator deletion on transcription of the human cytomegalovirus major immediate-early genes in infected undifferentiated and differentiated cells." J. Virol. 71: 1246-1255.

Nevels, M., W. Brune, et al. (2004). "SUMOylation of the human cytomegalovirus 72-kilodalton IE1 protein facilitates expression of the 86-kilodalton IE2 protein and promotes viral replication." J Virol 78(14): 7803-12.

Nevels, M., C. Paulus, et al. (2004). "Human cytomegalovirus immediate-early 1 protein facilitates viral replication by antagonizing histone deacetylation." Proc Natl Acad Sci U S A 101(49): 17234-9. Epub 2004 Nov 30.

Pari, G. S. and D. G. Anders (1993). "Eleven loci encoding trans-acting factors are required for transient complementation of human cytomegalovirus oriLyt-dependent DNA replication." J. Virol. 67: 6979-6988.

Pari, G. S., M. A. Kacica, et al. (1993). "Open reading frames UL44, IRS1/TRS1, and UL36-38 are required for transient complementation of human cytomegalovirus oriLyt-dependent DNA synthesis." J. Virol. 67(5): 2575-2582.

Park, M. Y., Y. E. Kim, et al. (2006). "Interactions among four proteins encoded by the human cytomegalovirus UL112-113 region regulate their intranuclear targeting and the recruitment of UL44 to prereplication foci." J Virol 80(6): 2718-27.

Penfold, M. E. and E. S. Mocarski (1997). "Formation of cytomegalovirus DNA replication compartments defined by localization of viral proteins and DNA synthesis." Virology 239(1): 46-61.

Ponjavic, J., B. Lenhard, et al. (2006). "Transcriptional and structural impact of TATA-initiation site spacing in mammalian core promoters." Genome Biol 7(8): R78.

Ripalti, A., M. C. Boccuni, et al. (1995). "Cytomegalovirus-mediated induction of antisense mRNA expression to UL44 inhibits virus replication in an astrocytoma cell line: identification of an essential gene." J. Virol. 69(4): 2047-2057.

Stinski, M. F. (1978). "Sequence of protein synthesis in cells infected by human cytomegalovirus: early and late virus-induced polypeptides." J. Virol. 26: 686-701.

Taylor, T. J. and D. M. Knipe (2004). "Proteomics of herpes simplex virus replication compartments: association of cellular DNA replication, repair, recombination, and chromatin remodeling proteins with ICP8." J. Virol. 78(11): 5856-5866.

Wang, D. and T. Shenk (2005). "Human cytomegalovirus UL131 open reading frame is required for epithelial cell tropism." J. Virol. 79(16): 10330-8.

Wang, S. K., C. Y. Duh, et al. (2004). "Human cytomegalovirus UL76 encodes a novel virion-associated protein that is able to inhibit viral replication." J. Virol. 78(18): 9750-9762.

Weiland, K. L., N. L. Oien, et al. (1994). "Functional analysis of human cytomegalovirus polymerase accessory protein." Virus Res. 34(3): 191-206.

White, E. A., C. L. Clark, et al. (2004). "Small internal deletions in the human cytomegalovirus IE2 gene result in nonviable recombinant viruses with differential defects in viral gene expression." J. Virol. 78(4): 1817-1830.

Wing, B. A. and E. S. Huang (1995). "Analysis and mapping of a family of 3'-coterminal transcripts containing coding sequences for human cytomegalovirus open reading frames UL93 through UL99." J. Virol. 69(3): 1521-1531.

Yu, D., M. C. Silva, et al. (2003). "Functional map of human cytomegalovirus AD169 defined by global mutational analysis." Proc. Natl. Acad. Sci. U. S. A. 100(21): 12396-12401.

Zuccola, H. J., D. J. Filman, et al. (2000). "The crystal structure of an unusual processivity factor, herpes simplex virus UL42, bound to the C terminus of its cognate polymerase." Mol. Cell 5(2): 267-278.

9

Protein-Primed Replication of Bacteriophage Φ29 DNA

Miguel de Vega and Margarita Salas
Instituto de Biología Molecular "Eladio Viñuela" (CSIC), Centro de Biología Molecular "Severo Ochoa" (CSIC-UAM), Madrid, Spain

1. Introduction

Unlike circular genomes in which the conventional replication fork machinery can accomplish the copy of the complete molecule, the requirement of a DNA/RNA molecule to prime DNA synthesis imposes replication strategies to avoid the loss of genetic information contained at the very end of the lagging strand in linear chromosomes since DNA polymerases are unable to start *de novo* DNA synthesis. Thus, once the most terminal primer is removed, a short region of unreplicated single-stranded DNA (ssDNA) will remain at the end of the chromosome that would eventually lead to a continuous shortening of the daughter DNA molecule after successive rounds of DNA replication (the end-replication problem). Therefore, it is essential to guarantee replication of the chromosome ends, that otherwise would cause cell death. Organisms containing linear genomes have developed novel replication strategies to overcome such a problem by either yielding head-tail concatemers, most of them making use of terminal redundancies as phages T4, T7 and SPP1, or by the circularisation and further rolling circle replication of their chromosomes, as it occurs in phage λ [reviewed in (Salas & de Vega, 2008)]. In higher eukaryotes telomerase extends directly the 3´ end, producing an overhanged ssDNA end (Kornberg & Baker, 1992) that finally can invade homologous double-stranded telomeric tracts, enlarging and protecting chromosome ends (Verdun & Karlseder, 2007).
Other organisms, as bacteriophages, animal viruses as adenovirus and human hepatitis B virus, mitochondrial plasmids, linear chromosomes and plasmids of *Streptomyces* (Salas, 1999), as well as several virus infecting Archaea, as halovirus (Bamford et al., 2005; Bath et al., 2006), possess replication origins, constituted by inverted terminal repetitions (ITR) together with a terminal protein (TP), placed at both ends of their linear chromosomes (Salas, 1991). In these cases, the location of the two replication origins allows both strands to be replicated continuously, without requiring asymmetric complexes of the replicative DNA polymerase with other accessory proteins to control the different mechanics of continuous and discontinuous synthesis (Blanco et al., 1989). The TP provides the OH- group of a specific serine, threonine or tyrosine to prime initiation of DNA replication from the ends of the linear chromosome, circumventing the end replication problem, the TP remaining covalently linked to such 5´-termini of the genome (TP-DNA) (Salas, 1991, 1999; Salas et al., 1996).

2. The protein-primed replication mechanism

The development of a soluble *in vitro* replication system with highly purified proteins and TP-DNA from bacteriophage ϕ29 of *Bacillus subtilis* has allowed us to lay the foundations of the so-called protein-primed mechanism of DNA replication (Salas et al., 1995; Salas et al., 1996).

Figure 1 shows a summary of the protein-priming mechanism of ϕ29 DNA replication (Salas, 1991). Initiation of replication starts by the formation of a TP/DNA polymerase heterodimer that recognises the TP-containing DNA ends which are the origins of replication. On the other hand, the formation of a nucleoprotein complex of the ϕ29-encoded double-stranded (ds)DNA binding protein p6 (DBP) at the DNA ends has been proposed to facilitate opening of the latter (see below) and, in the presence of the initiating nucleotide, dATP, stimulates the formation of the covalent linkage between dAMP and the OH group of a specific serine residue in the TP, catalysed by the ϕ29 DNA polymerase (hereafter ϕ29 DNApol). Afterwards, the same polymerase molecule starts the elongation step (DNA-primed) of replication. This results in the formation of the type I replication intermediates that consist in full-length dsDNA molecules with one or more ssDNA tails of different

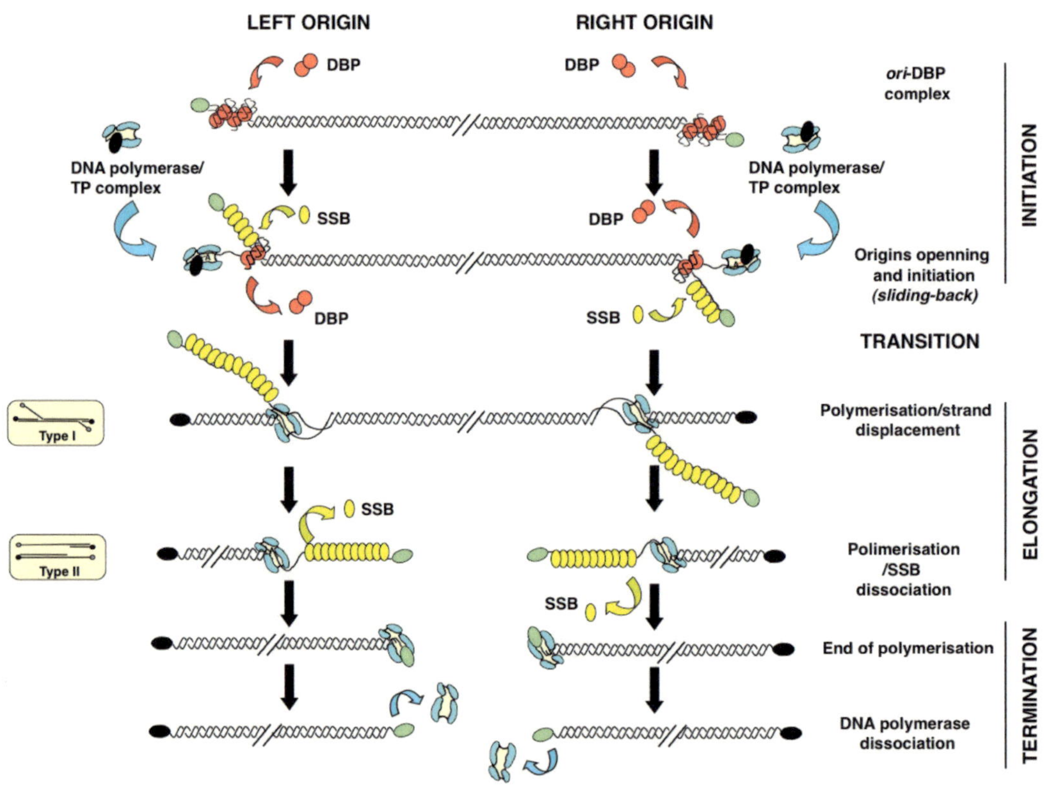

Fig. 1. Schematic representation of bacteriophage ϕ29 TP-DNA replication. Primer and parental TP are shown in black and green, respectively. ϕ29 DNApol, DBP and SSB are coloured in blue, red and yellow, respectively. An scheme of the type-I and type-II replication intermediates is shown at the left. See text for details.

lengths that are stretched by the binding of the phage-encoded single-stranded DNA binding protein (SSB). When the two replication forks, that have been initiated at each DNA end, are encountered, type I molecules give rise to two type II molecules that consist of a full-length ϕ29 DNA molecule in which a portion of the DNA, starting from one end, is double-stranded and the portion spanning to the other end is single-stranded. Type II molecules are elongated by the ϕ29 DNApol with concomitant dissociation of the SSB protein to yield two fully replicated ϕ29 TP-DNA molecules. The final dissociation of the DNA polymerase from each DNA molecule should allow the formation of new heterodimers with free TP molecules to initiate a new round of replication.

These steps and the proteins involved are dissected in the following sections.

2.1 Replication origins of TP containing genomes

ϕ29 is a lytic phage that infects the gram-positive bacterium *B. subtilis* (Anderson et al., 1966). It has a linear dsDNA genome 19.3 kbp long, with a 6 bp ITR (3´-TTTCAT) (Escarmís & Salas, 1982; Yoshikawa & Ito, 1982) and a 31 kDa TP covalently linked to each 5´ end by a phosphoester bond between Ser^{232} and 5´-dAMP (the initiator nucleotide) (Salas et al., 1978), forming the minimal replication origin.

Other *B. subtilis* phages related to ϕ29 that also contain linear dsDNA and TP of similar size are classified in three groups: 1) ø15, PZA and PZE that belong to the ϕ29 group; 2) Nf, M2 and B103; and 3) GA-1. The DNA of all these phages has a short ITR six nucleotides long (3´-TTTCAT) for ϕ29, ø15, PZA and B103, eight nucleotides long (3´-TTTCATTC) for Nf and M2, and seven nucleotides long (3´-TTTATCT) for GA-1 (Salas, 1991).

Phage Cp-1, that infects the Gram-positive bacterium *Streptococcus pneumoniae,* contains a 19.3 kbp linear dsDNA (Martín et al., 1996b) with a TP of 28 kDa covalently linked to the 5′ DNA ends by a phosphoester bond between a still undetermined Thr and 5′-dAMP (García et al., 1983; García et al., 1986). Cp-1 DNA has an ITR of 236 bp with the reiteration 3´-TTT (Martín et al., 1996a).

TP-DNA genomes have also been observed in phages infecting Gram-negative bacteria as it is the case of phage PRD1, a member of a family of lipid-containing phages that infect *Escherichia coli*. The 5′ termini of the 15 kbp long linear dsDNA of PRD1 (Bamford et al., 1991) are linked to a 28 kDa TP by a phosphoester bond between Tyr^{190} and 5′-dGMP (Bamford & Mindich, 1984; Shiue et al., 1991). The TP-DNA of PRD1 and related phages has 110 bp long ITR and the reiteration 3′-CCCC at the ends.

Adenoviruses also contain a linear dsDNA genome 36 kbp long with two replication origins located at the 100 bp long ITRs. The Adenovirus type-5 origin sequence starts with the reiteration 3´-GTAGTA. The 5´ ends are covalently linked to the 55 kDa TP by a phosphoester bond between Ser^{580} and 5´-dCMP [reviewed in (Coenjaerts & van der Vliet, 1995; Van der Vliet, 1995)].

The product of ϕ29 early gene 6 is a DBP that binds preferentially to the ϕ29 DNA ends every 24 nucleotides and with a defined phase, being essential for the activation of the initiation of DNA replication (Serrano et al., 1990). This protein has been described as a histone-like protein that self-associates into elongated oligomers doughnut-shaped that grow into right-handed double-helical filaments (Abril et al., 1999). These filaments form a scaffold tightly wrapped by a DNA right-handed superhelix (Serrano et al., 1990) restraining its positive supercoiling (Prieto et al., 1988; Serrano et al., 1993b) and helping to open the DNA ends, activating initiation of TP-DNA replication most probably by allowing replication origin recognition by the DNA polymerase/primer TP heterodimer (Serrano et al., 1993a). In support of this hypothesis, ϕ29 DBP is absolutely required for the *in vitro* formation of the TP-dAMP complex at low temperature (Serrano et al., 1994). Our results were pioneers in proposing the structural basis for the activation of replication origins, a biological event shown later to be universally conserved in both prokaryotic and eukaryotic initiators (Clarey et al., 2006; Erzberger et al., 2006; O'Donnell & Jeruzalmi, 2006).

By site-directed and deletion mutagenesis we showed that the N-terminal region of p6 is involved in DNA binding. Specifically, mutation in residues Lys^2 or Arg^6 resulted in p6 proteins impaired in DNA binding (Freire et al., 1994; Otero et al., 1990). On the other hand, residues critical for the dimerization of protein p6, identified by random mutagenesis, are Ile^8 and Ala^{44}. In addition to impaired dimer formation ability, mutations at these two residues showed reduced DNA binding affinity and they were affected in the initiation of ϕ29 DNA replication. Thus, dimers seem to be the active form of ϕ29 DBP for DNA binding (Abril et al., 2000).

2.2 Initiation of ϕ29 TP-DNA replication

The first step in ϕ29 TP-DNA replication is the recognition of the replication origins by a heterodimer formed by two viral encoded proteins: the replicative DNA polymerase and a free molecule of TP.

2.2.1 ϕ29 DNApol

ϕ29 DNApol is a monomeric enzyme of only 66 kDa, fully responsible for viral DNA replication (Blanco & Salas, 1985a). Based on amino acid sequence similarities and its sensitivity to specific inhibitors, we included ϕ29 DNApol in the family B (eukaryotic-type) of DNA-dependent DNA polymerases (Bernad et al., 1987). As any of them, it accomplishes sequential template-directed addition of dNMP units onto the 3´-OH group of a growing DNA chain, with insertion discrimination values ranging from 10^4 to 10^6 and with an efficiency of mismatch elongation 10^5 to 10^6-fold lower than that of a properly paired primer terminus (Esteban et al., 1993). In addition, ϕ29 DNApol catalyses 3´-5´ exonucleolysis, i.e., the release of dNMP units from the 3´ end of a DNA strand (Blanco & Salas, 1985b), showing a preferential degradation of a mismatched primer-terminus, in agreement with a role in proofreading of DNA insertion errors that enhances replication fidelity 10^2-fold (Esteban et al., 1994; Garmendia et al., 1992), as it occurs in most DNA replicases.

An extensive mutational analysis of individual residues contained in regions of high amino acid similarity among family B DNA polymerases, as well as the construction of deletion mutants (Blanco & Salas, 1996) allowed us to identify the ϕ29 DNApol catalytic residues required for these activities and those responsible for the stabilisation of the primer-terminus at both active sites. As these residues are evolutionarily conserved the results obtained with ϕ29 DNApol could be extrapolated to most DNA polymerases [reviewed in (Blanco & Salas, 1995, 1996)]. Thus, sequence alignments and site-directed mutagenesis served to identify the catalytic and ssDNA ligand residues responsible for the 3´-5´ exonuclease activity, located at the N-terminal one-third of the enzyme (exonuclease domain), and to propose the hypothesis, widely demonstrated later, of an evolutionary conserved 3´-5´ exonuclease active site among distantly related DNA-dependent DNA polymerases (Bernad et al., 1989). Such an active site is formed by three N-terminal amino acid motifs, named ExoI, ExoII, and ExoIII, invariantly containing four carboxylate groups that bind two metal ions and one tyrosine residue that orients the attacking water molecule (Bernad et al., 1989), as it had been shown to occur in *E. coli* Pol I (Derbyshire et al., 1991). In addition, these analyses led us to identify a new motif (Kx_2h) whose lysine residue plays an auxiliary role in catalysis, specifically in family B DNA polymerases (de Vega et al., 1997). Similarly, our site-directed mutagenesis studies of ϕ29 DNApol pioneered the functional analyses of specific amino acids at motifs YxGG, Dx_2SLYP, Kx_3NSxYG, Tx_2GR, YxDTDS, and KxY, highly conserved at the C-terminal two-thirds of eukaryotic DNA polymerases from family B. These investigations demonstrated the overlapping between polymerisation and protein-primed initiation domains, and served to identify the amino acids involved in metal binding and catalysis, as well as DNA, TP and dNTP ligands (Blanco & Salas, 1995, 1996; Pérez-Arnaiz et al., 2010).

We have shown that ϕ29 DNApol has three distinctive functional features compared to most replicases. First, it initiates DNA replication at the origins located at both ends of the linear genome by catalysing the addition of the initial dAMP onto the hydroxyl group of Ser^{232} of the phage TP, which acts as primer (see below) [reviewed in (Salas 1991, 1999; Salas & de Vega, 2006)]. Second, unlike most replicases that rely on accessory proteins to be stably bound to the DNA, as thioredoxin in the case of T7 DNA polymerase (Huber et al., 1987; Tabor et al., 1987), the β-subunit of *E. coli* Pol III holoenzyme (Kong et al., 1992), or the eukaryotic clamp protein, PCNA (Jonsson & Hübscher, 1997; Kelman, 1997), ϕ29 DNApol performs DNA synthesis without the assistance of processivity factors, displaying the highest processivity described for a DNA polymerase [>70 kb; (Blanco et al., 1989)]. A third distinctive property of ϕ29 DNApol is the efficient coupling of processive DNA polymerisation to strand displacement. This capacity enables the enzyme to replicate the double-stranded genome without the need for a helicase (Blanco et al., 1989). These two features, high processivity and intrinsic strand displacement activity, are currently being exploited for the use of ϕ29 DNApol in isothermal multiple displacement amplification (MDA) (Dean et al., 2002; Dean et al., 2001). These amplification technologies based on ϕ29 DNApol have two main advantages respect to classical PCR DNA amplification: first, no previous sequence information is required, due to the use of random hexamer primers, any DNA being susceptible to be amplified, and second, amplicons performed by the ϕ29 DNApol are much larger than those obtained with PCR. On the other hand, the ability displayed by ϕ29 DNApol to use circular multiply primed ssDNA as template has led to the development of the multiply primed rolling circle amplification, one of the most robust technologies to amplify circular templates of variable size (Dean et al., 2001). This amplification technology is being widely used for genome sequencing, efficient amplification and detection of known and unknown circular viral genomes (Johne et al., 2009), genotyping of single nucleotide polymorphisms (Qi, et al., 2001), whole genome analysis of noncultivable viruses (Johne et al., 2009), detection and identification of circular plasmids in zoonotic pathogens (Xu et al., 2008), and for the description of new metagenomes (López-Bueno et al., 2009). Recently we have achieved improvements of isothermal MDA by fusing DNA binding domains to the C-terminus of ϕ29 DNApol (de Vega et al., 2010). The results showed that the addition of Helix-hairpin-Helix domains increases DNA binding of the hybrid DNA polymerases without hindering their replication rate. In addition, the chimerical DNA polymerases displayed an improved DNA amplification efficiency on both circular plasmids and genomic DNA and are unique ϕ29 DNApol variants with enhanced amplification performance. These chimerical DNA polymerases will contribute to make ϕ29 DNA amplification technology one of the most powerful tools for genomics, consolidating MDA technology as the alternative to PCR for many applications.

Despite the exhaustive mutational analyses carried out throughout ϕ29 DNApol, they did not provide a structural rationale for both the intrinsic processivity and strand displacement capacity of the enzyme. Instead, resolution of the ϕ29 DNApol structure gave the insights into these two unique properties of the enzyme. These structural studies, carried out in collaboration with Tom Seitz's lab (Yale University), showed ϕ29 DNApol formed by an N-terminal exonuclease domain, containing the 3´-5´ exonuclease active site, and a C-terminal polymerisation domain that, like in other DNA polymerases, is subdivided into the universally conserved palm (containing the catalytic and DNA ligand residues), fingers (containing the dNTP ligands) and thumb (which confers stability to the primer) subdomains (Kamtekar et al., 2004) (see Figure 2A). 3D-structural comparisons indicated that the main difference between other family B DNA polymerases and ϕ29 DNApol was the presence in the latter of two additional subdomains, both corresponding to sequence insertions that we had previously identified as specifically conserved in the protein-primed subgroup of DNA polymerases, called TPR1 and TPR2 (Blasco et al., 1990; Dufour et al., 2000). TPR1 lies at the edge of the palm, while TPR2 contains a β-hairpin structure just facing the apex of the thumb subdomain. Palm, thumb, TPR1, and TPR2 subdomains form a doughnut-shaped structure that encircles the upstream duplex DNA at the polymerisation active site (Berman et al., 2007), constituting an internal clamp that provides the enzyme with the maximal DNA-binding stability required for its intrinsic processivity, mimicking and making unnecessary the sliding clamp used in other replisomes. On the other hand, TPR2, palm and fingers subdomains, together with the exonuclease domain, surround the downstream template strand (Berman et al., 2007), forming another tunnel whose narrow dimensions (~10 Å) do not allow dsDNA binding. Thus, downstream dsDNA has to be unwound to enable threading of the template strand through this tunnel to reach the polymerisation site, using the same topological mechanism as hexameric helicases to open dsDNA regions, and providing a structural basis for the strand displacement capacity of ϕ29 DNApol (Kamtekar et al., 2004; Rodríguez et al., 2005).

3D resolution of ϕ29 DNApol structure also gave us the clues about how primer-terminus switches between polymerisation and exonuclease active sites during proofreading of polymerisation errors. Comparison of the structures of many apo DNA polymerases with their corresponding binary complexes showed that the major conformational changes occur mainly in their thumb subdomains, composed of two microdomains with a clear helicoidal character linked by a flexible region (Beese et al., 1993; Doubliè et al., 1998; Eom et al., 1996; Franklin et al., 2001; Li et al., 1998; Shamoo & Steitz, 1999). Conversely, the ϕ29 DNApol thumb subdomain has an unusual structure since it is small and mainly constituted by a long β-hairpin without identifiable microdomains (Kamtekar et al., 2004). Moreover, comparison of the apo enzyme with the binary complexes showed that the thumb subdomain does not rotate upon DNA binding (Berman et al., 2007). We have shown that the prevention of a potential thumb movement by crosslinking the tips of the TPR2 and thumb subdomains did not affect the partitioning of the primer-terminus between the polymerisation and editing active sites (Rodríguez et al., 2009). The impeded motion of the TPR2 subdomain suggests that rotation of the DNA is not required to transfer the primer-terminus between the polymerisation and editing active sites in ϕ29 DNApol, most likely as there is not any structural barrier in between. Then, how does the frayed terminus travel to the exonuclease active site? Considering the ϕ29 DNApol thumb subdomain as a nearly static structure, the primer switching would be accomplished by a passive diffusion of the frayed primer-terminus. The energetically unfavourable gradual melting of three-four base pairs should be progressively offset by new and specific interactions established with DNA ligands of the thumb subdomain, as suggested (Pérez-Arnaiz et al., 2006). Such interactions would also channel the primer-terminus in the appropriate orientation to contact with ssDNA ligands of the exonuclease domain responsible for the stabilisation of the primer-terminus at the editing active site (de Vega et al., 1996, 1998b; Kamtekar et al., 2004; Pérez-Arnaiz et al., 2006; Rodríguez et al., 2009).

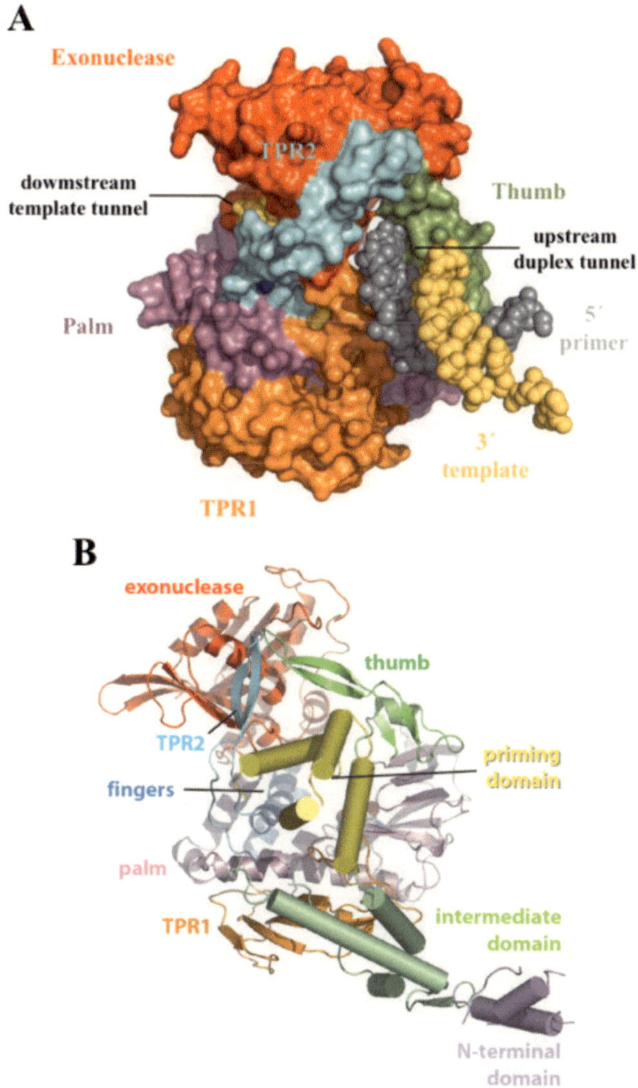

Fig. 2. (A) ϕ29 DNApol-DNA complex. (B) Structure of the ϕ29 DNApol-Terminal Protein complex. Reproduced with permission from Kamtekar, S., Berman, A.J., Wang, J., Lázaro, J.M., de Vega, M., Blanco, L., Salas, M. & Steitz, T.A. (2006). The phi29 DNA polymerase:protein-primer structure suggests a model for the initiation to elongation transition. *EMBO J.* Vol. 25, No. 6, pp. 1335-1343.

Additionally, recent resolution of ϕ29 DNApol tertiary complex structures has allowed us to dissect the subtle changes in the polymerisation active site that take place upon dNTP binding, providing the structural basis for the mechanism of translocation. Thus, once the catalysis of the phosphoester bond formation between the α-phosphate of the incoming dNTP and the OH- group of the priming nucleotide takes place, the pyrophosphate produced leaves the DNA polymerase, breaking the electrostatic crosslink that kept the fingers subdomain in the closed state. Concomitantly to the fingers opening, residues Tyr^{254} and Tyr^{390} move back into the nucleotide insertion site, leading to one position backwards translocation of the nascent base pair out of the binding pocket, as now the nucleotide insertion site is sterically inaccessible (Berman et al., 2007). This translocation allows the 3′ OH-group of the newly added nucleotide to be in a competent position to attack nucleophylically the α-phosphate of the incoming nucleotide during the next nucleotide insertion event (Berman et al., 2007) (see Figure 3).

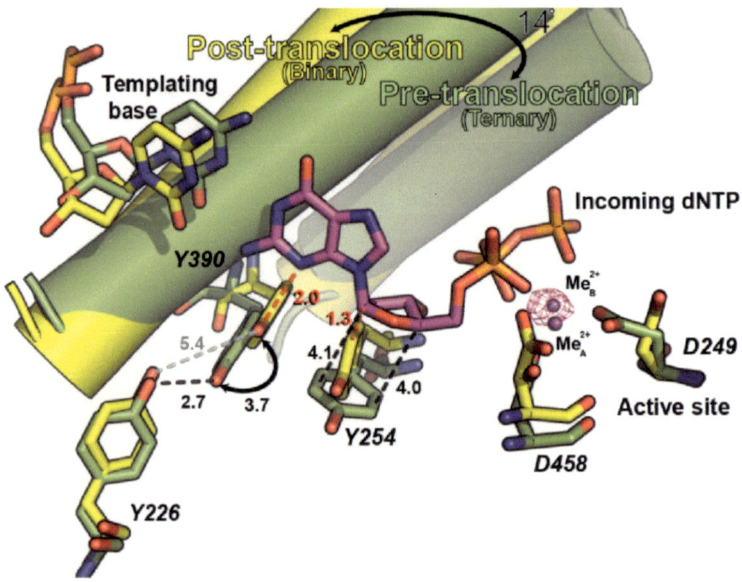

Fig. 3. Comparison of the binary (yellow) and ternary (green) complex structures of ϕ29 DNApol. The mechanistically significant amino acid movements are indicated. Reproduced with permission from Berman, A.J., Kamtekar, S., Goodman, J.L., Lázaro, J.M., de Vega, M., Blanco, L., Salas, M. & Steitz, T.A. (2007). Structures of phi29 DNA polymerase complexed with substrate: the mechanism of translocation in B-family polymerases. *EMBO J.* Vol. 26, No. 14, pp. 3494-3505.

2.2.2 ϕ29 Terminal protein

As already mentioned, the primer TP forms a heterodimer with the DNA polymerase for recognition and further initiation of TP-primed DNA replication. To discriminate between the two different functions, the TP molecule linked to the 5′ DNA ends is called parental TP and the TP present in the complex with DNA polymerase is called primer TP. Crystallographic resolution of the structure of ϕ29 DNApol/primer TP heterodimer has shown that the TP has an elongated three-domain structure (Figure 2B) (Kamtekar et al.,

2006). The N-terminal domain (residues 1–73) is structurally disordered likely because it is not interacting with the polymerase (Kamtekar et al., 2006; Pérez-Arnaiz et al., 2007). The intermediate domain (residues 74–172) contains two long α-helices and a short β-turn-β structure and makes extensive contacts with the TPR1 subdomain of the polymerase. This interface has many charged residues and includes two salt bridges between arginine residues in the TP and glutamic acid residues in the TPR1 subdomain (R158:E291; R169:E322). It is connected through a hinge region to the C-terminal priming domain (residues 173–266), a region highly electronegative that has a four-helix bundle topology. Ser^{232}, which provides the priming hydroxyl group for DNA synthesis, lies in a disordered loop (residues 227–233) at the end of the priming domain close to the active site of the DNA polymerase (see Figure 4, left panel). The priming domain structure shows interactions between many of their acidic residues and positively charged residues of the thumb subdomain of the polymerase (e.g., between E191:K575 and D198:K557), with residue R96 of the exonuclease domain and with TPR2 subdomain residues (Kamtekar et al., 2006; Rodríguez et al., 2004). Thus, the upstream duplex DNA "tunnel" of ϕ29 DNApol encircles the TP priming domain whose overall dimensions and its negative charge mimics DNA in

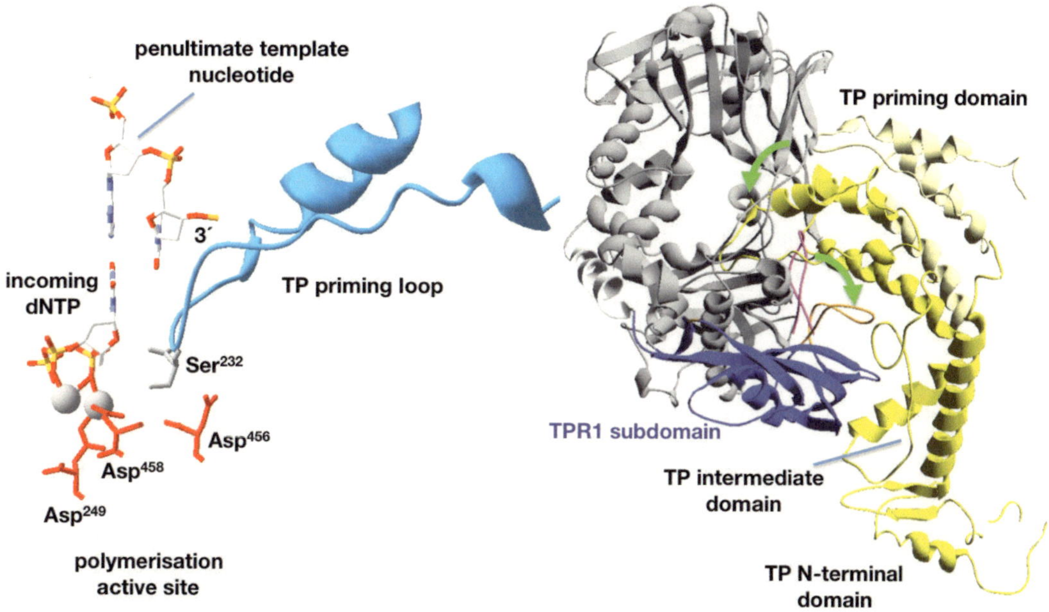

Fig. 4. Left, placement of TP priming residue Ser^{232} (in grey) and penultimate template nucleotide at the ø29 DNApol active site (catalytic aspartates are shown in red). Right, flexible orientations of TPR1 loop in the apoenzyme (coloured in magenta) and its stable and moved out structural conformation shown in the DNA polymerase/TP complex (coloured in orange). TP is coloured in yellow. Green arrows indicate the suggested conformational changes of both, the DNA polymerase TPR1 loop and the TP priming domain to allow the formation of a stable heterodimer. Reproduced with permission from Pérez-Arnaiz, P., Longás, E., Villar, L., Lázaro, J.M., Salas, M. & de Vega, M. (2007). Involvement of phage ϕ29 DNA polymerase and terminal protein subdomains in conferring specificity during initiation of protein-primed DNA replication. *Nucleic Acids Research.* Vol. 35, No. 21, pp. 7061-7073.

its interactions with the polymerase during initiation (de Vega et al., 1998a; Kamtekar et al., 2006). This explains why DNA synthesis by the heterodimer cannot begin at internal sites of the phage genome, as the upstream 3´ template would sterically clash with the TP (Kamtekar et al., 2006).

Our previous studies showed that ϕ29, GA-1 and Nf DNA polymerases display a great specificity for their corresponding primer TPs, as the heterologous systems did not give any detectable initiation product (González-Huici et al., 2000a; Longás et al., 2006). By means of chimerical proteins, constructed by swapping the priming domain of the related ϕ29 and GA-1 TPs, we showed that DNA polymerase can form catalytically active heterodimers exclusively with that chimerical TP containing the N-terminal and intermediate domains of the homologous TP, suggesting that the interaction between the polymerase TPR1 subdomain and the TP intermediate domain is the one main responsible for the specificity between both proteins (Pérez-Arnaiz et al., 2007).

In addition, the independent expression of the ϕ29 TP priming domain and intermediate plus N-terminal domains showed that the former can only prime initiation in the presence of the latter that assists the TP-dAMP formation most probably by inducing a conformational change in the DNA polymerase (Pérez-Arnaiz et al., 2007). The structure of the ϕ29 DNApol forming a complex with the TP is very similar to that of the apo enzyme, the main conformational changes being restricted to TPR1 residues 304-315 (Kamtekar et al., 2006). Such residues form loops with a high degree of flexibility in the apo enzyme. By the contrary, the ϕ29 heterodimer structure shows that this loop moves out to allow the TP to access the polymerase active site. Altogether, these results led to propose a model for the DNA polymerase-TP interaction in which the TP intermediate domain would recognise specifically and interact with the DNA polymerase TPR1 subdomain. Such interaction would promote the change of the TPR1 loop from a flexible to the stable moved out conformation that now would allow the proper (prone to catalysis) placement of the TP priming domain into the DNA polymerase structure (Pérez-Arnaiz et al., 2007) (see Figure 4, right panel).

2.2.3 Recognition of replication origins by the DNA polymerase/TP heterodimer

The ϕ29 DNApol/TP heterodimer recognises the replication origins at the genome ends (see Figure 1). Blunt-ended DNA fragments containing the left or right ϕ29 DNA ends, but not internal ϕ29 DNA fragments, were active as templates in *in vitro* initiation reactions (García et al., 1984; Gutiérrez et al., 1986a; Gutiérrez et al., 1986b). However, the activity was 6- to 10-fold lower than that obtained with TP-DNA (Gutiérrez, et al. 1986a; Gutiérrez et al., 1986b). These results indicated on the one hand, that specific DNA sequences located at the ϕ29 DNA ends are involved in origin recognition and on the other hand, that the parental TP is a major signal in the template for such a recognition, strongly suggesting that the heterodimer is recruited to the origin through interactions with the parental TP. In agreement with this, detection of initiation activity by using heterologous systems in which DNA polymerase, primer TP and TP-DNA came from ϕ29 and Nf related phages, showed that initiation was selectively enhanced when the DNA polymerase and the TP-DNA were from the same phage, implying a specific interaction between DNA polymerase and parental TP (González-Huici et al., 2000a). In line with this, a chimerical ϕ29 DNApol containing the GA-1 DNA polymerase TPR1 subdomain was capable of catalysing the initiation reaction primed by GA-1 TP but solely in the presence of ϕ29 TP-DNA, supporting the hypothesis that a major contribution to the parental TP recognition is carried out by the DNA polymerase (Pérez-Arnaiz et al., 2007). Similarly, mutations introduced at several TP-intermediate domain residues rendered TP mutants that could not support DNA replication when they acted as parental TP, indicating also a contribution of the primer TP in the specific recognition of the replication origins (Illana et al., 1998; Serna-Rico et al., 2000). Furthermore, measurement of the ability of the different DBPs coming from ϕ29, Nf and GA-1 bacteriophages to activate homologous and heterologous replication origins showed also a specific recognition of each nucleoprotein complex by the homologous DNA polymerase/TP heterodimer (Freire et al., 1996). The fact that ϕ29 DBP stimulates the initiation activity of the heterodimer formed by GA-1 primer TP and a chimerical ϕ29 DNApol containing the TPR1 subdomain of GA-1 DNA polymerase to a similar extent as that of the ϕ29 heterodimer, favours the hypothesis of a main and specific recognition of the DBP by the DNA polymerase (Pérez-Arnaiz et al., 2007).

2.2.4 A sliding-back mechanism for protein-primed DNA replication

As already indicated, the DNA ends of ϕ29 and those of the ϕ29-related phages have a reiteration of three nucleotides (3′-TTT.... 5′). Once the replication origins are specifically recognised by the heterodimer formed by the DNA polymerase and the primer TP (Blanco et al., 1987; Freire et al., 1996; González-Huici et al., 2000a; González-Huici et al., 2000b; Pérez-Arnaiz et al., 2007), the DNA polymerase catalyses the formation of a phosphoester bond between the initiator dAMP and the hydroxyl group of Ser^{232} of the TP (see Figure 1), a reaction directed by the second T at the 3´ end of the template strand (Méndez et al., 1992) and performed by the same catalytic residues responsible for canonical polymerisation (Blanco & Salas, 1995, 1996). Modelling of an incoming dNTP and a template strand onto the ϕ29 DNApol/primer TP complex shows that the priming Ser^{232} of TP is placed at the catalytic site of the DNA polymerase in line to attack nucleophylically the α-phosphate of the incoming nucleotide to form the phosphoester bond (Figure 4, left panel). The model also suggests that the 3´ end of the template strand goes deep into the catalytic site of the DNA polymerase through the downstream template strand tunnel until it positions the penultimate 3´ dTMP of the template strand at the catalytic site, allowing it to direct insertion of the initiator dAMP. To perform TP-DNA full-length synthesis, the TP-dAMP initiation product translocates backwards one position to recover the template information corresponding to the first 3´-T, the so-called sliding-back mechanism that requires a terminal repetition of 2 bp. This reiteration permits, prior to DNA elongation, the asymmetric translocation of the initiation product, TP-dAMP, to be paired with the first T residue (Méndez et al., 1992) (see scheme in Figure 5).

Our studies have shown how the sliding-back mechanism, or variations on it, seems to be a common feature of protein-priming systems to restore full-length DNA. Thus, in the case of the ϕ29-related phage GA-1, initiation also occurs at the 3´ second nucleotide of the template (3´-TTT) and, to a lesser extent, at the third nucleotide (Illana et al., 1996). The ϕ29-related phage Nf and the *Streptococcus pneumoniae* phage Cp-1 initiate at the 3´ third nucleotide of their terminal repetition (3´-TTT) (Longás et al., 2008; Martín et al., 1996b), whereas the *E. coli* phage PRD1 initiates at the fourth nucleotide (3´-CCCC) (Caldentey et al., 1993), requiring two and three consecutive sliding-back steps, respectively, to recover the DNA end information (stepwise sliding-back). The adenovirus genome ends present a more complex reiteration (3'-GTAGTA), the 3´ fourth to six template positions directing the formation of the TP-CAT initiation product. Thus, recovery of the 3´ ends is performed by a single jump, after which TP-CAT is paired with the terminal 3'-GTA (jumping-back) (King & van der Vliet, 1994) (see scheme in Figure 5).

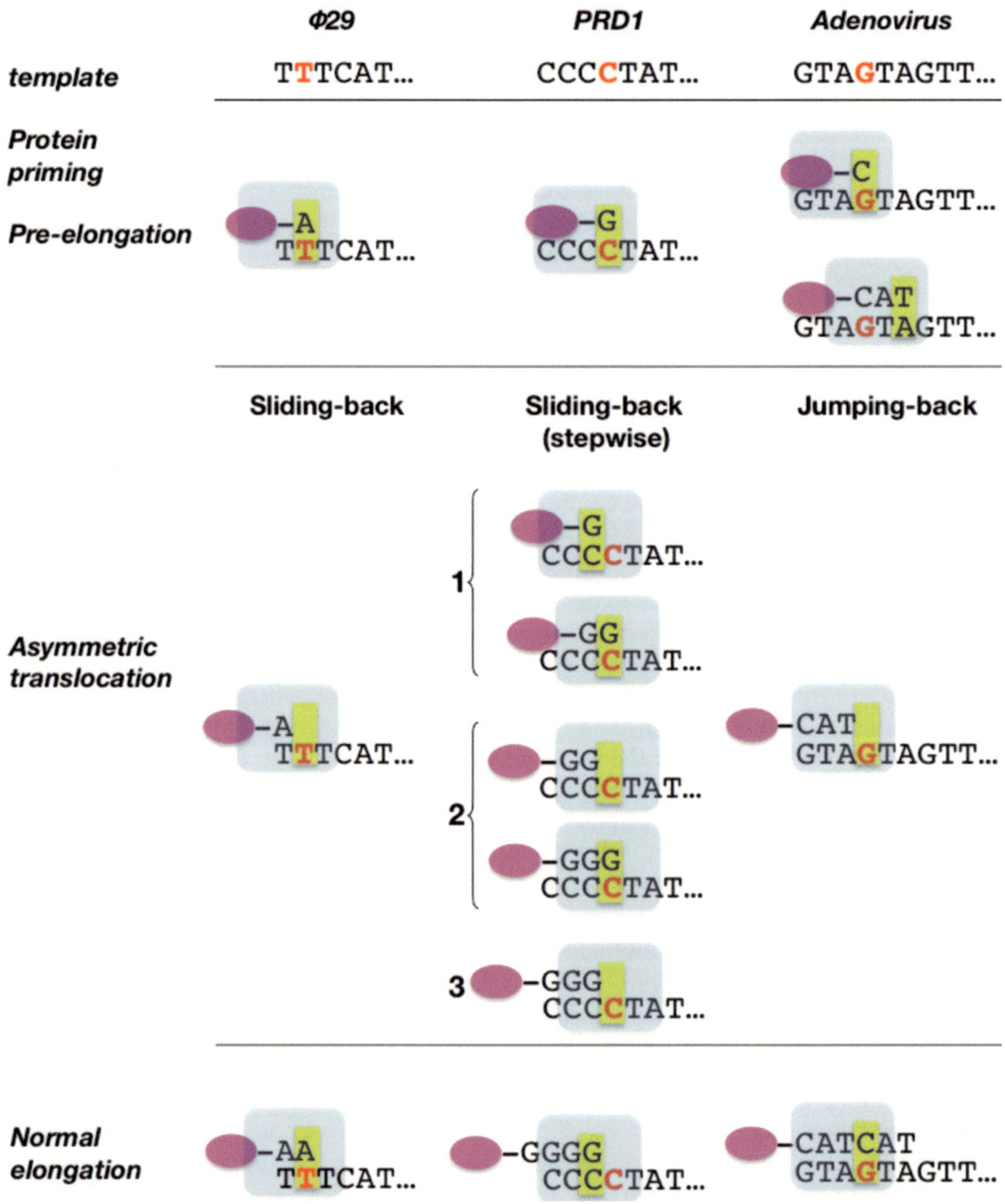

Fig. 5. Sliding-back (jumping-back) model for the transition from initiation to elongation. TP is represented as a pink oval and DNA polymerase as a grey square. The internal template nucleotide that directs the insertion of the initiator nucleotide is shown in bold red letter. Yellow box represents the catalytic active site of the DNA polymerase.

2.2.4.1 Why sliding-back during genome replication?

Protein-primed initiation can be predicted to be an inaccurate reaction. The insertion fidelity of protein-primed initiation in ϕ29 has been shown to be quite low, the insertion discrimination factor being about 10^2. Even more, the 3´-5´ exonuclease activity of ϕ29 DNApol is unable to act on the TP-dNMP initiation complex, precluding the possibility that a wrong dNMP covalently linked to TP could be proofread (Esteban et al., 1993). If misincorporation during the initiation reaction takes place, a mismatch would be produced with the terminal 3'-T on the template after the sliding-back of the incorrect TP-dNMP complex, unfavouring the further elongation step. If an incorrect TP-dNMP product were elongated it would be corrected in the next round of replication, because it would not serve as a template (Esteban et al., 1993). Thus, the sliding-back and its variations are envisaged to increase the fidelity during the initiation reaction, as several base pairing checking steps have to occur before elongation of the initiation product takes place (King & van der Vliet, 1994; Méndez et al., 1992). The fact that other TP-containing genomes also contain some kind of sequence repetitions at their ends supports the hypothesis that the sliding-back type of mechanism could be a common feature of protein-primed replication systems (Méndez et al., 1992).

2.3 Transition from protein-primed to DNA-primed replication

Our functional analyses established that the ϕ29 DNApol/primer TP heterodimer do not dissociate immediately after initiation or after sliding-back (Méndez et al., 1997). The same DNA polymerase molecule incorporates 5 nucleotides to the primer TP while is still complexed with the latter (initiation mode), undergoes some structural change during incorporation of nucleotides 6-9 (transition) and finally dissociates from the primer TP when nucleotide 10 is incorporated into the nascent DNA chain (elongation mode) (Méndez et al., 1997). These results probably reflect the polymerase requirement for a DNA primer of a minimum length to catalyse DNA elongation efficiently.

We have shown that the strength of the ϕ29 DNA pol-primer TP interaction is differently contributed by the TP priming and intermediate domains (Pérez-Arnaiz et al., 2007), supporting the model proposed for the transition from the protein-primed initiation to the DNA-primed elongation modes (Kamtekar et al., 2006). Thus, the TP intermediate domain would be in a fixed orientation on the polymerase by means of stable contacts with the TPR1 subdomain. The weak interaction observed with the DNA polymerase would facilitate the TP priming domain to rotate following the helicoidal pathway as DNA is synthesized. The relative motion of the TP priming domain with respect to the fixed TP intermediate domain would be possible due to the flexibility of the hinge region that connects both domains. After incorporation of 6-7 nucleotides the proximity of the priming Ser to the hinge region would impede a further priming domain rotation, promoting complex dissociation (Kamtekar et al., 2006) (see Figure 6).

2.4 DNA-primed elongation

Once the initiation, sliding-back and transition steps have been fulfilled and ϕ29 DNApol has separated from the primer TP, the DNA polymerase resumes TP-DNA replication; therefore, the same DNA polymerase molecule accounts for complete genome replication from a single binding event (Blanco et al., 1989). As mentioned before, the high stability of the ϕ29 DNApol/DNA complex, by virtue of the "internal sliding-clamp-like" structure

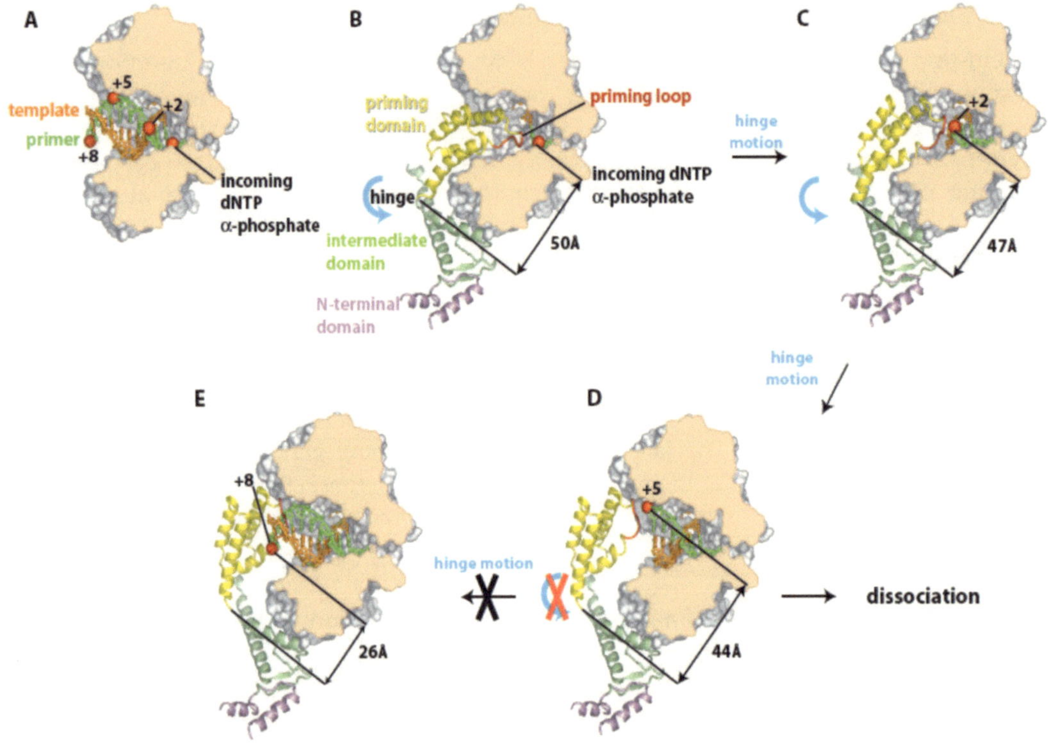

Fig. 6. A model for the transition from initiation of replication to elongation (see main text for details). Reproduced with permission from Kamtekar, S., Berman, A.J., Wang, J., Lázaro, J.M., de Vega, M., Blanco, L., Salas, M. & Steitz, T.A. (2006). The phi29 DNA polymerase:protein-primer structure suggests a model for the initiation to elongation transition. *EMBO J.* Vol. 25, No. 6, pp. 1335-1343.

formed by thumb, palm, TPR1 and TPR2 subdomains, allows the polymerase to perform complete DNA replication without the assistance of processivity factors, in contrast to most replicative DNA polymerases. In addition, the singular TPR2 subdomain enables the ϕ29 DNApol to couple polymerisation to the unwinding of the downstream dsDNA regions (strand displacement capacity) making unnecessary the intervention of a helicase-like protein (Blanco et al., 1989).

As mentioned above, since replication starts at both ϕ29 DNA ends and is coupled to strand displacement, this results in the generation of so-called type-I replication intermediates (see Figure 1). The ssDNA stretches generated are bound by the viral SSB, essential for elongation of replication *in vivo* (Mellado et al., 1980). Binding of ϕ29 SSB to ϕ29 DNA replicative intermediates has been demonstrated to occur *in vitro* (Gutiérrez et al., 1991b). The protein binds in a cooperative way (Soengas, et al., 1994) stimulating dNMP incorporation during ϕ29 DNA replication (Gutiérrez et al., 1991a), and increasing the elongation rate, mainly when ϕ29 DNApol mutants impaired in strand displacement are used, probably due to the helix destabilising activity of the ϕ29 SSB (Soengas et al., 1995). When the two converging DNA polymerases merge, a type-I replication intermediate becomes physically separated into two type-II replication intermediates (Gutiérrez et al., 1991b; Inciarte et al., 1980). Continuous elongation by the DNA polymerase completes replication of the parental strand.

2.5 Termination of TP-DNA replication

For termination of genome replication, the ϕ29 DNApol encounters a covalently linked TP molecule (see Figure 7, upper panel), terminating DNA replication by an as yet unknown mechanism. As already indicated, the TPR2 insertion of the ϕ29 DNApol, together with the exonuclease domain and the fingers and palm subdomains form a downstream tunnel whose narrow dimensions precludes the passage of a dsDNA through it. Considering that the terminal base of the template is covalently linked to the Ser^{232} of TP, the priming loop of the parental TP has to enter the downstream template-binding tunnel of ϕ29 DNApol to allow the last 5´-dAMP (covalently linked to the parental TP) to be replicated. However, the dimensions of such a tunnel do not allow the TP to pass through it to reach the catalytic active site, so a disruption of the interactions of TPR2 with the exonuclease domain and the thumb subdomain of the polymerase is required to get an opened tunnel (see Figure 7, lower

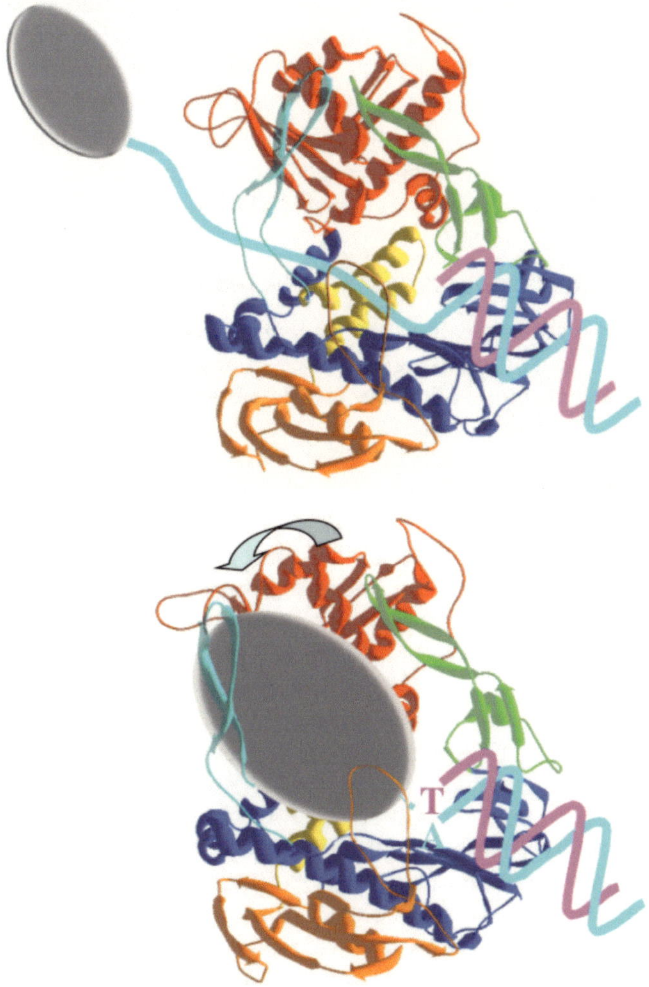

Fig. 7. Hypothetical partial opening of the TPR2 and thumb subdomains to allow the last 5´-template nucleotide to reach the polymerisation active site of the DNA polymerase. Template and primer strands are coloured in blue and magenta, respectively.

panel). By using primer/5´-streptavidine-bound template DNA to mimic the parental TP, we showed that all but 4 terminal nucleotides were replicated by the ϕ29 DNApol (de Vega et al., 1999). This situation could be parallel to the physiological one, in which ϕ29 DNApol has to finish the replication of a DNA template strand that contains a TP molecule covalently linked at its 5´ end. It is tempting to speculate that during termination of replication, a specific interaction between DNA polymerase and TP is required to allow synthesis of the terminal nucleotide.

2.6 Terminal protein-primed DNA amplification

By using appropriate amounts of the four ϕ29 DNA replication proteins described above, primer TP, DNA polymerase, the double-stranded DNA-binding protein, and the single-stranded DNA-binding protein, we were able to amplify limited amounts of the ϕ29 TP-DNA molecule by three orders of magnitude after 1 hr of incubation at 30 °C. Moreover, the quality of the amplified DNA was demonstrated by transfection experiments, in which infectivity of the synthetic (amplified) ϕ29 TP-DNA, measured as the ability to produce phage particles, was identical to that of the natural ϕ29 TP-DNA obtained from virions (Blanco et al., 1994), leading us to establish some of the requisites for the development of isothermal DNA amplification strategies based on the ϕ29 DNA replication machinery to amplify very large (> 70 kb) segments of exogenous DNA.

3. *In vivo* compartmentalisation of ϕ29 DNA replication

It is well established that replication of phage genomes occurs at specific intracellular locations by the use of large organising structures that bring together replication factors to enhance the efficiency of the replication process. Some lines of evidence support that replication of phage DNA takes place in close association with the bacterial membrane (Firshein, 1989; Mosig & Macdonald, 1986; Siegel & Schaechter, 1973). Our recent investigations have also given evidences concerning compartmentalization of phage ϕ29 DNA replication in *B. subtilis* cells.

We have shown that ϕ29 TP binds to dsDNA through its N-terminal domain in a non-sequence dependent way, both *in vitro* and *in vivo* (Muñoz-Espín et al., 2010; Zaballos & Salas, 1989). This capacity enables the parental TP, and therefore the viral TP-DNA, to associate with the bacterial nucleoid early after injection of the ϕ29 genome (see scheme in Figure 8) where the *B. subtilis* RNA polymerase is also located (Muñoz-Espín et al., 2010). There, synthesis of the ϕ29 early proteins DNA polymerase, primer TP, SSB and DBP, essential for *in vivo* ϕ29 DNA replication takes place. Once synthesized, primer TP binds the bacterial chromosome and recruits the DNA polymerase to form the heterodimer that will recognise TP-DNA replication origins. At this stage, replication of TP-DNA will start from both terminal origins giving rise to the replicative intermediates type I and II, as it has been observed by electron microscopy (Harding & Ito, 1980; Inciarte et al., 1980; Sogo et al., 1982) (see scheme in Figure 8).

By fluorescence microscopy, we have shown that at middle infection times, the DNA polymerase, TP, and viral TP-DNA are reorganised adopting a peripheral helix-like distribution toward the poles of the cell (Muñoz-Espín et al., 2009; Muñoz-Espín et al., 2010). Although the pathway followed by the ϕ29 replicative machinery from the nucleoid to bacterial peripherical regions remains to be determined, it has been proposed that it could travel associated to the replication of bacterial chromosome (Muñoz-Espín et al., 2010), as newly synthesized bacterial DNA is translocated towards the cell poles *via* a helical structure (Berlatzky et al., 2008).

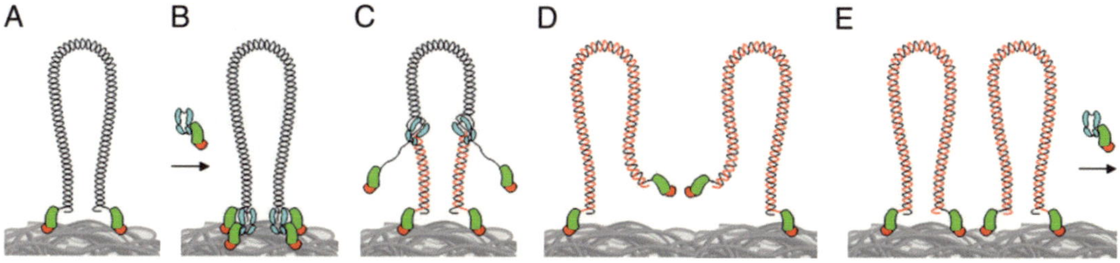

Fig. 8. Model of nucleoid-associated early ϕ29 DNA replication organised by the TP. (A) Attachment of ϕ29 TP-DNA to the bacterial nucleoid surface (gray mass at bottom) through the N-terminal domain (red) of the parental TPs (red and green). (B) Recruitment of the ϕ29 DNApol/primer TP heterodimer to the replication origins of TP-DNA. (C) Processive elongation of the nascent DNA strands (red lines) coupled to strand displacement. (D and E) Once DNA replication is completed, two ϕ29 TP-DNA molecules are ready for another round of replication. For simplicity, other viral proteins involved in DNA replication are not drawn. Reproduced with permission from Muñoz-Espín, D., Holguera, I., Ballesteros-Plaza, D., Carballido-López, R. & Salas, M. (2010). Viral terminal protein directs early organisation of phage DNA replication at the bacterial nucleoid. *Proceedings of the National Academy of Sciences of USA*. Vol. 107, No. 38, pp. 16548-16553.

The ϕ29 membrane protein p16.7 has a non-sequence specific DNA binding capacity (Meijer et al., 2001) that enables it to interact with the ϕ29 replication origins through recognition of the parental TP (Serna-Rico et al., 2003). This protein also shows a helix-like pattern at the membrane of infected cells, most probably being involved in the compartmentalization of *in vivo* membrane-associated ϕ29 DNA replication through a direct contact with TP-DNA, organising the viral replicating intermediates at numerous peripheral locations (Albert et al., 2005; Muñoz-Espín et al., 2009) (see Figure 9). Different experimental approaches have demonstrated that protein p16.7 interacts directly with the *B. subtilis* actin-like cytoskeleton protein MreB (Muñoz-Espín et al., 2009). This protein forms helix-like filamentous structures *in vivo* essential for the control of the bacterial rod-shaped morphology (Jones et al., 2001), suggesting that MreB would contribute to efficient ϕ29 DNA replication by recruiting protein p16.7 to the appropriate sites at the cell membrane allowing simultaneous replication of multiple templates at numerous peripheral locations. Further evidence is the finding that ϕ29 DNA replication is severely affected in ΔMreB cytoskeleton mutants (Muñoz-Espín et al., 2009).

ϕ29 gene 1 codes for a small protein (p1) that assembles into long protofilaments forming bidimensional sheets (Bravo & Salas, 1998) in association with the bacterial membrane *in vivo* (Serrano-Heras et al., 2003). Cell fractionation studies indicated that protein p1 is membrane-associated both during synthesis of ϕ29 DNA and after blocking ϕ29 DNA replication (Bravo & Salas, 1997). Membrane-association of p1 also occurs in the absence of other viral components, suggesting that protein p1 contacts the bacterial membrane directly (Bravo & Salas, 1997; Serrano-Heras et al., 2003). Phage ϕ29 DNA replication was shown to be significantly reduced when non-suppressor *B. subtilis* cells were infected with mutant phage sus*1*(629) at 37ºC (Bravo & Salas, 1997; Prieto et al., 1988). In addition, protein p1 was

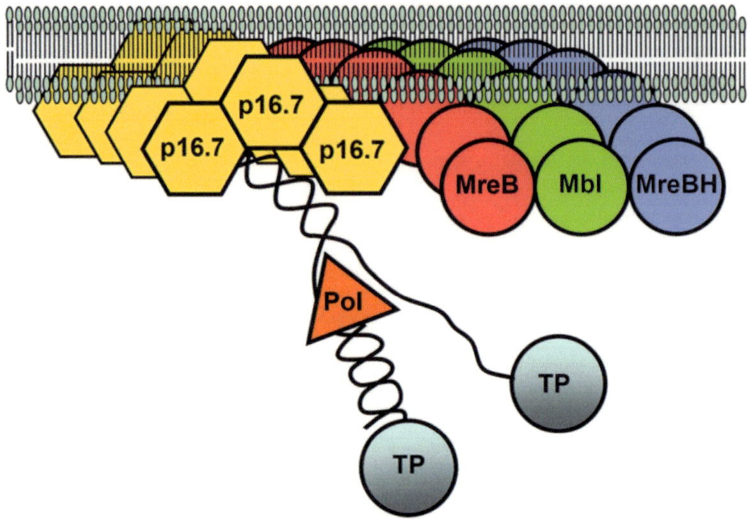

Fig. 9. Model of membrane-associated late ϕ29 DNA replication organised by the MreB cytoskeleton. MreB, Mbl, and MreBH are shown to form a putative triple helical structure closely associated with the inner surface of the membrane. Each dimeric unit of protein p16.7 is represented by a yellow hexagon. The tridimeric p16.7 units form oligomers in a helix-like localisation at the cell membrane. For simplicity, other viral proteins involved in DNA replication are not drawn. Reproduced with permission from Muñoz-Espín, D., Daniel, R., Kawai, Y., Carballido-López, R., Castilla-Llorente, V., Errington, J., Meijer, WJ & Salas, M. (2009). The actin-like MreB cytoskeleton organises viral DNA replication in bacteria. *Proceedings of the National Academy of Sciences of USA*. Vol. 106, No. 32, pp. 13347-13352.

also shown to interact with the viral TP *in vitro* (Bravo et al., 2000). These results suggest that protein p1 is a component of a membrane-associated structure which would play, in addition to p16.7, a role in the organisation of ϕ29 DNA replication by providing an anchoring site for the replication machinery.

4. ϕ29 codes for a *B.subtilis* uracil-DNA glycosylase inhibitor.

Downstream to ϕ29 gene 1 there is an open reading frame (ORF56) encoding an acidic protein of 56 amino acids (protein p56) that shows a dimeric state in solution and that accumulates throughout the ϕ29 infective cycle (Serrano-Heras et al., 2006). Chemical crosslinking assays showed that viral p56 interacts, both during the infective process and in the absence of viral components, with *B. subtilis* uracil-DNA glycosylase (UDG), a key enzyme that eliminates uracil residues from the DNA during the Base Excision Repair (BER) pathway (Serrano-Heras et al., 2006). *In vitro* assays demonstrated that such an interaction inhibits UDG. In agreement with this, extracts from ϕ29-infected cells showed a dramatic drop in bacterial UDG activity, in contrast to the nearly 90% of the activity that remained after incubation with extracts from non-infected cells.

4.1 Role of protein p56 in ϕ29 DNA replication

Inhibition of the cellular UDG activity after phage infection was established previously in two systems. The first was the inhibition of the host UDG after infection of *B. subtilis* with

the uracil-containing phage PBS2 (Friedberg et al., 1975). In this case, inhibition of cellular UDG was crucial to prevent the elimination of uracils from the viral genome. Similarly, bacteriophage T5 inhibits *E. coli* UDG, although the physiological role of this inhibition is still unclear, as its genome does not contain uracils (Warner et al., 1980).
Both, *in vitro* and *in vivo* assays have recently demonstrated the ability of ϕ29 DNApol to insert, extend and use as template dUMP residues with nearly the same efficiency that dTMP to give full-length DNA (Serrano-Heras et al., 2008). Whereas removal by the UDG of the uracil residues incorporated into the phage genome caused a drastic reduction in the efficiency of ϕ29 DNA replication, as ϕ29 DNApol is unable to use as template the resulting abasic sites (de Vega & Salas, unpublished results), such an inhibitory effect caused in replication by UDG was counteracted by the addition (*in vitro*) or expression (*in vivo*) of protein p56 (Serrano-Heras et al., 2008).
As in the case of bacteriophage T5, ϕ29 TP-DNA does not contain uracils, then, why does phage ϕ29 synthesize a UDG inhibitor? It has been suggested that this inhibition is related to the mechanism of ϕ29 DNA replication. As illustrated in Figure 1, during ϕ29 TP-DNA replication replicative intermediates (type-I and type-II) with long stretches of single-stranded DNA are generated. The presence of uracil in the replicative intermediates could recruit components of the cellular BER pathway, such as UDGs and AP endonucleases. Further removal of the uracil moiety would render an abasic site that cannot be used as template by the ϕ29 DNApol. By the contrary, the AP site will be further recognised by the cellular AP endonuclease that would introduce a nick into the phosphodiester backbone with accompanying loss of the terminal DNA region, giving rise to shorter viral DNA molecules lacking one parental TP. Therefore, the action of the cellular UDG on single-stranded DNA regions of the ϕ29 replicative intermediates would be harmful for viral replication (Serrano-Heras et al., 2008).

5. Conclusions and future research

The availability of an efficient *in vitro* ϕ29 TP-DNA replication system, as well as the biochemical characterisation of the different proteins involved, have greatly contributed to lay the foundations of the different steps in the protein-priming mechanism of DNA replication. In this, a specific DNA polymerase catalyses the formation of a phosphoester bond between the initiator dNMP and the OH group of a specific residue in the TP. *In vitro* systems have been also developed for the replication of adenovirus and bacteriophages GA1, Nf, PRD1 and Cp1, showing that they use a similar protein-priming mechanism for the initiation of replication. Thus, the mechanism of initiation of ϕ29 DNA replication can be extrapolated to other organisms containing a TP covalently linked to the 5′-ends of their genomes, as human hepatitis B virus, mitochondrial plasmids, linear chromosomes and plasmids of *Streptomyces*, as well as several virus infecting Archaea, as halovirus.
Despite of the advances in the knowledge of the protein-priming process, several questions regarding the initiation at internal positions of the TP-containing genomes remain to be elucidated, as the basis for the specificity for the templating nucleotide. In this respect, the use of chimerical TPs, constructed by swapping the priming domains of the related ϕ29 and Nf proteins, allowed us to conclude that this domain is one of the structural determinants that dictates the internal 3′ nucleotide used as template during initiation. On the other hand, the backwards motion of the primer TP with respect to the fixed template molecule, implies a breakage of the pair TP-A:T (in the case of bacteriophages ϕ29, Cp1, Nf and GA-1) or, most

drastically the triple base pairing TP-CAT:GTA, as in the case of adenovirus. This energetically unfavoured step should be explained by a power stroke mechanism, by which the energy released after dissociation of the pyrophosphate could drive the backwards movement of the TP-dNMP initiation product with respect to the DNA polymerase and template strand with the consequent correct base pairing with the preceding 3´ nucleotide, to reach a more energetically favoured situation. The elucidation of the conformational changes that govern the sliding-back mechanism will give the clues to understand such a special way to initiate genome replication.

Termination of replication of TP-containing genomes is still an unresolved matter. We have shown that protein-primed DNA polymerases exhibit an exquisite specificity for their TP counterparts during the initiation step of TP-DNA replication. Based on the ϕ29 DNApol structure, it seems obvious that to let the last 5´dAMP to be copied during termination, at least the parental TP priming loop of the template strand has to access the catalytic site of the polymerase following the downstream template tunnel pathway. The question that arises is whether there is also specificity between the DNA polymerase and the parental TP during termination, and how the DNA polymerase performs this step.

We are starting to understand how replication of ϕ29 is organised and compartmentalised into the bacterium, acting in concert with cellular factors to increase the efficiency of this biological process. Thus, early after ϕ29 infection TP-DNA replication takes place at the bacterial nucleoid by means of a non-specific interaction between the parental TP and the bacterial chromosome. Later during infection, the ϕ29 DNA replication machinery is organised in peripheral helix-like structures through an interaction of the phage protein p16.7, which recognises the dsDNA of replicating TP-DNA molecules, with the actin-like MreB cytoskeleton.

In addition, phage ϕ29 protein p56 is essential in the viral DNA replication cycle since it prevents the impairment caused by the host UDG. Inhibition of UDG has been proposed to be a defence mechanism developed by ϕ29 to prevent formation of abortive replicative intermediates. This is the first case reported of an UDG inhibitor encoded by a non-uracil containing DNA.

The mechanistic details of how *B. subtilis* MreB is specifically employed by phage ϕ29, and how they are temporally and spatially organized may be main directions for future experiments. Since bacteriophages contain genomes with a limited size due to their small dimensions, it is expected that new bacterial proteins interacting with viral components may be discovered. A major challenge is to identify these novel targets that might be used by bacteriophages to optimize the production of high numbers of progeny.

6. Acknowledgements

This work has been supported by grants BFU2008-00215 and Consolider-Ingenio 2010 24717 from the Spanish Ministry of Science and Innovation, and grant S2009/MAT-1507 from the Autonomous Community of Madrid to MS and by an Institutional grant from Fundación Ramón Areces to the Centro de Biología Molecular "Severo Ochoa".

7. References

Abril, A.M., Marco, S., Carrascosa, J.L., Salas, M. & Hermoso, J.M. (1999). Oligomeric structures of the phage ϕ29 histone-like protein p6. *J Mol Biol*. Vol. 292, No. 3, pp. 581-588

Abril, A.M., Salas, M. & Hermoso, J.M. (2000). Identification of residues within two regions involved in self-association of viral histone-like protein p6 from phage ϕ29. *J Biol Chem*. Vol. 275, No. 34, pp. 26404-26410, ISSN 0021-9258 (Print) 0021-9258 (Linking)

Albert, A., Muñoz-Espín, D., Jiménez, M., Asensio, J.L., Hermoso, J.A., Salas, M. & Meijer, W.J. (2005). Structural basis for membrane anchorage of viral ϕ29 DNA during replication. *J Biol Chem* Vol. 280, No. 52, pp. 42486-42488, ISSN 0021-9258 (Print) 0021-9258 (Print).

Anderson, D.L., Hickman, D.D. & Reilly, B.E. (1966). Structure of *Bacillus subtilis* bacteriophage ϕ29 and the length of ϕ29 deoxyribonucleic acid. *J Bacteriol*. Vol. 91, No. 5, pp. 2081-2089, ISSN 0021-9193 (Print) 0021-9193 (Linking)

Bamford, D.H. & Mindich, L. (1984). Characterization of the DNA-protein complex at the termini of the bacteriophage PRD1 genome. *J Virol*. Vol. 50, No. 2, pp. 309-315, ISSN 0022-538X (Print) 0022-538X (Linking)

Bamford, D.H., Ravantti, J.J., Ronnholm, G., Laurinavicius, S., Kukkaro, P., Dyall-Smith, M., Somerharju, P., Kalkkinen, N. & Bamford, J.K. (2005). Constituents of SH1, a novel lipid-containing virus infecting the halophilic euryarchaeon *Haloarcula hispanica*. *J Virol*. Vol. 79, No. 14, pp. 9097-9107, ISSN 0022-538X (Print)

Bamford, J.K., Hanninen, A.L., Pakula, T.M., Ojala, P.M., Kalkkinen, N., Frilander, M. & Bamford, D.H. (1991). Genome organization of membrane-containing bacteriophage PRD1. *Virology*. Vol. 183, No. 2, pp. 658-676, ISSN 0042-6822 (Print) 0042-6822 (Linking)

Bath, C., Cukalac, T., Porter, K. & Dyall-Smith, M.L. (2006). His1 and His2 are distantly related, spindle-shaped haloviruses belonging to the novel virus group, *Salterprovirus*. *Virology*. Vol. 350, No. 1, pp. 228-239, ISSN 0042-6822 (Print)

Beese, L.S., Derbyshire, V. & Steitz, T.A. (1993). Structure of DNA polymerase I Klenow fragment bound to duplex DNA. *Science*. Vol. 260, No. 5106, pp. 352-355

Berlatzky, I.A., Rouvinski, A. & Ben-Yehuda, S. (2008). Spatial organization of a replicating bacterial chromosome. *Proc Natl Acad Sci U S A*. Vol. 105, No. 37, pp. 14136-14140, ISSN 1091-6490 (Electronic) 0027-8424 (Linking)

Berman, A.J., Kamtekar, S., Goodman, J.L., Lázaro, J.M., de Vega, M., Blanco, L., Salas, M. & Steitz, T.A. (2007). Structures of phi29 DNA polymerase complexed with substrate: the mechanism of translocation in B-family polymerases. *EMBO J*. Vol. 26, No. 14, pp. 3494-3505, ISSN 0261-4189 (Print)

Bernad, A., Zaballos, A., Salas, M. & Blanco, L. (1987). Structural and functional relationships between prokaryotic and eukaryotic DNA polymerases. *EMBO J*. Vol. 6, No. 13, pp. 4219-4225

Bernad, A., Blanco, L., Lázaro, J.M., Martín, G. & Salas, M. (1989). A conserved 3'-5' exonuclease active site in prokaryotic and eukaryotic DNA polymerases. *Cell*. Vol. 59, No. 1, pp. 219-228

Blanco, L. & Salas, M. (1985a). Replication of phage ϕ29 DNA with purified terminal protein and DNA polymerase: synthesis of full-length ϕ29 DNA. *Proc Natl Acad Sci USA*. Vol. 82, No. 19, pp. 6404-6408

Blanco, L. & Salas, M. (1985b). Characterization of a 3'-5' exonuclease activity in the phage ϕ29-encoded DNA polymerase. *Nucleic Acids Res*. Vol. 13, No. 4, pp. 1239-1249

Blanco, L., Prieto, I., Gutiérrez, J., Bernad, A., Lázaro, J.M., Hermoso, J.M. & Salas, M. (1987). Effect of NH4+ ions on ϕ29 DNA-protein p3 replication: formation of a complex between the terminal protein and the DNA polymerase. *J. Virol*. Vol. 61, No. 12, pp. 3983-3991

Blanco, L., Bernad, A., Lázaro, J.M., Martín, G., Garmendia, C. & Salas, M. (1989). Highly efficient DNA synthesis by the phage ϕ29 DNA polymerase. Symmetrical mode of DNA replication. *J Biol Chem*. Vol. 264, No. 15, pp. 8935-8940

Blanco, L., Lázaro, J.M., de Vega, M., Bonnin, A. & Salas, M. (1994). Terminal protein-primed DNA amplification. *Proc Natl Acad Sci USA*. Vol. 91, No. 25, pp. 12198-12202

Blanco, L. & Salas, M. (1995). Mutational analysis of bacteriophage ϕ29 DNA polymerase. *Methods Enzymol*. Vol. 262, No. pp. 283-294

Blanco, L. & Salas, M. (1996). Relating structure to function in ϕ29 DNA polymerase. *J Biol Chem* Vol. 271, No. 15, pp. 8509-8512

Blasco, M.A., Blanco, L., Parés, E., Salas, M. & Bernad, A. (1990). Structural and functional analysis of temperature-sensitive mutants of the phage ϕ29 DNA polymerase. *Nucleic Acids Res*. Vol. 18, No. 16, pp. 4763-4770

Bravo, A. & Salas, M. (1997). Initiation of bacteriophage ϕ29 DNA replication in vivo: assembly of a membrane-associated multiprotein complex. *J. Mol. Biol*. Vol. 269, No. 1, pp. 102-112

Bravo, A. & Salas, M. (1998). Polymerization of bacteriophage ϕ29 replication protein p1 into protofilament sheets. *EMBO J*. Vol. 17, No. 20, pp. 6096-6105

Bravo, A., Illana, B. & Salas, M. (2000). Compartmentalization of phage ø29 DNA replication: interaction between the primer terminal protein and the membrane associated protein p1. *EMBO J*. Vol. 19, No. 20, pp. 5575-5584

Caldentey, J., Blanco, L., Bamford, D.H. & Salas, M. (1993). *In vitro* replication of bacteriophage PRD1 DNA. Characterization of the protein-primed initiation site. *Nucleic Acids Res*. Vol. 21, No. 16, pp. 3725-3730

Clarey, M.G., Erzberger, J.P., Grob, P., Leschziner, A.E., Berger, J.M., Nogales, E. & Botchan, M. (2006). Nucleotide-dependent conformational changes in the DnaA-like core of the origin recognition complex. *Nat Struct Mol Biol*. Vol. 13, No. 8, pp. 684-690, 1545-9993 (Print) 1545-9985 (Linking)

Coenjaerts, F.E. & van der Vliet, P.C. (1995). Adenovirus DNA replication in a reconstituted system. *Methods Enzymol*. Vol. 262, No. pp. 548-560, ISSN 0076-6879 (Print) 0076-6879 (Linking)

de Vega, M., Lázaro, J.M., Salas, M. & Blanco, L. (1996). Primer-terminus stabilization at the 3'-5' exonuclease active site of ϕ29 DNA polymerase. Involvement of two amino acid residues highly conserved in proofreading DNA polymerases. *EMBO J*. Vol. 15, No. 5, pp. 1182-1192

de Vega, M., Ilyina, T., Lázaro, J.M., Salas, M. & Blanco, L. (1997). An invariant lysine residue is involved in catalysis at the 3'-5' exonuclease active site of eukaryotic-type DNA polymerases. *J Mol Biol* Vol. 270, No. 1, pp. 65-78

de Vega, M., Blanco, L. & Salas, M. (1998a). ϕ29 DNA polymerase residue Ser122, a single-stranded DNA ligand for 3'-5' exonucleolysis, is required to interact with the terminal protein. *J Biol Chem*. Vol. 273, No. 44, pp. 28966-28977

de Vega, M., Lázaro, J.M., Salas, M. & Blanco, L. (1998b). Mutational analysis of ϕ29 DNA polymerase residues acting as ssDNA ligands for 3'-5' exonucleolysis. *J Mol Biol* Vol. 279, No. 4, pp. 807-822

de Vega, M., Blanco, L. & Salas, M. (1999). Processive proofreading and the spatial relationship between polymerase and exonuclease active sites of bacteriophage ϕ29 DNA polymerase. *J Mol Biol* Vol. 292, No. 1, pp. 39-51 de Vega, M., Lázaro, J.M., Mencía, M., Blanco, L. & Salas, M. (2010). Improvement of ϕ29 DNA polymerase amplification performance by fusion of DNA binding motifs. *Proc Natl Acad Sci U S A*. Vol. 107, No. 38, pp. 16506-16511, 1091-6490 (Electronic) 0027-8424 (Linking)

Dean, F.B., Nelson, J.R., Giesler, T.L. & Lasken, R.S. (2001). Rapid amplification of plasmid and phage DNA using Phi29 DNA polymerase and multiply-primed rolling circle amplification. *Genome Res*. Vol. 11, No. 6, pp. 1095-1099

Dean, F.B., Hosono, S., Fang, L., Wu, X., Faruqi, A.F., Bray-Ward, P., Sun, Z., Zong, Q., Du, Y., Du, J., Driscoll, M., Song, W., Kingsmore, S.F., Egholm, M. & Lasken, R.S. (2002). Comprehensive human genome amplification using multiple displacement amplification. *Proc Natl Acad Sci USA*. Vol. 99, No. 8, pp. 5261-5266

Derbyshire, V., Grindley, N.D. & Joyce, C.M. (1991). The 3'-5' exonuclease of DNA polymerase I of *Escherichia coli*: contribution of each amino acid at the active site to the reaction. *EMBO J*. Vol. 10, No. 1, pp. 17-24

Doublié, S., Tabor, S., Long, A.M., Richardson, C.C. & Ellenberger, T. (1998). Crystal structure of a bacteriophage T7 DNA replication complex at 2.2 Å resolution. *Nature*. Vol. 391, No. 6664, pp. 251-258

Dufour, E., Méndez, J., Lázaro, J.M., de Vega, M., Blanco, L. & Salas, M. (2000). An aspartic acid residue in TPR-1, a specific region of protein-priming DNA polymerases, is required for the functional interaction with primer terminal protein. *J Mol Biol*. Vol. 304, No. 3, pp. 289-300

Eom, S.H., Wang, J. & Steitz, T.A. (1996). Structure of Taq polymerase with DNA at the polymerase active site. *Nature*. Vol. 382, No. 6588, pp. 278-281

Erzberger, J.P., Mott, M.L. & Berger, J.M. (2006). Structural basis for ATP-dependent DnaA assembly and replication-origin remodeling. *Nat Struct Mol Biol*. Vol. 13, No. 8, pp. 676-683, ISSN 1545-9993 (Print) 1545-9985 (Linking)

Escarmís, C. & Salas, M. (1982). Nucleotide sequence of the early genes 3 and 4 of bacteriophage ϕ29. *Nucleic Acids Res*. Vol. 10, No. 19, pp. 5785-5798

Esteban, J.A., Salas, M. & Blanco, L. (1993). Fidelity of ϕ29 DNA polymerase. Comparison between protein-primed initiation and DNA polymerization. *J Biol Chem*. Vol. 268, No. 4, pp. 2719-2726

Esteban, J.A., Soengas, M.S., Salas, M. & Blanco, L. (1994). 3'-5' exonuclease active site of ϕ29 DNA polymerase. Evidence favoring a metal ion-assisted reaction mechanism. *J Biol Chem*. Vol. 269, No. 50, pp. 31946-31954

Firshein, W. (1989). Role of the DNA/membrane complex in prokaryotic DNA replication. *Annu Rev Microbiol*. Vol. 43, No. pp. 89-120, ISSN 0066-4227 (Print) 0066-4227 (Linking)

Franklin, M.C., Wang, J. & Steitz, T.A. (2001). Structure of the replicating complex of a pol α family DNA polymerase. *Cell*. Vol. 105, No. 5, pp. 657-667

Freire, R., Salas, M. & Hermoso, J.M. (1994). A new protein domain for binding to DNA through the minor groove. *EMBO J*. Vol. 13, No. 18, pp. 4353-4360, ISSN 0261-4189 (Print) 0261-4189 (Linking)

Freire, R., Serrano, M., Salas, M. & Hermoso, J.M. (1996). Activation of replication origins in ϕ29-related phages requires the recognition of initiation proteins to specific nucleoprotein complexes. *J Biol Chem* Vol. 271, No. 48, pp. 31000-31007

Friedberg, E.C., Ganesan, A.K. & Minton, K. (1975). N-Glycosidase activity in extracts of *Bacillus subtilis* and its inhibition after infection with bacteriophage PBS2. *J Virol*. Vol. 16, No. 2, pp. 315-321, ISSN 0022-538X (Print) 0022-538X (Linking)

García, E., Gómez, A., Ronda, C., Escarmís, C. & López, R. (1983). Pneumococcal bacteriophage Cp-1 contains a protein bound to the 5' termini of its DNA. *Virology*. Vol. 128, No. 1, pp. 92-104, 0042-6822 (Print) 0042-6822 (Linking)

García, J.A., Peñalva, M.A., Blanco, L. & Salas, M. (1984). Template requirements for initiation of phage ϕ29 DNA replication in vitro. *Proc Natl Acad Sci USA*. Vol. 81, No. 1, pp. 80-84

García, P., Hermoso, J.M., García, J.A., García, E., López, R. & Salas, M. (1986). Formation of a covalent complex between the terminal protein of pneumococcal bacteriophage Cp-1 and 5'-dAMP. *J Virol*. Vol. 58, No. 1, pp. 31-35, ISSN 0022-538X (Print) 0022-538X (Linking)

Garmendia, C., Bernad, A., Esteban, J.A., Blanco, L. & Salas, M. (1992). The bacteriophage ϕ29 DNA polymerase, a proofreading enzyme. *J Biol Chem* Vol. 267, No. 4, pp. 2594-2599

González-Huici, V., Lázaro, J.M., Salas, M. & Hermoso, J.M. (2000a). Specific recognition of parental terminal protein by DNA polymerase for initiation of protein-primed DNA replication. *J Biol Chem* Vol. 275, No. 19, pp. 14678-14683

González-Huici, V., Salas, M. & Hermoso, J.M. (2000b). Sequence requirements for protein-primed initiation and elongation of phage ϕ29 DNA replication. *J Biol Chem* Vol. 275, No. 51, pp. 40547-40553

Gutiérrez, C., Martín, G., Sogo, J.M. & Salas, M. (1991a). Mechanism of stimulation of DNA replication by bacteriophage ϕ29 single-stranded DNA-binding protein p5. *J Biol Chem*. Vol. 266, No. 4, pp. 2104-2111, ISSN 0021-9258 (Print) 0021-9258 (Linking)

Gutiérrez, C., Sogo, J.M. & Salas, M. (1991b). Analysis of replicative intermediates produced during bacteriophage ϕ29 DNA replication in vitro. *J Mol Biol*. Vol. 222, No. 4, pp. 983-994, ISSN 0022-2836 (Print) 0022-2836 (Linking)

Gutiérrez, J., García, J.A., Blanco, L. & Salas, M. (1986a). Cloning and template activity of the origins of replication of phage ϕ29 DNA. *Gene*. Vol. 43, No. 1-2, pp. 1-11

Gutiérrez, J., Vinós, J., Prieto, I., Méndez, E., Hermoso, J.M. & Salas, M. (1986b). Signals in the ϕ29 DNA-terminal protein template for the initiation of phage ϕ29 DNA replication. *Virology*. Vol. 155, No. 2, pp. 474-483

Harding, N.E. & Ito, J. (1980). DNA replication of bacteriophage ϕ29: characterization of the intermediates and location of the termini of replication. *Virology*. Vol. 104, No. 2, pp. 323-338, 0042-6822 (Print) 0042-6822 (Linking)

Huber, H.E., Tabor, S. & Richardson, C.C. (1987). *Escherichia coli* thioredoxin stabilizes complexes of bacteriophage T7 DNA polymerase and primed templates. *J Biol Chem* Vol. 262, No. 33, pp. 16224-16232

Illana, B., Blanco, L. & Salas, M. (1996). Functional characterization of the genes coding for the terminal protein and DNA polymerase from bacteriophage GA-1. Evidence for a sliding-back mechanism during protein-primed GA-1 DNA replication. *J Mol Biol* Vol. 264, No. 3, pp. 453-464

Illana, B., Zaballos, A., Blanco, L. & Salas, M. (1998). The RGD sequence in phage ϕ29 terminal protein is required for interaction with ϕ29 DNA polymerase. *Virology*. Vol. 248, No. 1, pp. 12-19

Inciarte, M.R., Salas, M. & Sogo, J.M. (1980). Structure of replicating DNA molecules of *Bacillus subtilis* bacteriophage ϕ29. *J Virol*. Vol. 34, No. 1, pp. 187-199, 0022-538X (Print) 0022-538X (Linking)

Johne, R., Müller, H., Rector, A., van Ranst, M. & Stevens, H. (2009). Rolling-circle amplification of viral DNA genomes using phi29 polymerase. *Trends Microbiol.* Vol. 17, No. 5, pp. 205-211, ISSN 1878-4380 (Electronic) 0966-842X (Linking)

Jones, L.J., Carballido- López, R. & Errington, J. (2001). Control of cell shape in bacteria: helical, actin-like filaments in *Bacillus subtilis*. *Cell*. Vol. 104, No. 6, pp. 913-922, ISSN 0092-8674 (Print) 0092-8674 (Linking)

Jonsson, Z.O. & Hübscher, U. (1997). Proliferating cell nuclear antigen: more than a clamp for DNA polymerases. *Bioessays*. Vol. 19, No. 11, pp. 967-975

Kamtekar, S., Berman, A.J., Wang, J., Lázaro, J.M., de Vega, M., Blanco, L., Salas, M. & Steitz, T.A. (2004). Insights into strand displacement and processivity from the crystal structure of the protein-primed DNA polymerase of bacteriophage ϕ29. *Mol Cell.* Vol. 16, No. 4, pp. 609-618

Kamtekar, S., Berman, A.J., Wang, J., Lázaro, J.M., de Vega, M., Blanco, L., Salas, M. & Steitz, T.A. (2006). The phi29 DNA polymerase:protein-primer structure suggests a model for the initiation to elongation transition. *EMBO J.* Vol. 25, No. 6, pp. 1335-1343, ISSN 0261-4189 (Print)

Kelman, Z. (1997). PCNA: structure, functions and interactions. *Oncogene*. Vol. 14, No. 6, pp. 629-640

King, A.J. & van der Vliet, P.C. (1994). A precursor terminal protein-trinucleotide intermediate during initiation of adenovirus DNA replication: regeneration of molecular ends in vitro by a jumping back mechanism. *EMBO J.* Vol. 13, No. 23, pp. 5786-5792

Kong, X.P., Onrust, R., O'Donnell, M. & Kuriyan, J. (1992). Three-dimensional structure of the beta subunit of *E. coli* DNA polymerase III holoenzyme: a sliding DNA clamp. *Cell.* Vol. 69, No. 3, pp. 425-437

Kornberg, A. & Baker, T.A. 81992) *DNA replication* (2nd edition), Freeman, W.H., ISBN 978-1-891389-44-3, New York

Li, Y., Kong, Y., Korolev, S. & Waksman, G. (1998). Crystal structures of the Klenow fragment of *Thermus aquaticus* DNA polymerase I complexed with deoxyribonucleoside triphosphates. *Protein Sci.* Vol. 7, No. 5, pp. 1116-1123

Longás, E., de Vega, M., Lázaro, J.M. & Salas, M. (2006). Functional characterization of highly processive protein-primed DNA polymerases from phages Nf and GA-1, endowed with a potent strand displacement capacity. *Nucleic Acids Res.* Vol. 34, No. 20, pp. 6051-6063

Longás, E., Villar, L., Lázaro, J.M., de Vega, M. & Salas, M. (2008). Phage ϕ29 and Nf terminal protein-priming domain specifies the internal template nucleotide to initiate DNA replication. *Proc Natl Acad Sci U S A.* Vol. 105, No. 47, pp. 18290-18295, 1091-6490 (Electronic) 0027-8424 (Linking)

López-Bueno, A., Tamames, J., Velázquez, D., Moya, A., Quesada, A. & Alcamí, A. (2009). High diversity of the viral community from an Antarctic lake. *Science*. Vol. 326, No. 5954, pp. 858-861, 1095-9203 (Electronic) 0036-8075 (Linking)

Martín, A.C., Blanco, L., García, P., Salas, M. & Méndez, J. (1996a). *In vitro* protein-primed initiation of pneumococcal phage Cp-1 DNA replication occurs at the third 3' nucleotide of the linear template: a stepwise sliding-back mechanism. *J Mol Biol* Vol. 260, No. 3, pp. 369-377

Martín, A.C., López, R. & García, P. (1996b). Analysis of the complete nucleotide sequence and functional organization of the genome of *Streptococcus pneumoniae* bacteriophage Cp-1. *J Virol.* Vol. 70, No. 6, pp. 3678-3687, ISSN 0022-538X (Print) 0022-538X (Linking)

Meijer, W.J., Serna-Rico, A. & Salas, M. (2001). Characterization of the bacteriophage ϕ29-encoded protein p16.7: a membrane protein involved in phage DNA replication. *Mol Microbiol.* Vol. 39, No. 3, pp. 731-746

Mellado, R.P., Peñalva, M.A., Inciarte, M.R. & Salas, M. (1980). The protein covalently linked to the 5' termini of the DNA of *Bacillus subtilis* phage ϕ29 is involved in the initiation of DNA replication. *Virology.* Vol. 104, No. 1, pp. 84-96

Méndez, J., Blanco, L., Esteban, J.A., Bernad, A. & Salas, M. (1992). Initiation of φ 29 DNA replication occurs at the second 3' nucleotide of the linear template: a sliding-back mechanism for protein-primed DNA replication. *Proc Natl Acad Sci USA.* Vol. 89, No. 20, pp. 9579-9583

Méndez, J., Blanco, L. & Salas, M. (1997). Protein-primed DNA replication: a transition between two modes of priming by a unique DNA polymerase. *EMBO J.* Vol. 16, No. 9, pp. 2519-2527

Mosig, G. & Macdonald, P. (1986). A new membrane-associated DNA replication protein, the gene 69 product of bacteriophage T4, shares a patch of homology with the *Escherichia coli* dnaA protein. *J Mol Biol.* Vol. 189, No. 1, pp. 243-248, ISSN 0022-2836 (Print) 0022-2836 (Linking)

Muñoz-Espín, D., Daniel, R., Kawai, Y., Carballido-López, R., Castilla-Llorente, V., Errington, J., Meijer, W.J. & Salas, M. (2009). The actin-like MreB cytoskeleton organizes viral DNA replication in bacteria. *Proc Natl Acad Sci U S A.* Vol. 106, No. 32, pp. 13347-13352, ISSN 1091-6490 (Electronic) 0027-8424 (Linking)

Muñoz-Espín, D., Holguera, I., Ballesteros-Plaza, D., Carballido-López, R. & Salas, M. (2010). Viral terminal protein directs early organization of phage DNA replication at the bacterial nucleoid. *Proc Natl Acad Sci U S A.* Vol. 107, No. 38, pp. 16548-16553, ISSN 1091-6490 (Electronic) 0027-8424 (Linking)

O'Donnell, M. & Jeruzalmi, D. (2006). Helical proteins initiate replication of DNA helices. *Nat Struct Mol Biol.* Vol. 13, No. 8, pp. 665-667, ISSN 1545-9993 (Print) 1545-9985 (Linking)

Otero, M.J., Lázaro, J.M. & Salas, M. (1990). Deletions at the N-terminus of bacteriophage ϕ29 protein p6: DNA binding and activity in ϕ29 DNA replication. *Gene.* Vol. 95, No. 1, pp. 25-30, ISSN 0378-1119 (Print) 0378-1119 (Linking)

Pérez-Arnaiz, P., Lázaro, J.M., Salas, M. & de Vega, M. (2006). Involvement of ϕ29 DNA polymerase thumb subdomain in the proper coordination of synthesis and degradation during DNA replication. *Nucleic Acids Res.* Vol. 34, No. 10, pp. 3107-3115

Pérez-Arnaiz, P., Longás, E., Villar, L., Lázaro, J.M., Salas, M. & de Vega, M. (2007). Involvement of phage ϕ29 DNA polymerase and terminal protein subdomains in conferring specificity during initiation of protein-primed DNA replication. *Nucleic Acids Res.* Vol. 35, No. 21, pp. 7061-7073, ISSN 1362-4962 (Electronic)

Pérez-Arnaiz, P., Lázaro, J.M., Salas, M. & de Vega, M. (2010). ϕ29 DNA polymerase active site: role of residue Val250 as metal-dNTP complex ligand and in protein-primed initiation. *J Mol Biol.* Vol. 395, No. 2, pp. 223-233, ISSN 1089-8638 (Electronic) 0022-2836 (Linking)

Prieto, I., Serrano, M., Lázaro, J.M., Salas, M. & Hermoso, J.M. (1988). Interaction of the bacteriophage ϕ29 protein p6 with double-stranded DNA. *Proc Natl Acad Sci USA.* Vol. 85, No. 2, pp. 314-318

Qi, X., Bakht, S., Devos, K.M., Gale, M.D. & Osbourn, A. (2001). L-RCA (ligation-rolling circle amplification): a general method for genotyping of single nucleotide polymorphisms (SNPs). *Nucleic Acids Res.* Vol. 29, No. 22, pp. E116, ISSN 1362-4962 (Electronic) 0305-1048 (Linking)

Rodríguez, I., Lázaro, J.M., Salas, M. & de Vega, M. (2004). ϕ29 DNA polymerase-terminal protein interaction. Involvement of residues specifically conserved among protein-primed DNA polymerases. *J Mol Biol* Vol. 337, No. 4, pp. 829-841

Rodríguez, I., Lázaro, J.M., Blanco, L., Kamtekar, S., Berman, A.J., Wang, J., Steitz, T.A., Salas, M. & de Vega, M. (2005). A specific subdomain in ϕ29 DNA polymerase confers both processivity and strand-displacement capacity. *Proc Natl Acad Sci USA.* Vol. 102, No. 18, pp. 6407-6412

Rodríguez, I., Lázaro, J.M., Salas, M. & de Vega, M. (2009). Involvement of the TPR2 subdomain movement in the activities of ϕ29 DNA polymerase. *Nucleic Acids Res.* Vol. 37, No. 1, pp. 193-203, ISSN 1362-4962 (Electronic)

Salas, M., Mellado, R.P., Viñuela, E. & Sogo, J.M. (1978). Characterization of a protein covalently linked to the 5' termini of the DNA of *Bacillus subtilis* phage ϕ29. *J Mol Biol.* Vol. 119, No. 2, pp. 269-291, ISSN 0022-2836 (Print)

Salas, M. (1991). Protein-priming of DNA replication. *Annu Rev Biochem.* Vol. 60, No. pp. 39-71

Salas, M., Freire, R., Soengas, M.S., Esteban, J.A., Méndez, J., Bravo, A., Serrano, M., Blasco, M.A., Lázaro, J.M., Blanco, L. & et al. (1995). Protein-nucleic acid interactions in bacteriophage ϕ29 DNA replication. *FEMS Microbiol. Rev.* Vol. 17, No. 1-2, pp. 73-82

Salas, M., Miller, J.T., Leis, J., DePamphilis, M.L. (1996) Mechanisms for priming DNA. In *DNA replication in eukaryotic cells,* DePamphilis, M.L., pp. 131-176, Cold Spring Harbor Laboratory Press, ISBN 0-87969-459-9, New York

Salas, M. (1999). Mechanisms of initiation of linear DNA replication in prokaryotes. *Genet. Eng. (N Y).* Vol. 21, pp. 159-171

Salas, M. & de Vega, M. (2006). Bacteriophage protein-primed DNA replication. In *Recent advances in DNA virus replication.* Hefferon, K.L., pp. 259-288, Research Signpost, ISBN 81-308-0042-X, Kerala (India)

Salas, M. & de Vega, M. (2008). Replication of bacterial viruses. In *Encyclopedia of Virology, 3rd edition.* Mahy, B.W.J. and van Regenmortel, M.H.V., Vol. 4, pp. 339-406, Elsevier, ISBN 978-0-12-374410-4, Oxford

Serna-Rico, A., Illana, B., Salas, M. & Meijer, W.J. (2000). The putative coiled coil domain of the ϕ29 terminal protein is a major determinant involved in recognition of the origin of replication. *J Biol Chem* Vol. 275, No. 51, pp. 40529-40538

Serna-Rico, A., Muñoz-Espín, D., Villar, L., Salas, M. & Meijer, W.J. (2003). The integral membrane protein p16.7 organizes in vivo ϕ29 DNA replication through interaction with both the terminal protein and ssDNA. *EMBO J.* Vol. 22, No. 9, pp. 2297-2306

Serrano, M., Salas, M. & Hermoso, J.M. (1990). A novel nucleoprotein complex at a replication origin. *Science.* Vol. 248, No. 4958, pp. 1012-1016

Serrano, M., Gutiérrez, C., Salas, M. & Hermoso, J.M. (1993a). Superhelical path of the DNA in the nucleoprotein complex that activates the initiation of phage ϕ29 DNA replication. *J Mol Biol* Vol. 230, No. 1, pp. 248-259, ISSN 0022-2836 (Print)

Serrano, M., Salas, M. & Hermoso, J.M. (1993b). Multimeric complexes formed by DNA-binding proteins of low sequence specificity. *Trends Biochem. Sci.* Vol. 18, No. 6, pp. 202-206, ISSN 0968-0004 (Print)

Serrano, M., Gutiérrez, C., Freire, R., Bravo, A., Salas, M. & Hermoso, J.M. (1994). Phage ϕ29 protein p6: a viral histone-like protein. *Biochimie*. Vol. 76, No. 10-11, pp. 981-991

Serrano-Heras, G., Salas, M. & Bravo, A. (2003). In vivo assembly of phage ϕ29 replication protein p1 into membrane-associated multimeric structures. *J Biol Chem* Vol. 278, No. 42, pp. 40771-40777

Serrano-Heras, G., Salas, M. & Bravo, A. (2006). A uracil-DNA glycosylase inhibitor encoded by a non-uracil containing viral DNA. *J. Biol. Chem.* Vol. 281, No. 11, pp. 7068-7074

Serrano-Heras, G., Bravo, A. & Salas, M. (2008). Phage ϕ29 protein p56 prevents viral DNA replication impairment caused by uracil excision activity of uracil-DNA glycosylase. *Proc Natl Acad Sci U S A*. Vol. 105, No. 49, pp. 19044-19049, ISSN 1091-6490 (Electronic) 0027-8424 (Linking)

Shamoo, Y. & Steitz, T.A. (1999). Building a replisome from interacting pieces: sliding clamp complexed to a peptide from DNA polymerase and a polymerase editing complex. *Cell*. Vol. 99, No. 2, pp. 155-166, ISSN 0092-8674 (Print)

Shiue, S.Y., Hsieh, J.C. & Ito, J. (1991). Mapping of the DNA linking tyrosine residue of the PRD1 terminal protein. *Nucleic Acids Res*. Vol. 19, No. 14, pp. 3805-3810, ISSN 0305-1048 (Print) 0305-1048 (Linking)

Siegel, P.J. & Schaechter, M. (1973). The role of the host cell membrane in the replication and morphogenesis of bacteriophages. *Annu Rev Microbiol*. Vol. 27, No. pp. 261-282, ISSN 0066-4227 (Print) 0066-4227 (Linking)

Soengas, M.S., Esteban, J.A., Salas, M. & Gutiérrez, C. (1994). Complex formation between phage ϕ29 single-stranded DNA binding protein and DNA. *J Mol Biol*. Vol. 239, No. 2, pp. 213-226, ISSN 0022-2836 (Print) 0022-2836 (Linking)

Soengas, M.S., Gutiérrez, C. & Salas, M. (1995). Helix-destabilizing activity of ϕ29 single-stranded DNA binding protein: effect on the elongation rate during strand displacement DNA replication. *J Mol Biol* Vol. 253, No. 4, pp. 517-529

Sogo, J.M., García, J.A., Peñalva, M.A. & Salas, M. (1982). Structure of protein-containing replicative intermediates of *Bacillus subtilis* phage ϕ29 DNA. *Virology*. Vol. 116, No. 1, pp. 1-18, ISSN 0042-6822 (Print) 0042-6822 (Linking)

Tabor, S., Huber, H.E. & Richardson, C.C. (1987). *Escherichia coli* thioredoxin confers processivity on the DNA polymerase activity of the gene 5 protein of bacteriophage T7. *J Biol Chem* Vol. 262, No. 33, pp. 16212-16223, ISSN 0021-9258 (Print) 0021-9258 (Linking)

Van der Vliet, P.C. (1995). Adenovirus DNA replication. *Curr Top Microbiol Immunol*. Vol. 199 (Pt 2), No. pp. 1-30, ISSN 0070-217X (Print) 0070-217X (Linking)

Verdun, R.E. & Karlseder, J. (2007). Replication and protection of telomeres. *Nature*. Vol. 447, No. 7147, pp. 924-931, ISSN 1476-4687 (Electronic)

Warner, H.R., Johnson, L.K. & Snustad, D.P. (1980). Early events after infection of *Escherichia coli* by bacteriophage T5. III. Inhibition of uracil-DNA glycosylase activity. *J Virol*. Vol. 33, No. 1, pp. 535-538, ISSN 0022-538X (Print) 0022-538X (Linking)

Xu, Y., Gao, S., Bruno, J.F., Luft, B.J. & Dunn, J.J. (2008). Rapid detection and identification of a pathogen's DNA using Phi29 DNA polymerase. *Biochem Biophys Res Commun*. Vol. 375, No. 4, pp. 522-525, ISSN 1090-2104 (Electronic) 0006-291X (Linking)

Yoshikawa, H. & Ito, J. (1982). Nucleotide sequence of the major early region of bacteriophage ϕ29. *Gene*. Vol. 17, No. 3, pp. 323-335, ISSN 0378-1119 (Print)

Zaballos, A. & Salas, M. (1989). Functional domains in the bacteriophage ϕ29 terminal protein for interaction with the ϕ29 DNA polymerase and with DNA. *Nucleic Acids Res*. Vol. 17, No. 24, pp. 10353-10366

10

Meiotic DNA Replication

David T. Stuart
University of Alberta Department of Biochemistry, Edmonton, Alberta, Canada

1. Introduction

Chromosome replication is a basic biological process that is essential for cellular proliferation. Owing to its fundamental nature the process of DNA replication is highly conserved among eukaryotic organisms. In the course of a typical somatic cell cycle, cells are "born" in G1 phase. Throughout this phase the cells grow in size increasing their mass and their protein synthetic capacity. As cells grow during G1 they monitor their size and protein synthetic capacity along with a variety of parameters in the external milieu including nutrient availability (Hartwell, 1974). When the internal and external environments are deemed to be suitable, the cell will commit to a cell division cycle. Initiating a cell cycle is a serious matter for yeast cells in that once they initiate the program they are committed to its completion (Hartwell, 1974). Should the cell have insufficient resources or capacity to successfully complete division the result is arrest and inevitable loss of viability. The decision to initiate a division cycle is taken at START in the budding yeast *Saccharomyces cerevisiae*; this event is referred to as R, the restriction point in mammalian cells (Hartwell, 1974; Pardee, 1974). If conditions are appropriate for proliferation, G1 phase cells will make the transition to S-phase where DNA replication ensues followed by progression through G2 and chromosome segregation at mitosis followed by completion of the cycle at cytokinesis.

Prior to completing the START transition and committing to a round of cell division *S. cerevisiae* can adopt several alternative fates. Haploid cells can conjugate with a partner of the opposite mating type to form diploids (Cross et al., 1988). Alternatively, both haploid and diploid cells are capable of entering a quiescent state in response to deprivation of some nutrients (Gray et al., 2004). Under the appropriate conditions diploid *MAT*a/α cells can exit the mitotic cell cycle and initiate the meiotic differentiation program leading to sporulation (Kupiec et al., 1997). This differentiation program is triggered by starvation for nitrogen and glucose. Upon encountering these conditions diploid *S. cerevisiae* will arrest in G1 phase with unreplicated DNA. The meiotic differentiation process initiates from G1 phase where the starved cells accumulate, and progresses through premeiotic DNA replication followed by extensive homologous recombination. Meiotic recombination is followed by two consecutive rounds of chromosome segregation, the meiosis I (reductional) division, and meiosis II (equational) division. Significantly, these two rounds of chromosome division occur without an intervening S-phase hence the meiotic progeny are haploid and the haploid nuclei are encapsulated in spores that are highly resistant to environmental insult. Hence, with regard to chromosome metabolism, the meiotic program resembles a somatic cell cycle but many aspects of the process are modified to achieve the desired developmental aim of ploidy reduction, increased genetic diversity, and spore formation.

2. The transition to premeiotic S-phase

In mitotically proliferating *S. cerevisiae* cells, progression past START and entry into S-phase is dependent upon the Cyclin Dependent kinase Cdk1 (formerly known as Cdc28) (Reed, 1992). Cdk1 is activated in G1-phase by the three G1 cyclins Cln1, Cln2, and Cln3 (Richardson et al., 1989). The Cln-Cdk1 complexes serve multiple functions in promoting entry into a mitotic cell cycle (Levine et al., 1995). Starvation for nitrogen and glucose causes diploid cells to arrest in G1 and precludes progression into a mitotic cell division cycle. Under these conditions the *CLN1, CLN2* and *CLN3* genes are repressed (Gallego et al., 1997). The *CLN* cyclins are not required for entry into or progression through meiotic differentiation and indeed enforced expression of *CLN* cyclins under starvation conditions impedes the initiation of meiotic differentiation (Dirick et al., 1998; Colomina et al., 1999). It has been proposed that *CLN* expression acts as the switch that determines whether a cell initiates a mitotic division cycle or enters meiotic differentiation (Colomina et al., 1999).
Nitrogen deprivation, the condition that represses the expression of the *CLN* genes and precludes entry into a mitotic cell division cycle, induces the expression of a cascade of meiosis-specific genes (Kassir et al., 2003). *MAT*a/α diploid cells respond to starvation for nitrogen and glucose by activating expression of *IME1* (Inducer of Meiosis) (Kassir et al., 1988). The induction of *IME1* requires input from a complex signaling pathway that integrates nutritional signals (nitrogen and glucose) and ploidy *MAT*a and *MAT*α mating type genes (Kassir et al., 2003). *MAT*a/α diploids will respond to this condition by initiating the program of meiotic differentiation, whereas haploids, *MAT*a/a or *MAT*α/α diploids will arrest in G1 and enter a quiescent state. *IME1* is a meiosis-specific transcription factor that activates the expression of a large family of early meiotic genes many of which encode proteins that function in DNA replication and recombination (Mitchell, 1994). One of the key targets of Ime1 protein is the *IME2* gene (Smith et al., 1990). Ime2 encodes a meiosis-specific protein kinase with amino acid sequence similarity to Cdks. Indeed it has been proposed that Ime2 may replace the functions of Cln-Cdk1 complexes in meiosis (Dirick et al., 1998). While Ime2 may share some of the roles played by G1 cyclins it is unlikely that Ime2 directly replaces Cdk function in meiosis (Honigberg, 2004). However, Ime2 does play many roles in the meiotic differentiation program including driving the induction of early and middle phase meiosis-specific genes, and promoting inactivation of both APC^{CDH1} (Anaphase Promoting Complex) and the Cdk inhibitor Sic1 (Dirick et al., 1998; Bolte et al., 2002; Sedgwick et al., 2006; Holt et al., 2007). The latter two functions are essential to allow the accumulation of active B-type cyclin-Cdk1 complexes as APC^{CDH1} targets the cyclins for proteolytic degradation and Sic1 binds to the cyclin-Cdk1 complexes and inhibits their catalytic activity.
Ime1 and Ime2 are key regulators of the meiotic differentiation program. Loss of Ime1 function causes diploid cells to arrest in G1 phase in response to starvation, and precludes initiation of the meiotic program (Kassir et al., 1988; Smith et al., 1990). Mutations that inactivate Ime2 result in diploid cells undergoing a prolonged G1-phase arrest in response to starvation followed by delayed and defective DNA replication that leads to loss of viability (Foiani et al., 1996).

3. Initiation of premeiotic DNA replication

The initiation of DNA replication is a tightly regulated process that begins with the stepwise assembly of a protein complex that ultimately recruits a DNA helicase and the DNA polymerases required for replication of the chromosomal DNA (Remus & Diffley, 2009). Although meiotic differentiation differs from mitotic proliferation, in some cases drastically, the fundamental aspects of the premeiotic DNA replication mirror the processes that occur during mitotic proliferation.

DNA replication initiates from specific chromosomal locations referred to as origins of replication (Ori). These sequences are distributed along each of the chromosomes so that DNA replication can initiate from multiple sites. The relatively compact Oris of *S. cerevisiae* have been well defined and have an essential core sequence 5′-TTTTATGTTTA-3′ and a set of three less well conserved accessory sequences that stimulate the efficiency of Ori activation (Marahrens & Stillman, 1992; Marahrens & Stillman, 1994). Data from numerous investigations support the contention that origins of replication are activated with variable efficiency in mitotically proliferating cells. Additionally, not every Ori is activated in every S-phase (McCune et al., 2008; Patel et al., 2008). Thus, Oris that are activated more efficiently have a higher probability of being activated at higher frequency.

Origin of DNA replication usage has been less rigorously investigated during premeiotic DNA replication. Analysis of origin activation by two-dimensional gel electrophoresis suggested that in *S. cerevisiae* the same origins that are activated during mitotic proliferation are also utilized during premeiotic DNA replication (Collins & Newlon, 1994). This study did not investigate the efficiency or frequency of origin activation. A more recent investigation of origin usage in the fission yeast *Schizosaccharomyces pombe* using microarray technology revealed that the same origins of DNA replication are used during mitosis and meiosis in this yeast (Heichinger et al., 2006). These authors found an overall reduction in the efficiency of origin utilization in premeiotic DNA replication relative to proliferation and they speculated that this might at least in part explain why premeiotic DNA replication takes so much longer than mitotic DNA replication (2 hours for premeiotic S-phase vs. 20 minutes for mitotic S-phase in *S. cerevisiae)* (Cha et al., 2000; Heichinger et al., 2006). Transcription initiating near or proceeding through Ori sequences can influence the efficiency of origin utilization (Donato et al., 2006; Mori & Shirahige, 2007). Additionally, the state of histone modification, in particular acetylation, has been correlated with the efficiency of Ori assembly and activation (Vogelauer et al., 2002; Weber et al., 2008; Unnikrishnan et al., 2010). Some of these conclusions were reached by using chemical inhibition of histone deacetylases (HDACs) to alter the modification state of the chromatin. These conclusions are controversial since altering HDAC activity can affect many aspects of gene regulation and one effect of HDAC inhibition is to reduce the supply of pyrimidine nucleotide precursors for DNA replication resulting in reduced fork speed and the recruitment of latent origins of DNA replication: (Gay et al., 2010).

Since transcription patterns and the landscape of protein binding to DNA changes dramatically when cells transition from mitotic proliferation to meiotic differentiation it is not surprising that there would be a change in the usage of origins. It is unclear why there is an overall reduction in origin firing in meiotic cells but one possibility is that that some factor required for origin firing is limited during meiosis. Owing to the fact that meiotic differentiation initiates under starvation conditions where there may be no exogenous source of amino acids or nitrogen and that the total number of ribosomes decreases by 50%

or more (Hopper et al., 1974; Magee & Hopper, 1974) it is likely that the overall rate of protein synthesis is reduced in cells undergoing meiosis (Esposito et al., 1969). Under these conditions labile factors such as Dbf4 may become limiting to origin activation (Patel et al., 2008). During mitotic proliferation Ori activation is temporally regulated with a subset of origins being activated early and another subset being activated later in S-phase (Raghuraman & Brewer, 2010). Activation of these origins displays distinct properties, early firing origins are activated even in the presence of hydroxyurea which inhibits or reduces activation of late origins (Santocanale et al., 1999). S-phase initiation requires Cdk1, and the S-phase form of *S. cerevisiae* Cdk1 is activated by the cyclins Clb5 and Clb6. Early origins are activated in the absence of the S-phase cyclin Clb5 whereas late activated origins depend upon Clb5 (Donaldson et al., 1998). This particular characteristic has been attributed to the fact that Clb6-Cdk1 complexes are present early in S-phase but Clb6 is rapidly degraded as cells progress through S-phase (Jackson et al., 2006). The role of cyclin Cdk complexes in triggering DNA replication will be considered in section 5 of this chapter. The mechanisms governing this temporal pattern of origin activation have been speculated upon but have yet to be clarified. Recent investigations suggest that earlier firing origins are more efficient and have a higher probability of firing in any given cell cycle. It has not yet been determined whether temporal regulation is imposed upon Ori activation during premeiotic DNA replication.

4. Assembling the prereplication complex

DNA replication is initiated from specific origins of replication by assembling complex multiprotein machines on origins of replication and then activating those complexes. PreReplication Complex (PreRC) assembly at origins of DNA replication has been extensively investigated in mitotically proliferating cells (Diffley, 2001). Contributions from several laboratories have revealed that assembly of the complex proceeds in a step-wise fashion (Diffley et al., 1995). In yeast the Ori sequence is constitutively bound by the Origin Recognition Complex (Orc) composed or the proteins Orc1 – Orc6 (Rowley et al., 1995). In contrast the Orc proteins assemble on the origins in G1-phase in metazoans and Orc1 is destabilized as the cells pass through S-phase (DePamphilis, 2005). The Orc complex marks the chromosomal origins of DNA replication, and serves as a nucleation site for the assembly of a functional PreRC (Diffley et al., 1995; Rowley et al., 1995).

A key cell cycle regulated step in promoting further assembly of the PreRC is the accumulation of Cdc6 and Cdt1 in late G1 phase. Transcription of the Cdc6 gene is induced in late G1 phase by the MBF transcription factor (Zhou & Jong, 1990). In mitotically proliferating cells the accumulating Cdc6 in conjunction with Cdt1 binds to Orc complexes tethered to Ori DNA (Devault et al., 2002). The ATPase activity associated with Cdc6 is then required to promote loading of the Mcm (Mini Chromosome Maintenance) complex on to the ORC complex (Stillman, 2005). The loading of Mcm is a key step in assembling the origin complex. Failure of this loading or loss of Cdc6 function precludes further assembly of PreRCs and blocks the initiation of DNA replication (Piatti et al., 1995). Surprisingly, loss of Cdc6 function does not arrest chromosome metabolism. Rather, cells depleted of Cdc6 simply skip over S-phase and progress to a reductional chromosome division leading to loss of viability (Piatti et al., 1995).

The Cdc6 gene is subject to regulated transcription during meiotic differentiation where it accumulates during G1 phase (Ofir et al., 2004). Cdc6 is essential for progression through premeiotic S-phase and meiotic recombination in both yeast and higher eukaryotes (Lemaitre et al., 2002; Lemaitre et al., 2004; Ofir et al., 2004). Loss of Cdc6 in meiotic differentiation precludes the initiation of premeiotic DNA replication but allows an attempted chromosome division without having replicated the DNA or forming a synaptonemal complex, leading to loss of viability (Hochwagen et al., 2005). Current thinking ascribes progression to meiotic chromosome divisions in the absence of S-phase to the idea that progression through G1 – S – M phases is restrained by the S-phase checkpoint which detects single stranded DNA or some aspect of DNA replication fork structure. A failure to initiate DNA replication results in no signal that could be detected by the checkpoint and so the checkpoint is not activated. Under these conditions the transcriptional program that drives meiotic differentiation proceeds and the cells progress to attempt the segregation of unreplicated chromosomes (Stuart & Wittenberg, 1998).

The primary role of Cdc6 is to promote the association of the hexameric Mcm complex with DNA bound Orc complexes (Tanaka et al., 1997). The Mcm proteins Mcm 2 - 7 form sub-complexes that can subsequently be loaded on to the Orc complex as a dimer of hexamers (Stillman, 2005). The Mcm complex functions as an ATP-dependent DNA helicase (Ishimi, 1997). By loading a dimer of Mcm hexamers on to Orc complexes the hexamers can drive unwinding of the duplex DNA leading to bidirectional DNA replication. In addition to their role in DNA unwinding, the Mcm helicase also provides binding sites for the recruitment of other factors that form the replication forks such as DNA polymerases (Forsburg, 2004).

Components of the Mcm complex accumulate cooperatively in the nucleus during G1-phase and are required for activation not only of S-phase but also of the S-phase checkpoint (Labib et al., 2001). Surprisingly, it has been reported that Mcm proteins are not required for premeiotic DNA replication in yeast (Forsburg & Hodson, 2000). This study made use of a set of yeast strains harboring temperature sensitive mutations in a subset of the *MCM* genes. The opposite conclusion was reached by investigators using temperature sensitive degron mutants that eliminated or profoundly reduced the abundance of the Mcm proteins upon activation of the degron (Lindner et al., 2002). The difference between these two investigations may simply have been the degree to which the Mcm proteins could be depleted from the cells.

Subsequent to the loading of the hexameric Mcm complex in late G1-phase, assembly of the PreRC continues with the recruitment of several additional factors Cdc45, Dpb11, Sld2, Sld3, and the GINS complex (Remus & Diffley, 2009; Tanaka & Araki, 2010). Cdc45 has no identified catalytic activity but it makes specific contacts with the Mcm complex and is essential for mitotic DNA replication (Hopwood & Dalton, 1996). Cdc45 is essential for premeiotic DNA replication and meiosis in plants (Stevens et al., 2004), and it is assumed to be essential for premeiotic DNA synthesis in yeast although this has never been formally reported.

Cdc45 binding to the Mcm complex at the preRC is linked to binding of Dpb11, Sld2, and Sld3. Dpb11 is thought to act as a scaffold to allow association of Sld2, Sld3 and the replicative DNA polymerases Pol1 (DNA polymerase alpha) and Pol2 (DNA polymerase epsilon) with the preRC (Masumoto et al., 2000; Tanaka et al., 2007; Zegerman & Diffley, 2007). Sld2, Sld3, and Dpb11 are all essential for the initiation of DNA replication in proliferating cells (Araki et al., 1995; Kamimura et al., 1998; Kamimura et al., 2001). Stable assembly of Sld2 and Sld3 with Dpb11 and the preRC is dependent upon Cdk activity. Phosphorylation of Sld2 and Sld3 on multiple Cdk sites promotes their stable binding to Dpb11 and the preRC (Tanaka et al., 2007; Zegerman & Diffley, 2007). Temperature sensitive *sld2*, and mutants display a profound defect in premeiotic DNA replication implying that they serve the same essential role in meiotic cells that they play in proliferating cells (Figure 1).

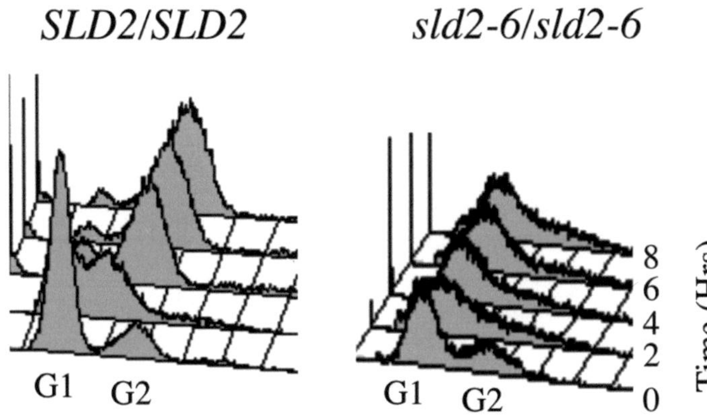

Fig. 1. Flow cytometry profiles of *SLD2/SLD2* and *sld2-6/sld2-6* mutant cells that have been induced to initiate meiotic differentiation at the non-permissive temperature of 36°C. The *sld2-6* mutant arrests in G1-phase - early S-phase and does not complete S-phase. The *sld2-6* temperature sensitive allele was provided by Dr. H. Araki and was introduced into the *S. cerevisiae* SK1 genetic background by gene replacement.

The GINS complex is a tetrameric protein assembly whose name derives from Go-Ichi-Ni-San; the Japanese numbers 5,1,2,3, in reference to Sld5, Psf1, Psf2, Psf3, the components of the complex (Takayama et al., 2003). GINS associates with Sld2, Dpb11, and Pol2 in a sub-complex that is loaded on to the preRC (Muramatsu et al., 2010). The GINS complex is essential for the initiation of DNA replication and replication fork progression in proliferating cells (Takayama et al., 2003). The function of GINS in premeiotic S-phase has not been directly investigated, however the finding that *psf2* mutants display meiotic chromosome segregation defects in *S. pombe* suggests that Psf2 and GINS also play a role in meiotic DNA replication (Gómez et al., 2005).

The assembly of the correct preRC architecture is important for regulating the initiation of DNA replication and the ultimate function of this complex is to recruit and position the replicative DNA polymerases to the Ori where the chromosomal DNA will be unwound by the Mcm complex and bidirectional DNA synthesis will initiate. Pol1, the catalytic subunit of DNA polymerase alpha-primase is essential for meiotic DNA replication and likely serves the purpose of synthesizing the lagging strand as it does in proliferating cells (Budd et al., 1989). Not unexpectedly, subunits of the DNA primase, Pri1 and Pri2, are also required for the synthesis of the lagging strand (Longhese et al., 1993). The leading strand DNA polymerase Pol3 (DNA polymerase delta) plays a role in meiotic DNA replication and meiotic homologous DNA recombination (Schild & Byers, 1978; Maloisel et al., 2008). Pol2 (DNA polymerase epsilon) is also found at the replication fork and has a role as leading strand DNA polymerase in proliferating cells (Calzada et al., 2005). Surprisingly the catalytic activity of Pol2 is not essential in mitotically proliferating cells likely owing to redundancy with Pol3 activity (Kesti et al., 1999; Ohya et al., 2002). Both of the leading strand polymerases are expected to be required for premeiotic DNA replication but this has not been formally demonstrated.

Thus, while preRCs are composed of primarily the same components during the initiation of S-phase in meiotic and proliferating cells, it should be noted that the composition of meiotic preRC has not been formally investigated and may have components remaining to be identified that impart meiosis-specific regulation to the activation of premeiotic DNA synthesis.

5. Activating premeiotic DNA synthesis: the role of Cyclin-Cdk and Dbf4-Cdc7

In proliferating cells the activation of DNA synthesis is dependent upon B-type cyclin-Cdk1 and Dbf4-Cdc7. *S. cerevisiae* has a single cell cycle regulating Cdk, referred to as Cdk1. Cdk1 is essential for all the major cell cycle transitions in *S. cerevisiae* (Nasmyth, 1993). Cdk1 can bind to and is activated by nine different cyclins. *CLN1, CLN2,* and *CLN3* are expressed in proliferating G1 phase cells. Six B-type cyclins *CLB1 - CLB6* are expressed in S-phase, G2 and mitosis (Lew & Reed, 1992). Cyclin binding to Cdk1 serves the purposes of activating the catalytic function of the kinase through promoting a change in the conformation of Cdk1 and they direct the Cdk1 kinase activity against specific substrates (Morgan, 1995; Loog & Morgan, 2005). Cdk1 is essential for activating S-phase in proliferating cells and during meiotic development (Reed, 1980; Benjamin et al., 2003). Cdk1 in complex with the cyclins Clb5 and Clb6 is the primary Cdk1 complex that drives the initiation of DNA replication. Clb5 is the dominant cyclin of the Clb5, Clb6 pair as it is more stable and accumulates to greater abundance (Jackson et al., 2006). Although other B-type cyclins can activate Cdk1 to promote S-phase in proliferating cells none do so as efficiently as Clb5 (Donaldson et al., 1998; Cross et al., 1999; Hu et al., 2008). This is in part due to the consideration that Clb5 and Clb6 accumulate in late G1 whereas the other B-type cyclins Clbs1 - 4, normally accumulate later in G2 and M-phase (Fitch et al., 1992; Richardson et al., 1992; Schwob & Nasmyth, 1993). However, even when other cyclins are ectopically expressed in G1 they can induce DNA replication but with a significant delay relative Clb5 (Donaldson, 2000; Hu & Aparicio, 2005). It is likely that this is due to substrate specificity. Clb5 and Clb6 have an amino acid motif (MRAIL) that has affinity for the substrate sequence RxL that is present in proteins like Sld2 and Sld3 that are high affinity substrates for Clb5 (Cross & Jacobson, 2000; Ubersax et al., 2003; Loog & Morgan, 2005). Hence Clb5 and Clb6 are referred to as S-phase cyclins.

The key and possibly only essential role for Cdk1 in activating DNA replication is to phosphorylate Sld2 and Sld3 to allow them to bind Dpb11 and the preRC complex or stabilize their binding through creation of high affinity sites (Tanaka et al., 2007; Zegerman & Diffley, 2007). There may be additional roles in supporting DNA polymerase binding since the DNA polymerase epsilon subunit Dpb2 is also Cdk substrate (Kesti et al., 1999).

Cdk1 activity is required for several aspects of chromosome metabolism in the early stages of meiotic differentiation. Cdk1 is strictly required for premeiotic DNA replication as demonstrated by the meiotic G1 arrest when mutants expressing an analog sensitive version of Cdk1 are treated with the inhibitor 1-NM-PP1 (Benjamin et al., 2003). Cdk1 is also required for the initiation of meiotic DNA recombination and synaptonemal complex formation (Henderson et al., 2006; Zhu et al., 2010). Both of these processes are dependent upon successful completion of premeiotic DNA replication.

Temperature sensitive alleles of Cdk1 cannot be inactivated sufficiently to block premeiotic DNA replication, which led to the idea that Cdk1 activity was not required for progression through meiotic differentiation (Shuster & Byers, 1989). It is unclear why proliferating cells need more Cdk1 activity to initiate S-phase than do meiotically differentiating cells. One possibility is that in proliferating cells Cdk1 is required to activate the transcription factors MBF (MluI binding factor) and SBF (SCB binding factor) (deBruin et al., 2004). These transcription factors induce the expression of the genes whose products function to promote S-phase and DNA replication *CLB5, POL1, RNR1* etc. (Koch & Nasmyth, 1994). In contrast, many of the genes whose products are required for premeiotic S-phase are regulated by the meiosis-specific transcription factor Ime1 (Mitchell, 1994). SBF is not active in meiotic cells; however, MBF is active during meiotic G1 and promotes G1-specific transcription; however, inactivation of MBF does not eliminate expression of the genes required for DNA replication and does not cause any defect in premeiotic DNA replication (Raithatha & Stuart, 2005). Additionally, there is evidence that a subset of MBF regulated genes are differentially regulated during mitotic and meiotic G1-phase (Raithatha & Stuart, 2005).

In mitotically proliferating *S. cerevisiae* the S-phase cyclins *CLB5* and *CLB6* are not essential for S-phase activation, indeed cells will only arrest in G1 when all six of the B-type cyclins are inactivated (Schwob et al., 1994). In contrast *CLB5* and *CLB6* are strictly required for the initiation of premeiotic S-phase (Dirick et al., 1998; Stuart & Wittenberg, 1998). During the course of unperturbed meiotic differentiation Clb5 and Clb6 are the first cyclins to accumulate and these trigger DNA replication whereas the other B-type cyclin genes are regulated by Ndt80 and only accumulate during the middle phase of sporulation during pachytene (Chu et al., 1998). Even if Clb1 or Clb3 is expressed early in meiosis under the regulation of a *CLB5* promoter these cyclins fail to trigger premeiotic S-phase in a *clb5 clb6* mutant (J. DeCesare & D. Stuart unpublished observation). Suggesting that Clb5 and Clb6 have some particular property that allows them to activate DNA synthesis during meiosis. Possibilities include subcellular localization, recruitment to specific substrates or substrate specificity. Clb5 accumulates in the nucleus both in proliferating and sporulating cells as expected since it effectively phosphorylates components of the preRC. The fact that any B-type cyclin can induce DNA replication in proliferating cells implies that all cyclin-Cdk1 complexes can gain access to the appropriate substrates at least in proliferating cells. However, it is unlikely that simple subcellular localization gives Clb5 its specific ability to activate premeiotic DNA replication because Clb3 has been localized to the nucleus in both proliferating and sporulating cells so in principle it should have access to the same suite of substrates as Clb5-Cdk1 complexes. The S-phase cyclins Clb5 and Clb6 display homology with other B-type cyclins in their Cdk1 binding domain however the amino-terminal portions of each cyclin are highly diverged from each other as well as other B-type cyclins and it is not clear what sequences direct these cyclins to their proper nuclear location.

Even though all cyclin-Cdk1 complexes can enter the nucleus they may not all have access to the same substrates. The potential remains for compartmentalization within the nucleus or sequestration of cyclin-Cdk1 complexes to locations within the nucleus where they may not have access to the critical substrates required to initiate premeiotic DNA replication. It is very likely that the architectural organization of the nucleus differs between mitosis and meiosis owing to the unique demands for synaptonemal complex formation, extensive homologous recombination, and the reductional meiosis I chromosome division. Within this altered nuclear landscape Clb5 and Clb6-Cdk1 complexes may have a unique ability to interact efficiently with the substrate proteins required to assemble and fire origins of DNA replication.

The molecular mechanisms that confer substrate specificity to cyclins have yet to be fully resolved (Miller & Cross, 2001). It is clear that Clb5 has a preference for a specific collection of protein substrates that can interact with the cyclin MRAIL motif. Indeed Clb5 may harbor additional substrate interaction motifs that confer increased affinity to one or more meiosis-specific substrates. The cyclins that are shown to have specific functions in S-phase: *S. cerevisae* Clb5, and Clb6 and *C. albicans* Clb4, have a conserved motif of charged amino acids at their carboxyl-terminus that is not present in other cyclins (Figure 2). This sequence may have a role in the S-phase functions of these cyclins but no analysis of mutations in this motif have been reported. Premeiotic S-phase is influenced by proteins that are only expressed during meiotic differentiation (see next section) and it may well be that Clb5-Cdk1 can specifically phosphorylate or interact with those substrates. While it is not surprising that there would be cyclins with specialized roles in meiotic differentiation the mechanism by which that specificity is conferred remain to be elucidated.

```
Sc. Clb5: 374 IHDEAFQSLCIDLVKDIASSKTHLDSLILKYKKPRYGS
Sc. Clb6: 330 ESDPAFKDFISELVEDIAVPDTNLDSLRLKYKKPKHGM
Kl. Clb : 340 DNEIELKELSQILINDIAKPTTQLNALIHKYKKIGTWN
Ca. Clb4: 433 YTEKQLQPLADVLLENCRHAEINHKAIFEKYKERRYRK
                +  +  +   L+           +  KYK
```

Fig. 2. A conserved cluster of charged amino acids near the carboxyl-terminus of the *S. cerevisae* S. phase cyclins Clb5 and Clb6. A similar cluster is present in the *C. albicans* Clb4 (an S-phase cyclin) and a cyclin from *K. lactis* (r_klactIV3887) whose function has not been confirmed. This charged cluster is not found in other *S. cerevisiae* cyclins.

In addition to cyclin-Cdk1, activation of DNA replication requires the kinase activity associated with the Dbf4-Cdc7 protein kinase (Masai et al., 1999). Cdc7 is the catalytic subunit of the protein kinase whereas Dbf4 is an activating and substrate targeting subunit similar to a cyclin (Jackson et al., 1993). The enzyme complex is referred to as DDK (Dbf4 Dependent Kinase). In *S. cerevisiae* Dbf4 accumulates in late G1 phase and binds Cdc7, which is constitutively expressed. The complex is then recruited to preRCs through interactions with both Mcm and Orc proteins (Dowell et al., 1994). The catalytic activity of Cdc7 is required to activate DNA replication in proliferating cells as inactivation of *cdc7* temperature sensitive mutants results in a strict G1-S-phase arrest (Newlon & Fangman, 1975). This phenotype is replicated by the analog sensitive alleles of Cdc7 that can be specifically inhibited by the small molecule PP1 [4-amino-1-tert-butyl-3-(p-methylyphenyl)pyrazolo [3,4-d]pyrimidine] (Wan et al., 2006). Recruitment of Dbf4 to the PreRC is essential for the activation of DNA replication, mutations that allow Dbf4 to bind Cdc7 but not the preRC cause a failure in DNA replication (Duncker et al., 2002).

The role of Cdc7 in premeiotic DNA replication has been controversial since both *cdc7* temperature sensitive mutants and analog sensitive mutants arrest post S-phase prior to the onset of meiotic recombination (Schild & Byers, 1978; Buck et al., 1991; Wan et al., 2006). In contrast the activating subunit Dbf4 is essential for premeiotic DNA replication (Valentin et al., 2006). Dbf4 is a highly unstable protein that can be rapidly depleted from cells unlike Cdc7, which is very stable (Ferreira et al., 2000). It may be the case that like Cdk, there is a lower threshold of Cdc7 kinase activity required in meiosis. Nonetheless the requirement for Dbf4 argues that Dbf4-Cdc7 activity is required for premeiotic DNA replication.

The essential substrates of Cdc7 have been intensively sought after. Genetic analysis revealed that a mutation in Mcm5 (Mcm5-$P^{83}L$) could bypass the need for Cdc7 or Dbf4 both during mitotic proliferation and for premeiotic DNA replication (Hardy et al., 1997; Matos et al., 2008). Interestingly DDK does not appear to phosphorylate Mcm5. Rather it seems likely that phosphorylation of other components of the MCM complex Mcm2, Mcm4 and Mcm6 by DDK leads to a conformational change in the complex allowing its activation (Hoang et al., 2007). The $P^{83}L$ mutation in Mcm5 may result in a similar change that allows activation of the complex in the absence of DDK phosphorylation (Hoang et al., 2007). Currently the best candidates for the essential substrates of Dbf4-Cdc7 are Mcm2, Mcm4 and Mcm6. DDK can phosphorylate these Mcm proteins both in vitro and in vivo (Lei et al., 1997; Masai et al., 2006; Francis et al., 2009). Indeed Cdc7 preferentially phosphorylates the Mcm proteins within the context of the PreRC and chromatin bound Mcms are much better Cdc7 substrates than the free Mcm proteins (Francis et al., 2009). The role of Mcm phosphorylation is not entirely clear but there is evidence that it stabilizes the binding of Cdc45 and perhaps other components of the preRC (Zou & Stillman, 2000). Additionally, it has been posed that phosphorylation of the Mcm complex may lead to a conformational change that relieves autoinhibition of the helicase activity (Sheu & Stillman, 2010).

DDK has additional roles in meiotic chromosome metabolism. Strains that harbor *cdc7* mutations are defective in the formation of DNA double strand breaks (DSBs) that initiate meiotic homologous recombination (Wan et al., 2006). DDK phosphorylates several residues on Mer2 protein allowing it to stably associate with the chromatin and trigger double stand breaks (Sasanuma et al., 2008; Wan et al., 2008). Phosphorylation of Mer2 by DDK is dependent upon prior phosphorylation of Mer2 by Cdk1 (Sasanuma et al., 2008; Wan et al., 2008). Thus, the initiation of DSB formation and homologous recombination requires integration of inputs from both Cdk1 and DDK kinases.

6. Does DNA replication differ between meiosis and mitosis?

The process of initiating DNA replication in proliferating cells and cells undergoing meiotic differentiation are fundamentally the same. All of the proteins required to initiate S-phase in mitotically proliferating cells seem to also be required for premeiotic S-phase although not all have been rigorously tested in meiotic cells (Simchen, 1974). Premeiotic S-phase displays a reduced requirement for Cdk and DDK activity but these enzymes are still required. Based upon genetic and molecular studies it appears that the preRC assembled in cells initiating premeiotic S-phase is similar to or the same as that assembled in proliferating cells. However, a variety of investigations have revealed significant differences between mitotic and premeiotic S-phase. One fundamental physiological difference between the two processes is that proliferating cells display a specific cell size requirement before they can transition from G1 to S-phase (Cook & Tyers, 2007). Premeiotic DNA replication and indeed the entire meiotic differentiation process in *S. cerevisiae* is independent of cell size control (Stuart, 2008). This issue is somewhat controversial as some investigators have observed cell size regulation of meiotic differentiation but the differences may be related to the genetic background of the strains used in the experiments (Calvert & Dawes, 1984; Day et al., 2004).

Genetic studies have revealed several genes whose products are required for meiotic but not mitotic S-phase: *SPO7, SPO9, MUM2*, and *CDC55* (Esposito & Klapholtz, 1981; Davis et al.,

2001; Nolt et al., 2011). *SPO7* and *CDC55* encode subunits of protein phosphatases and may be candidates for meiosis-specific regulators of DNA replication. *MUM2* displays genetic interactions with both the replicative DNA polymerase *POL1* and *ORC2* suggesting that this protein may participate in activating premeiotic origins of DNA replication; however, the basis for its requirement has yet to be reported (Davis et al., 2001). The function of *SPO9* remains to be characterized. Currently the molecular basis for the meiosis-specific requirement for these proteins remains unknown.

Premeiotic S-phase is also dependent upon Ime2, a meiosis-specific kinase whose amino acid sequence is similar to Cdks (Foiani et al., 1996). Loss of Ime2 function causes a profound delay in premeiotic S-phase. Ime2 may not directly regulate the initiation of premeiotic DNA replication because *ime2* mutants display a plethora of defects including reduced recombination, reduction in early and middle meiotic gene expression (Mitchell et al., 1990; Benjamin et al., 2003). Ime2 is implicated in the inactivation of the APC^{CDH1} an event necessary to allow accumulation of B-type cyclins (Bolte et al., 2002; Holt et al., 2007). Ime2 is also implicated in destabilizing Sic1 although this effect may not be direct (Dirick et al., 1998; Sedgwick et al., 2006).

One of the most easily observable differences between premeiotic S-phase and S-phase in proliferating cells is the prolonged time frame for premeiotic DNA replication. S-phase lasts for nearly 2 hours in meiotic cells whereas the process lasts a mere 20 minutes in proliferating cells (Cha et al., 2000). Since the same origins of replication are utilized in meiotic and mitotic S-phase the most likely explanation for the slow progress of DNA replication is that origins are activated with lower efficiency as observed in fission yeast (Heichinger et al., 2006). Alternatively, the rate of fork movement may be slower in meiotic cells. Experiments using metabolic labeling and DNA fiber autoradiography suggested that the rate of replication fork movement is the same in meiotic and mitotic cells (Johnston et al., 1982). However, during premeiotic DNA replication the replication forks must contend with the assembling Spo11 DSB complexes on the chromatin. Replication forks have been shown to pause when encountering stable protein-DNA complexes (Azvolinsky et al., 2009). It is possible that replication fork pausing caused by the DSB complexes slows the progression of premeiotic DNA replication. Indeed deletion of *SPO11* shortens premeiotic S-phase supporting this contention (Cha et al., 2000).

7. Premeiotic DNA replication and meiotic recombination: What's the connection?

The ultimate goal of the meiotic differentiation process is to produce the haploid progeny required for sexual reproduction. One of the hallmarks of the meiotic process is elevated rates of recombination that effectively "shuffle the genome" allowing for relatively unbiased assortment of the parental genetic material. The process of generating haploid progeny yields at least two significant advantages to *S. cerevisiae*. First the genetic assortment that occurs increases the likelihood of generating at least a subset of progeny that are in possession of increased fitness relative to the parent. Second by passing through a haploid stage any deleterious recessive mutations that have accumulated in the diploid parent may be eliminated since a haploid harboring this allele will be inviable, a type of genetic "quality control' mechanism.

Meiotic recombination has been extensively studied in *S. cerevisiae* owing to the ease with which meiotic progeny can be separated and tracked. Meiotic DNA recombination is generally predicated upon the successful completion of premeiotic DNA replication. The DNA double strand breaks (DSBs) that initiate meiotic recombination only form after the DNA has been replicated. This order of events is clearly important since the formation of DSBs prior to DNA replication would be catastrophic for genome integrity. This dependent relationship was elegantly demonstrated by a study that removed origins of DNA replication from the left arm of chromosome III, effectively delaying the completion of the replication of that arm of the chromosome. While DNA replication and DNA double strand break formation occurred with the expected normal timing on the right arm of chromosome III, DNA replication and DSB formation was profoundly delayed on the left arm (Borde et al., 2000).

A variety of possible mechanisms have been put forth to explain this relationship such as altered chromatin structure of the replicated DNA allowing DSB formation or access to the DSB forming complex (Berchowitz et al., 2009). Another potential explanation is that the DNA replication machinery may interact with and "license" or activate the protein complex that produces the meiotic DNA double strand breaks.

DNA DSBs are formed by a protein complex that binds to the chromatin in meiotic G1-phase. The complex is minimally composed of Spo11, Rec102, Rec104, Ski8 Mer2, Me14, Rec114, Mre11, and Rad50 (Keeney, 2001). Some of the integral components of the DSB formation complex are substrates for the S-phase protein kinases Clb5-Cdk1 and Dbf4-Cdc7. Mer2 is phosphorylated by Clb5-Cdk1 and this modification acts as a priming phosphorylation to trigger phosphorylation by Dbf4-Cdc7 (Henderson et al., 2006; Sasanuma et al., 2008; Wan et al., 2008). These phosphorylation events are essential for meiotic DSB formation and recombination. A mutated Mer2 lacking Cdk phosphorylation sites is defective in interacting with other components of the DSB forming complex (Henderson et al., 2006). Could Cdk1 and DDK be the connection between premeiotic DNA replication and meiotic recombination?

A parsimonious model to explain the temporal regulation of DSB formation and the involvement of Clb5-Cdk1 and Dbf4-Cdc7 could be that when Clb5-Cdk1 accumulates in premeiotic G1 phase it phosphorylates proteins required to assembly the PreRC (Sld2 and Sld3) as well as the DSB initiation complex (Mer2). Dbf4 accumulating in premeiotic G1-phase binds to Cdc7 and recruits the active Cdc7 to the PreRC. Upon the initiation of DNA replication the Mcm complex and other residents of the replication forks move along the chromosomes and Dbf4-Cdc7 moves along with the fork. As replication forks pass and possibly pause at sites of DSB initiation complexes Dbf4-Cdc7 phosphorylates members of the complex allowing for complete assembly or activation of the complex such that DSB formation can ensue following the passage of the replication fork.

This model is consistent with most published data however *cdc6* mutants that fail to assemble PreRCs form DSBs despite the absence of any detectable DNA replication (Hochwagen et al., 2005). Although this mutation decouples replication and recombination it is not inconsistent with the proposed model. The Dbf4-Cdc7 complex normally becomes tethered to the PreRC following loading of the Mcm complex by Cdc6. In the absence of Cdc6 the Mcm complex fails to load on to the DNA and Dbf4-Cdc7 complexes are thus not sequestered and can proceed to phosphorylate target proteins such as the DSB initiation complex factors hence allowing DSB formation. The localization and activity of Dbf4-Cdc7 has not been determined in *cdc6* mutants and so this model currently remains a matter of conjecture. Indeed it is also possible that the DNA replication checkpoint regulates the DSB formation complex and impedes the formation of DSBs until DNA replication is complete (Tonami et al., 2005).

8. Conclusion

DNA replication is an integral component of the meiotic differentiation program and is essential to the integrity of chromosome cohesion, meiotic recombination, and chromosome segregation. Defects in meiotic DNA replication have consequences that range from infertility and death of the progeny gametes to genomic instability and aneuploidy that can manifest as genetic diseases, birth defects and cancer. Despite our growing understanding of the mechanisms that govern DNA replication in mitotically proliferating cells, the regulation of premeiotic DNA replication remains largely uncharacterized. Several specific topics hold great promise for new discovery in the future, in particular the role of cyclin-Cdk1 in triggering premeiotic DNA synthesis, the regulation of preRC assembly in meiotic cells, and the relationship between DNA replication and homologous recombination.

Premeiotic DNA replication is subject to several distinct forms of regulation involving meiosis-specific regulatory proteins and meiosis-specific requirements for cyclin-Cdk and DDK. Future investigations will likely focus on clarification of substrate specificity, subcellular localization, and protein-protein interactions involving cyclin-Cdk1 and DDK. Additionally, premeiotic DNA replication requires some proteins that are meiosis-specific. Mum2 has no close orthologs in other organisms and as yet has no clearly defined role but that it is required for premeiotic DNA replication in *S. cerevisiae*. PreRC complexes have not yet been closely examined in cells undergoing meiotic differentiation. Biochemical characterization of these complexes through proteomic investigation may yield a wealth of new information about the components of meiotic replication complex and how premeiotic DNA replication is regulated. The biochemical relationship between the DNA replication machinery and the recombination machinery remains to be characterized and such investigations will certainly lead to an understanding of how DNA DSB formation is restrained until the DNA replication has been replicated. The molecular mechanisms governing the distinct regulation of premeiotic DNA replication remain to be elucidated but these will undoubtedly be geared to accomplishing the specific developmental aims of meiotic differentiation, namely the production of haploid gametes.

9. References

Araki, H., Leem, S. H., et al. (1995). Dpb11, which interacts with DNA polymerase II(epsilon) in *Saccharomyces cerevisiae*, has a dual role in S-phase progression and at a cell cycle checkpoint. Proc Natl Acad Sci U S A 92(25): pp.11791-11795.

Azvolinsky, A., Giresi, P. G., et al. (2009). Highly transcribed RNA polymerase II genes are impediments to replication fork progression in *Saccharomyces cerevisiae*. Mol Cell 34(6): pp.722-734.

Benjamin, K. R., Zhang, C., et al. (2003). Control of landmark events in meiosis by the CDK Cdc28 and the meiosis-specific kinase Ime2. Genes & Dev. 17: pp.1524-1539.

Berchowitz, L. E., Hanlon, S. E., et al. (2009). A positive but complex association between meiotic double-strand break hotspots and open chromatin in *Saccharomyces cerevisiae*. Genome Res 19(12): pp.2245-2257.

Bolte, M., Steigemann, P., et al. (2002). Inhibition of APC-mediated proteolysis by the meiosis-specific protein kinase Ime2. Proc. Natl. Acad. Sci. USA 99: pp.4385-4390.

Borde, V., Goldman. A. S. H., et al. (2000). Direct coupling between meiotic DNA replication and recombination initiation. Science 290: pp.806-809.

Buck, V., White, A., et al. (1991). *CDC7* protein kinase activity is required for mitosis and meiosis in *Saccharomyces cerevisiae*. Mol. Gen. Genet 227: pp.452-457.

Budd, M. E., Wittrup, K. D., et al. (1989). DNA polymerase I is required for premeiotic DNA replication and sporulation but not for X-ray repair in *Saccharomyces cerevisiae*. Mol. Cell. Biol. 9: pp.365-376.

Calvert, G. R. and Dawes, I. W. (1984). Cell size control of development in *Saccharomyces cerevisiae*. Nature 312: pp.61-63.

Calzada, A., Hodgson, B., et al. (2005). Molecular anatomy and regulation of a stable replisome at a paused eukaryotic DNA replication fork. Genes Dev. 19: pp.1905-1919.

Cha, R. S., Weiner, B. M., et al. (2000). Progression of meiotic DNA replication is modulated by interchromosomal interaction proteins, negatively by Spo11 and positively by Rec8. Genes & Dev. 14: pp.493-503.

Chu, S., DeRisi, J., et al. (1998). The transcriptional program of sporulation in budding yeast. Science 282: pp.699-705.

Collins, I. and Newlon, C. S. (1994). Chromosomal DNA replication initiates at the same origins in meiosis and mitosis. Mol. Cell. Biol. 14: pp.3524-3534.

Colomina, N., Gari, E., et al. (1999). G1 cyclins block the Ime1 pathway to make mitosis and meiosis incompatible in budding yeast. EMBO J. 18: pp.320-329.

Cook, M. and Tyers, M. (2007). Size control goes global. Curr Opin Biotechnol 18(4): pp.341-350.

Cross, F., Hartwell, L. H., et al. (1988). Conjugation in *Saccharomyces cerevisiae*. Annu Rev Cell Biol 4: pp.429-457.

Cross, F. R. and Jacobson, M. (2000). Conservation and function of a potential substrate-binding domain of the yeast Clb5 B-type cyclin. Mol. Cell. Biol. 20: pp.4782-4790.

Cross, F. R., Yuste-Rojas, M., et al. (1999). Specialization and targeting of B-type cyclins. Mol. Cell 4: pp.11-19.

Davis, L., Barbera, M., et al. (2001). The *Saccharomyces cerevisiae MUM2* gene interacts with the DNA replication machinery and is required for meiotic levels of double strand breaks. Genetics 157(3): pp.1179-1189.

Day, A., Markwardt, J., et al. (2004). Cell size and Cln-Cdc28 complexes mediate entry into meiosis by modulating cell growth. Cell cycle 3: pp.1433-1439.

deBruin, R. A. M., McDonald, W. H., et al. (2004). Cln3 activates G1-specific transcription via phosphorylation of the SBF bound repressor Whi5. Cell 117: pp.887-898.

DePamphilis, M. L. (2005). Cell cycle dependent regulation of the origin recognition complex. Cell Cycle 4(1): pp.70-79.

Devault, A., Vallen, E. A., et al. (2002). Identification of Tah11/Sid2 as the ortholog of the replication licensing factor Cdt1 in Saccharomyces cerevisiae. Curr Biol 12(8): pp.689-694.

Diffley, J. F. (2001). DNA replication: building the perfect switch. Curr Biol 11(9): pp.R367-370.

Diffley, J. F., Cocker, J. H., et al. (1995). Stepwise assembly of initiation complexes at budding yeast replication origins during the cell cycle. J Cell Sci Suppl 19: pp.67-72.

Dirick, L., Goetsch, L., et al. (1998). Regulation of meiotic S-phase by Ime2 and a Clb5,6-associated kinase in *Saccharomyces cerevisiae*. Science 281: pp.1854-1857.

Donaldson, A. (2000). Yeast mitotic cyclin *CLB2* cannot substitute for S-phase cyclins in replication origin firing. EMBO reports 1: pp.507-512.

Donaldson, A. D., Raghuraman, M. K., et al. (1998). Clb5-dependent activation of late replication origins in *Saccharomyces cerevisiae*. Mol. Cell 2: pp.173-182.

Donato, J. J., Chung, S. C., et al. (2006). Genome-wide hierarchy of replication origin usage in *Saccharomyces cerevisiae*. PLoS Genet 2(9): pp.e141.

Dowell, S. J., Romanowski, P., et al. (1994). Interaction of Dbf4, the Cdc7 protein kinase regulatory subunit, with yeast replication origins in vivo. Science 265(5176): pp.1243-1246.

Duncker, B. P., Shimada, K., et al. (2002). An N-terminal domain of Dbf4p mediates interaction with both origin recognition complex (ORC) and Rad53p and can deregulate late origin firing. Proc Natl Acad Sci U S A 99(25): pp.16087-16092.

Esposito, M. S., Esposito, R. E., et al. (1969). Acetate utilization and macromolecular synthesis during sporulation of yeast. J Bacteriol 100(1): pp.180-186.

Esposito, R. E. and Klapholtz, S. (1981). Meiosis and Ascospore Development. The Molecular Biology of the Yeast *Saccharomyces*: Life Cycle and Inheritance. J. Strathern, Jones, E. W. and Broach, J. Cold Spring Harbor, NY, Cold Spring Harbor Press: 211-287.

Ferreira, M. F., Santocanale, C., et al. (2000). Dbf4p, an essential S phase-promoting factor, is targeted for degradation by the anaphase-promoting complex. Mol Cell Biol 20(1): pp.242-248.

Fitch, I., Dahman, C., et al. (1992). Characterization of four B-type cyclin genes of the budding yeast *Saccharomyces cerevisiae*. Mol. Biol. Cell 3: pp.805-818.

Foiani, M., Nadgar-Boger, E., et al. (1996). A meiosis-specific protein kinase, Ime2, is required for the correct timing of DNA replication and for spore formation in yeast meiosis. Mol. Gen. Genetics 253: pp.278-288.

Forsburg, S. L. (2004). Eukaryotic MCM proteins: beyond replication initiation. Microbiol Mol Biol Rev 68(1): pp.109-131.

Forsburg, S. L. and Hodson, J. A. (2000). Mitotic replication initiation protein are not required for premeiotic S phase. Nature genetics 25: pp.263-268.

Francis, L. I., Randell, J. C., et al. (2009). Incorporation into the prereplicative complex activates the Mcm2-7 helicase for Cdc7-Dbf4 phosphorylation. Genes Dev 23(5): pp.643-654.

Gallego, C., Gari, E., et al. (1997). The Cln3 cyclin is down regulated by translational repression and degradation during G1 arrest caused by nitrogen deprivation in budding yeast. EMBO J. 16: pp.7196-7206.

Gay, S., Lachages, A. M., et al. (2010). Nucleotide supply, not local histone acetylation, sets replication origin usage in transcribed regions. EMBO Rep 11(9): pp.698-704.

Gómez, E. B., Angeles, V. T., et al. (2005). A screen for *Schizosaccharomyces pombe* mutants defective in rereplication identifies new alleles of rad4+, cut9+ and psf2+. Genetics 169(1): pp.77-89.

Gray, J. V., Petsko, G. A., et al. (2004). "Sleeping beauty": quiescence in *Saccharomyces cerevisiae*. Microbiol Mol Biol Rev 68(2): pp.187-206.

Hardy, C. F., Dryga, O., et al. (1997). *mcm5/cdc46-bob*1 bypasses the requirement for S phase activator Cdc7p. Proc. Nat. Acad. Sci. 94: pp.3151-3155.

Hartwell, L. H. (1974). *Saccharomyces cerevisiae* Cell Cycle. Bacteriol. Rev. 38: pp.164-198.

Heichinger, C., Penkett, C. J., et al. (2006). Genome-wide characterization of fission yeast DNA replication origins. Embo J 25(21): pp.5171-5179.
Henderson, K. A., Kee, K., et al. (2006). Cyclin-dependent kinase directly regulates initiation of meiotic recombination. Cell 125(7): pp.1321-1332.
Hoang, M. L., Leon, R. P., et al. (2007). Structural changes in Mcm5 protein bypass Cdc7-Dbf4 function and reduce replication origin efficiency in *Saccharomyces cerevisiae.* Mol Cell Biol 27(21): pp.7594-7602.
Hochwagen, A., Tham, W. H., et al. (2005). The FK506 binding protein Fpr3 counteracts protein phosphatase 1 to maintain meiotic recombination checkpoint activity. Cell 122(6): pp.861-873.
Holt, L. J., Hutti, J. E., et al. (2007). Evolution of Ime2 phosphorylation sites on Cdk1 substrates provides a mechanism to limit the effects of the phosphatase Cdc14 in meiosis. Mol Cell 25(5): pp.689-702.
Honigberg, S. M. (2004). Ime2p and Cdc28p: Co-pilots driving meiotic development. J. Cell. Biochem. 92: pp.1025-1033.
Hopper, A. K., Magee, P. T., et al. (1974). Macromolecule synthesis and breakdown in relation to sporulation and meiosis in yeast. J Bacteriol 119(2): pp.619-628.
Hopwood, B. and Dalton, S. (1996). Cdc45p assembles into a complex with Cdc46p/Mcm5p, is required for minichromosome maintenance, and is essential for chromosomal DNA replication. Proc. Natl. Acad. Sci. U S A. 93: pp.12309-12314.
Hu, F. and Aparicio, O. M. (2005). Swe1 regulation and transcriptional control restrict the activity of mitotic cyclins toward replication proteins in *Saccharomyces cerevisiae.* Proc Natl Acad Sci U S A 102(25): pp.8910-8915.
Hu, F., Gan, Y., et al. (2008). Identification of Clb2 residues required for Swe1 regulation of Clb2-Cdc28 in *Saccharomyces cerevisiae*. Genetics 179(2): pp.863-874.
Ishimi, Y. (1997). A DNA helicase activity is associated with an MCM4, -6, and -7 protein complex. J Biol Chem 272(39): pp.24508-24513.
Jackson, A. L., Pahl, P. M., et al. (1993). Cell cycle regulation of the yeast Cdc7 protein kinase by association with the Dbf4 protein. Mol. Cell. Biol. 13: pp.2899-2908.
Jackson, L. P., Reed, S. I., et al. (2006). Distinct mechanisms control the stability of the related S-phase cyclins Clb5 and Clb6. Mol Cell Biol 26(6): pp.2456-2466.
Johnston, L. H., Williamson, D. H., et al. (1982). On the mechanism of premeiotic DNA synthesis in the yeast *Saccharomyces cerevisiae*. Exp Cell Res 141(1): pp.53-62.
Kamimura, Y., Masumoto, H., et al. (1998). Sld2, which interacts with Dbp11 in *Saccharomyces cerevisiae*, is required for chromosomal DNA replication. Mol. Cell. Biol. 18: pp.6102-6109.
Kamimura, Y., Tak, Y.-S., et al. (2001). Sld3, which interacts with cdc45 (Sld4), functions for chromosomal DNA replication in *Saccharomyces cerevisiae*. EMBO J. 20: pp.2097-2107.
Kassir, Y., Adir, N., et al. (2003). Transcriptional regulation of meiosis in budding yeast. Int. Rev. Cytol 224: pp.11-71.
Kassir, Y., Granot, D., et al. (1988). *IME1*, a positive regulator gene of meiosis in *S. cerevisiae.* Cell 52: pp.853-862.
Keeney, S. (2001). Mechanism and control of meiotic recombination initiation. Curr Top Dev Biol 52: pp.1-53.

Kesti, T., Flick, K., et al. (1999). DNA polymerase epsilon catalytic domains are dispensable for DNA replication, DNA repair, and cell viability. Mol Cell 3(5): pp.679-685.

Koch, C. and Nasmyth, K. (1994). Cell cycle regulated transcription in yeast. Curr. Opin. in Cell Biology 6: pp.451-459.

Kupiec, M., Byers, B., et al. (1997). Meiosis and sporulation in *Saccharomyces cerevisiae*. Molecular and Cellular Biology of the Yeast *Saccharomyces cerevisiae*. Cell cycle and Cell Biology: pp.889-1036.

Labib, K., Kearsey, S. E., et al. (2001). MCM2-7 proteins are essential components of prereplicative complexes that accumulate cooperatively in the nucleus during G1-phase and are required to establish, but not maintain, the S-phase checkpoint. Mol Biol Cell 12(11): pp.3658-3667.

Lei, M., Kawasaki, Y., et al. (1997). Mcm2 is a target of regulation by Cdc7-Dbf4 during the initiation of DNA synthesis. Genes Dev 11(24): pp.3365-3374.

Lemaitre, J. M., Bocquet, S., et al. (2002). Competence to replicate in the unfertilized egg is conferred by Cdc6 during meiotic maturation. Nature 419(6908): pp.718-722.

Lemaitre, J. M., Bocquet, S., et al. (2004). The regulation of competence to replicate in meiosis by Cdc6 is conserved during evolution. Mol Reprod Dev 69(1): pp.94-100.

Levine, K., Tinklenberg, A. H., et al. (1995). The *CLN* gene family: central regulators of the cell cycle Start in budding yeast. Prog. Cell Cycle Res. 1: pp.101-114.

Lew, D. J. and Reed, S. I. (1992). A proliferation of cyclins. Trends Cell Biol. 2: pp.77-81.

Lindner, K., Gregan, J., et al. (2002). Essential role of MCM proteins in premeiotic DNA replication. Mol. Biol. Cell 13: pp.435-444.

Longhese, M. P., Jovine, L., et al. (1993). Conditional mutations in the yeast DNA primase genes affect different aspects of DNA metabolism and interactions in the DNA polymerase alpha-primase complex. Genetics 133(2): pp.183-191.

Loog, M. and Morgan, D. O. (2005). Cyclin specificity in the phosphorylation of cyclin-dependent kinase substrates. Nature 434: pp.104-108.

Magee, P. T. and Hopper, A. K. (1974). Protein synthesis in relation to sporulation and meiosis in yeast. J Bacteriol 119(3): pp.952-960.

Maloisel, L., Fabre, F., et al. (2008). DNA polymerase delta is preferentially recruited during homologous recombination to promote heteroduplex DNA extension. Mol Cell Biol 28(4): pp.1373-1382.

Marahrens, Y. and Stillman, B. (1992). A yeast chromosomal origin of DNA replication defined by multiple functional elements. Science 255(5046): pp.817-823.

Marahrens, Y. and Stillman, B. (1994). Replicator dominance in a eukaryotic chromosome. EMBO J 13(14): pp.3395-3400.

Masai, H., Sato, N., et al. (1999). CDC7 kinase complex as a molecular switch for DNA replication. Front Biosci 4: pp.D834-840.

Masai, H., Taniyama, C., et al. (2006). Phosphorylation of MCM4 by Cdc7 kinase facilitates its interaction with Cdc45 on the chromatin. J Biol Chem 281(51): pp.39249-39261.

Masumoto, H., Sugino, A., et al. (2000). Dpb11 controls the association between DNA polymerase α and ε and the autonomous replicating sequence region in budding yeast. Mol. Cell. Biol. 20: pp.2809-2817.

Matos, J., Lipp, J. J., et al. (2008). Dbf4-dependent CDC7 kinase links DNA replication to the segregation of homologous chromosomes in meiosis I. Cell 135(4): pp.662-678.

McCune, H. J., Danielson, L. S., et al. (2008). The Temporal Program of Chromosome Replication: Genomewide Replication in clb5Δ *Saccharomyces cerevisiae*. Genetics 180(4): pp.1833-1847.

Miller, M. E. and Cross, F. R. (2001). Cyclin specificity: how many wheels do you need on a unicycle? J Cell Sci 114(Pt 10): pp.1811-1820.

Mitchell, A. P. (1994). Control of meiotic gene expression in *Saccharomyces cerevisiae*. Microbiol. Rev. 58: pp.56-70.

Mitchell, A. P., Driscoll, S. E., et al. (1990). Positive control of sporulation specific genes by the *IME1* and *IME2* products in *Saccharomyces cerevisiae*. Mol. Cell. Biol. 10: pp.2104-2110.

Morgan, D. O. (1995). Principles of CDK regulation. Nature 374: pp.131-134.

Mori, S. and Shirahige, K. (2007). Perturbation of the activity of replication origin by meiosis-specific transcription. J Biol Chem 282(7): pp.4447-4452.

Muramatsu, S., Hirai, K., et al. (2010). CDK-dependent complex formation between replication proteins Dpb11, Sld2, Pol (epsilon), and GINS in budding yeast. Genes Dev 24(6): pp.602-612.

Nasmyth, K. (1993). Control of the yeast cell cycle by the Cdc28 protein kinase. Curr. Op. Cell Biol. 5: pp.166-179.

Newlon, C. S. and Fangman, W. L. (1975). Mitochondrial DNA synthesis in cell cycle mutants of *Saccharomyces cerevisiae*. Cell 5(4): pp.423-428.

Nolt, J. K., Rice, L. M., et al. (2011). PP2A (Cdc55) is required for multiple events during meiosis I. Cell Cycle 10(9).

Ofir, Y., Sagee, S., et al. (2004). The role and regulation of the preRC component Cdc6 in the initiation of premeiotic DNA replication. Mol. Biol. Cell 15: pp.2230-2242.

Ohya, T., Kawasaki, Y., et al. (2002). The DNA polymerase domain of pol(epsilon) is required for rapid, efficient, and highly accurate chromosomal DNA replication, telomere length maintenance, and normal cell senescence in Saccharomyces cerevisiae. J Biol Chem 277(31): pp.28099-28108.

Pardee, A. B. (1974). A restriction point for control of normal animal cell proliferation. Proc Natl Acad Sci U S A 71(4): pp.1286-1290.

Patel, P. K., Kommajosyula, N., et al. (2008). The Hsk1(Cdc7) replication kinase regulates origin efficiency. Mol Biol Cell 19(12): pp.5550-5558.

Piatti, S., Lengauer, C., et al. (1995). Cdc6 is an unstable protein whose de novo synthesis in G1 is important for the onset of S phase and for preventing a 'reductional' anaphase in the budding yeast *Saccharomyces cerevisiae*. EMBO J. 14: pp.3788-3799.

Raghuraman, M. K. and Brewer, B. J. (2010). Molecular analysis of the replication program in unicellular model organisms. Chromosome Res 18(1): pp.19-34.

Raithatha, S. A. and Stuart, D. T. (2005). Meiosis-specific regulation of the *Saccharomyces cerevisiae* S-phase cyclin CLB5 is dependent on MluI cell cycle box (MCB) elements in its promoter but is independent of MCB-binding factor. Genetics 169: pp.1329-1342.

Reed, S. I. (1980). The selection of S. cerevisiae mutants defective in the start event of cell division. Genetics 95: pp.561-577.

Reed, S. I. (1992). The role of p34 kinases in the G1 to S-phase transition. Annu. Rev. Cell Biol. 8: pp.529-561.

Remus, D. and Diffley, J. F. (2009). Eukaryotic DNA replication control: lock and load, then fire. Curr Opin Cell Biol 21(6): pp.771-777.

Richardson, H. E., Lew, D. J., et al. (1992). Cyclin-B homologs in *Saccharomyces cerevisiae* function in S phase and in G2. Genes Dev. 6: pp.2021-2034.

Richardson, H. E., Wittenberg, C., et al. (1989). An essential G1 function for cyclin-like proteins in yeast. Cell 59: pp.1127-1133.

Rowley, A., Cocker, J. H., et al. (1995). Initiation complex assembly at budding yeast replication origins begins with the recognition of a bipartite sequence by limiting amounts of the initiator, ORC. EMBO J 14(11): pp.2631-2641.

Santocanale, C., Sharma, K., et al. (1999). Activation of dormant origins of DNA replication in budding yeast. Genes Dev 13(18): pp.2360-2364.

Sasanuma, H., Hirota, K., et al. (2008). Cdc7-dependent phosphorylation of Mer2 facilitates initiation of yeast meiotic recombination. Genes Dev 22(3): pp.398-410.

Schild, D. and Byers, B. (1978). Meiotic effects of DNA-defective cell division cycle mutations of *Saccharomyces cerevisiae*. Chromosoma 70: pp.109-130.

Schwob, E., Boehm, T., et al. (1994). The B-type cyclin kinase inhibitor $p40^{SIC1}$ controls the G1/S transition in *Saccharomyces cerevisiae*. Cell 79: pp.233-244.

Schwob, E. and Nasmyth, K. (1993). *CLB5* and *CLB6*, a new pair of B cyclins involved in DNA replication in *Saccharomyces cerevisiae*. Genes Dev. 7: pp.1160-1175.

Sedgwick, C., Rawluk, M., et al. (2006). *Saccharomyces cerevisiae* Ime2 phosphorylates Sic1 at multiple PXS/T sites but is insufficient to trigger Sic1 degradation. Biochem J. 399: pp.151-160.

Sheu, Y. J. and Stillman, B. (2010). The Dbf4-Cdc7 kinase promotes S phase by alleviating an inhibitory activity in Mcm4. Nature 463(7277): pp.113-117.

Shuster, E. O. and Byers, B. (1989). Pachytene arrest and other meiotic effects of the start mutations in *Saccharomyces cerevisiae*. Genetics 123: pp.29-43.

Simchen, G. (1974). Are mitotic functions required in meiosis. Genetics 76: pp.745-753.

Smith, H. E., Su, S. Y. S., et al. (1990). Role of *IME1* expression in regulation of meiosis in *Saccharomyces cerevisiae*. Mol. Cell. Biol. 10: pp.6103-6113.

Stevens, R., Grelon, M., et al. (2004). A CDC45 homolog in *arabadopsis* is essential for meiosis, as shown by RNA interference-induced gene silencing. Plant Cell 16: pp.99-113.

Stillman, B. (2005). Origin recognition and the chromosome cycle. FEBS Lett 579(4): pp.877-884.

Stuart, D. and Wittenberg, C. (1998). *CLB5* and *CLB6* are required for premeiotic DNA replication and activation of the meiotic S/M checkpoint. Genes & Dev. 12: pp.2698-2710.

Stuart, D. T. (2008). The meiotic differentiation program uncouples S-phase from cell size control in *Saccharomyces cerevisiae*. Cell Cycle 7: pp.777-786.

Takayama, Y., Kamimura, Y., et al. (2003). GINS, a novel multiprotein complex required for chromosomal DNA replication in budding yeast. Genes & Dev. 17: pp.1153-1165.

Tanaka, S. and Araki, H. (2010). Regulation of the initiation step of DNA replication by cyclin-dependent kinases. Chromosoma 119(6): pp.565-574.

Tanaka, S., Umemori, T., et al. (2007). CDK-dependent phosphorylation of Sld2 and Sld3 initiates DNA replication in budding yeast. Nature 445(7125): pp.328-332.

Tanaka, T., Knapp, D., et al. (1997). loading of an Mcm protein onto DNA replication origins is regulated by Cdc6 and CDKs. Cell 90: pp.649-660.

Tonami, Y., Murakami, H., et al. (2005). A checkpoint control linking meiotic S phase and recombination initiation in fission yeast. Proc Natl Acad Sci U S A 102(16): pp.5797-5801.

Ubersax, J. A., Woodbury, E. L., et al. (2003). Targets of the cyclin-dependent kinase Cdk1. Nature 425: pp.859-864.

Unnikrishnan, A., Gafken, P. R., et al. (2010). Dynamic changes in histone acetylation regulate origins of DNA replication. Nat Struct Mol Biol 17(4): pp.430-437.

Valentin, G., Schwob, E., et al. (2006). Dual role of the Cdc7-regulatory protein Dbf4 during yeast meiosis. J Biol Chem 281(5): pp.2828-2834.

Vogelauer, M., Rubbi, L., et al. (2002). Histone acetylation regulates the time of replication origin firing. Mol Cell 10(5): pp.1223-1233.

Wan, L., Niu, H., et al. (2008). Cdc28-Clb5 (CDK-S) and Cdc7-Dbf4 (DDK) collaborate to initiate meiotic recombination in yeast. Genes Dev 22(3): pp.386-397.

Wan, L., Zhang, C., et al. (2006). Chemical inactivation of Cdc7 kinase in budding yeast results in a reversible arrest that allows efficient cell synchronization prior to meiotic recombination. Genetics 174(4): pp.1767-1774.

Weber, J. M., Irlbacher, H., et al. (2008). Control of replication initiation by the Sum1/Rfm1/Hst1 histone deacetylase. BMC Mol Biol 9: pp.100.

Zegerman, P. and Diffley, J. F. (2007). Phosphorylation of Sld2 and Sld3 by cyclin-dependent kinases promotes DNA replication in budding yeast. Nature 445(7125): pp.281-285.

Zhou, C. and Jong, A. (1990). CDC6 mRNA fluctuates periodically in the yeast cell cycle. J Biol Chem 265(32): pp.19904-19909.

Zhu, Z., Mori, S., et al. (2010). Cyclin-dependent kinase promotes formation of the synaptonemal complex in yeast meiosis. Genes Cells 15(10): pp.1036-1050.

Zou, L. and Stillman, B. (2000). Assembly of a complex containing Cdc45p, replication protein A, and Mcm2p at replication origins controlled by S-phase cyclin-dependent kinases and Cdc7p-Dbf4p kinase. Mol Cell Biol 20(9): pp.3086-3096.

11

Cell Cycle Modification in Trophoblast Cell Populations in the Course of Placenta Formation

Tatiana Zybina and Eugenia Zybina
Institute of Cytology RAS, Saint.-Petersburg, Russia

1. Introduction

It is well established that the presence of the diploid chromosome set in cell nuclei of the majority of tissues is a characteristic of vertebrates. This peculiarity was supplemented by the rule of the relative constancy of DNA in nuclei with diploid chromosome set (Boivin et al., 1948). However, some cells contain doubled or multiplied chromosome set as compared to other cells of the organism or other individuals of the species. As distinct from the generative polyploidy in which polyploidy covers all cell types including gametes, somatic polyploidy extents to cells of several tissues (Brodsky, Uryvaeva, 1985).

At present there are numerous data that the cells of some tissues of animal and plants appear to be polyploid. The incidence of polyploidy in the tissues of animals and plants as well as levels of ploidy is described in detail in quite a few books and reviews (Geitler, 1953; Tschermak-Woess, 1971; Nagl, 1978, 1981, 1995; Brodsky, Uryvaeva, 1985; Raikov, 1982; Zybina, 1986; D'Amato, 1989; Zybina, Zybina, 1996; Edgar, Orr-Weaver, 2001; Ravid et al., 2002). A large body of data on incidence of polyploidy in animal and plant tissues enabled W. Nagl to make a conclusion that polyploidy is a widespread phenomenon characteristic of the overwhelming majority of eukaryotes (Nagl, 1978; 1981; 1995). According to Nagl, Vertebrata represent a specific taxon that differs from other eukaryotes in the extent of polyploidy among the differentiated cells. Thus, in insects and higher plants, nearly all normal, differentiated cells are polyploid. The majority of Mammalia and, most probably, other Vertebrates, are characterized by the diploid chromosome set in most cells including both proliferative and the tissue-specific cells. Polyploidy in Vertebrata is present in many cell types, i.e., hepatocytes, cardyomyocytes, megakaryocytes and some others (Brodsky, Uryvaeva, 1985; Hancock et al, 1993; Kudryavtsev et al, 1993; Nagl, 1995; Anatskaya et al, 2001). It suggests that propagation of vertebrates is, probably, due to an advantage of the mitotic cycle that involves a machinery of accurate reproduction of diploid cells over other cell reproduction cycles that result in polyploidization. It cannot be ruled out that the biological advantage of mitosis has made it possible the wide distribution of Vertebrata. Nevertheless, genome multiplication characteristic of wide range of highly differentiated cells in different taxons suggests an undoubtedly important biological significance of polyploidy in the lifespan of some specific cell types.

Most of suggestions consider polyploidy as a factor promoting some tissue-specific functions of some cell types (Nagl, 1978, 1985; Brodsky, Uryvaeva, 1985; Edgar, Orr-Weaver, 2001; Lee et al., 2009). In some mammalian tissues the number of polyploid cells increases under conditions of the physiological stress: in cardiomyocytes in heart disease (Rumyantsev, 1991); in the aorta vascular smooth muscle cells of hypertensive animals (Owens, Schwartz, 1982; Ravid et al., 2002; Hixon, Gualberto, 2003; Nagata et al., 2005; Gui et al., 2007); in the smooth muscle cells of myometrium during pregnancy (Heiden, James, 1975), in thyrocytes and cells of the adrenal gland with age (Auer et al., 1985; Ravid et al., 2002). Besides, an increase in proportion of polyploidy cells correlates with aging and cell senescence (Yang et al., 2007; McCrann et al., 2008; Celton-Morizur, Desdoutes, 2010). Switching to polyploidy, as a rule, results in loss of capability for cell divisions that is also a characteristic of the differentiated cells. An increase of cell size leads to a change of cell metabolic characteristics. Switch to endoreduplication cycle in which cell growth is gained without periodic reorganization of cytoskeleton and cell contacts, concomitant to the entrance into mitosis allows cell to continue cell growth and proliferation without prominent structural transformation. Such a way of cell reproduction may be important for the highly specialized cell types. Therefore, it worth considering different types of cell cycle modification as possible ways to gain different levels of genome multiplication characteristic of different cell types of animals and plants.

1.1 Abbreviations

AER - agranular endoplasmic reticulum, GER - granular endoplasmic reticulum, NE - nuclear membrane; AL - annulate lamellae; BB - Barr body; GCB - gonosomal chromatin body

2. General considerations on the somatic polyploidization mechanisms

The clearest notions on ways of somatic polyploidization were developed basing on the cell cycle concept (Howard, Pelc, 1953; Nagl, 1978; Brodsky, Uryvaeva, 1985; Edgar, Orr-Weaver, 2001; Lee et al., 2009).

2.1 Restitution (uncompleted) mitoses

Switching off the last step of mitosis - cytotomy - may be the first step to polyploidy: binucleate cell is formed, each nucleus containing diploid chromosome set. In the next cell cycle and mitosis two metaphase plates may unite forming the common plate. If the mitosis comes to the end, it results in two mononucleated cells with tetraploid chromosome set. Such cycles may repeat and lead to formation of mono- and binucleate cells of the higher ploidy level:

$$2c - (2c \times 2) - 4c - (4c \times 2) - 8c - (8c \times 2)$$

Such a ploidy level was proved by V.Ja. Brodsky basing on the dynamics of transition of mono- and binucleate cells of different ploidy using combination of cytophotometry and ^{3}H-thymidine labeling of DNA replication (Brodsky, Uryvaeva, 1985). Acytokinetic mitoses with subsequent polyploidizing mitosis is rather widespread way of polyploidization, for example, in liver, myocardium, retina pigment epithelium (Rumyantsev, 1982). Similar ways were described later by using time-lapse video images in the aortic vascular smooth muscle cells, however, as one of different ways of polyploidy genome gaining (Nagata et al., 2005). An essential point, in our opinion, is "mitotic origin" of polyploid cells: rise of a polyploid nucleus requires a diploid cell to enter mitosis.

Block of mitosis may occur somewhat earlier - at the prophase, metaphase, and anaphase. The cells reaching these phases then undergo chromosome despiralization and return into interphase. As the chromosome do not move to the poles, the cells retain the doubled chromosome set and become polyploid. Such a cycle was called the restitution cycle (Nagl; 1978; 1995) or the incompleted polyploidizing mitosis (Uryvaeva, 1979). Prophase restitution was described in the root tip cells of onion *Alliun cepa* and *A. carinatum* (Nagl, 1978). In case of prophase restitution, the cells enter prophase, then return to interphase via telophasic decondensation.

Metaphase restitution was found in the onion root tip cells in which mitosis was blocked by colchicines; spontaneous metaphase restitution was observed in the pea endosperm (Nagl, 1978). The restitution mitoses can be recognized by overcontraction of chromosomes, their enhanced stickiness and failure of ordered arrangement being due to misfunction of the spindle (Nagl, 1978).

Anaphase restitution was also observed in the onion root tip cells under the colchicine treatment, and spontaneously - in the suspensor of *Lathyrus latifolius* (Nagl, 1978). In this case of chromosome bridges, these are probably responsible for non-disjunction of the daughter nuclei. In the next G1-phase a cell with a dumbbell-like nucleus or a binucleate cell with tightly attached nuclei is formed. Metaphase and anaphase restitution were also described in cancer cells (Therman et al., 1986).

Uncompleted polyploidizing mitoses were also found in the decidual cells in the rat endometrium - both in the normal pregnancy and in the induced deciduomata (Zybina, 1986). Uncompleted mitosis with delays of its middle phases was found in the vertebrate tissue, in particular, in megakaryocytes and cancer cells (Brodsky, Uryvaeva, 1985; Nagl, 1995).

Spontaneous polyploidization in human tissues often includes different types of restitution mitoses that seem to result from disorder in many mitotic events; these events also including reverse cytokinesis. Thus, the hypertensive aortic vascular smooth muscle cells (VSMC) at the time-lapse video showed delayed mitosis as compared to the normal one (Nagata et al., 2005). In most cases, sister chromatids were normally segregated and the cleavage furrow was also normally formed, but cytokinesis progression was stopped. Thereafter, reversion of cytokinesis occurred, and ultimately two nuclei were reversed into a single binucleate cell. In some cases, the cleavage furrow was formed again, and finally the VSMC were divided into two daughter cells. In other, rare, cases (4 times per 100 time-lapse images), there occurred exit from mitosis without cell division that resulted in polyploid mononuclear cell formation. In these cases, the cleavage furrow was formed even before sister chromatid disjunction and/or segregation that resulted in chromosome separation into two parts, the parts being bound by a chromosome bridge. These mitoses resulted in polyploid cells with single irregular-shaped lobular nuclei (Nagata et al., 2005). At last, there occurred some mitoses with a shallow cleavage furrow and missegregation of sister chromatids; thereafter the furrow disappeared and mononuclear polyploid cell with round nucleus was formed. Immunolabelling of β- and γ-tubulin proved that the cell retained mitotic spindle and centrosomes that allow mitosis progression, Aurora B was also found to be normally expressed, but another chromosome passenger protein Survivin was downregulated. Lack of Survivin expression was, probably, the reason for disturbance of the Aurora B/Survivin complex formation, Aurora B kinase dysfunction and failure of chromosome movement leading to polyploidization. Thus, failure of expression of one regulator of mitotic machinery may exert a pleiotropic effect on the proceeding and result of mitosis. Such a pleiotropic effect is the reason for various mitotic modifications and aberrations in cancer cells (Therman et al., 1986; Therman, Kuhn, 1989) and for numerous cases of spontaneous and induced mitotic restitution (Nagl, 1978).

Regulation of the tissue-specific restitution cycle is not quite clearly elucidated. At present, processes of transition to polyploidization similar to uncompleted mitoses are considered as overcoming of mitotic spindle assembly checkpoint (Cahill et al., 1998; Gualberto et al., 1998). The former delays the onset of anaphase and the exit from mitosis. The mitotic checkpoint accomplishes its function by controlling activity of the cell cycle regulatory machinery composed by the Mitosis Promoting Factor (MPF), the Anaphase Promoting Factor, and proteasome. MPF is a protein complex that consists of a cyclin-dependent kinase $p34^{cdc2}$, cyclin B, and associated proteins (Hixon, Gualberto, 2003). MPF induces formation of a mitotic spindle by phosphorylating components of the mitotic spindle including microtubule-based motor proteins. Cyclins B are known to be involved in the microtubule metabolism (Nurse, 1991; Ookata et al., 1995). Degradation of CyclinB/p**34** ^{cdc2} correlates with entrance into the normal ana- and telophase (Lehner, O'Farrel, 1990; Holloway et al., 1993). The Anaphase Promoting Complex (APC) and Proteasome control metaphase-anaphase transition and the exit from mitosis. At the onset of anaphase, the activity of separins contribute to release cohesins from chromosomes, allowing for segregation of bivalents to opposite poles. Separin activity is blocked by securins. At the karyokinesis the APC-complex promotes destruction of secutins and cyclin B leading to chromosome segregation and cytokinesis. Therefore, mutation in $p34^{cdc2}$ in the phosphorylation sites blocks mitosis progression (Compton et al., 1995).

Some data about regulation of transition to polyploidization cycles were obtained on the model of VSMC. The aortic VSMC of mice genetically prone to hypertension were treated with colcemid to estimate effect of the spindle checkpoint mechanism. While VSMC from normotensive animals were able to arrest the cell cycle progression in mitosis, VSMC isolated from hypertensive animals re-entered the cell cycle in the absence of chromosomal segregation and undervent polyploid rounds of DNA synthesis. While VSMC of normotensive rats accumulated Cyclin B (mitotic arrest) in response to a mitotic spindle inhibitor, unscheduled degradation of Cyclin B was observed in VSMC isolated from capacitance arteries of spontaneously hypertensive animals (Hixon, Gualberto, 2003). In this case, exit from mitosis may proceed in the absence of chromosome segregation and karyokinesis thereby leading to cell cycle re-entry and polyploidization.

2.2 Endocycles

More profound reduction of mitotic cycle, as compared to uncompleted mitosis, results in *endocycles.* This term covers all phenomena of genome multiplication that are accomplished without nuclear envelope disappearance (Nagl, 1978; 1981; 1995; Therman et al., 1983; 1986; Edgar, Orr-Weaver, 2001). The endocycles include *classic and angiospermal endomitosis,* and *endoreduplication or polyteny* (Geitler, 1953; Nagl, 1978; 1995; Kiknadze, Istomina, 1980; Zybina, Zybina, 1996; 2005).

2.2.1 Endomitosis

In the course of the classic endomitosis, chromosomes undergo successive modifications similar to that in mitosis, but without nuclear envelope disappearance, metaphase plate arrangement, and anaphase movement. In this case, there occur chromosome condensation, sister chromatid separation that is followed by their decondensation (Geitler, 1953; Nagl, 1978; 1995). Morphology of the endomitotic chromosomes is somewhat different from the mitotic ones by less sharp contours.

Classic endomitosis was described in invertebrate tissues: in a Heteropteran *Gerris lateralis* (Geitler, 1953); in the parietal cells of testicular follicle of grasshoppers (Kiknadze, Istomina, 1980), in the albumen gland and neurons of the snail *Succinea lauta* (Anisimov, 1997 a, b, c; Anisimov, Kirsanova, 2002; Anisimov, 2005). Recently, the latter case was studied in detail. In the transition from endointerphase to endoprophase and, then, to endometaphase, nuclear envelope was retained, autosomes did not reach the complete shortening and thickening like in mitosis; meantime, the spindle and chromosome movement were not observed. In endoanaphase there occurred splitting of chromosomes into chromatids without spindle formation. In the transition to endotelophase and endointerphase the split chromatids stayed to lie in parallel, meantime undergoing progressive decondensation, so in endointerphase, numerous paired chromocenters were seen in the nucleus. In DNA synthesis study using ^{3}H-thymidine, the cycle of endomitosis was revealed, and duration of phases of endointerphase - G1, S, and G2 - was determined (Anisimov, 1997a). Each phase of endomitotic cycle was characterized by specific chromosome structure and arrangement, and in G1-, S-, and G2-phases, numerous chromocenters were observed, the degree of their condensation being characteristic of each phase of the endointerphase.

Endomitosis was also observed in the trophoblast of placenta and hydatidiform mole (Sarto et al., 1982; Therman et al., 1983, 1986). In these cells there occurred pictures of endomitosis, the degree of chromosome condensation differing in different cells. In the ^{3}H-thymidine-labelled cells, paired endomitotic chromosomes were seen, their condensation was less pronounced than in the unlabelled cells. Therefore, at the endointerphase, a partial chromosome decondensation and replication occurred (Therman et al., 1986); different chromosome regions probably were decondensed at different intervals.

The transcriptional activity of endomitotic nuclei appeared to be sufficiently high (Anisimov, 1997c). The highest ^{3}H-uridine labelling in snail tissues was observed in G1-, S-, and G2-phase, i.e., during the whole endometaphase. In endointerphase and endoprophase the ^{3}H-uridine labeling decreased up to minimum, so that in endometaphase it accounts for 4% of the endointerphase level. In endotelophase a fast increase of the ^{3}H-uridine labeling was observed. We can conclude that transcriptional activity persists throughout the whole endomitotic cycle, but undergoes cyclic transformation, so that at the endometaphase it is minimal. Electron microscopic observation also demonstrated a certain degree of chromosome condensation at all endomitotic stages in cells of the albumen gland of the snail. The uncomplete condensation is accompanied by the radial looping of thin chromatin threads running from the endochromosome axis; perichromatin granules were seen at the loops. Such an organization of endochromosomes resembles lampbrush chromosomes found in diplotene oocytes in many vertebrates (Callan, 1986). The extent of looping also seems to undergo the condensation cycle: maximal number of loops was observed at endointerphase, minimal - at endometaphase (Anisimov, 1997b, c). Thus, classic endomitosis represents a variation of the cell cycle that retains cycle of replication, chromosome condensation, and transcriptional activity; however, this cycle is "shortened", some events corresponding to mitosis are omitted.

It seems to be of interest that throughout the endomitotic cycle not only the nuclear envelope, but also nucleolus persists; the level of transcription activity of nucleolar organizer varies at different phases of the endomitotic cycle (Anisimova, Anisimov, 2002). The nucleolar activity also varies depending on the functional state of the cell, in particular, of the differentiation rate and direction (Anisimova, Anisimov, 2002).

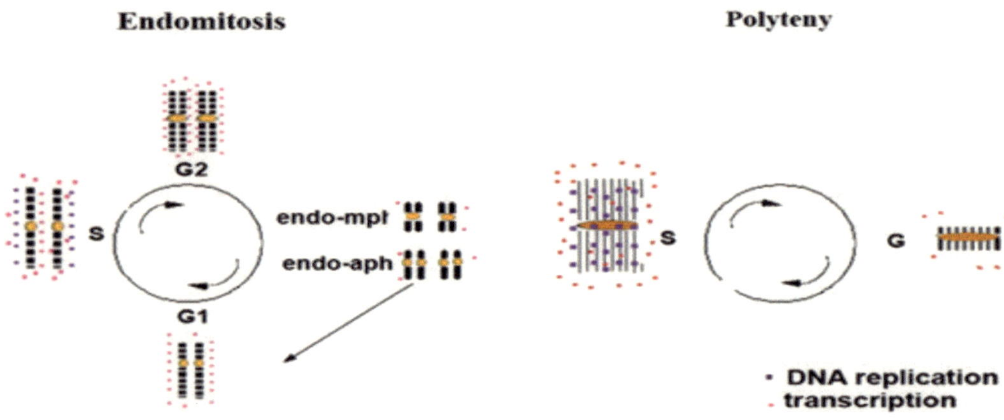

Fig. 1. Scheme of endocycles in endomitosis and polyteny. In the endomitotic cycle replication, chromosome condensation/decondensation and transcription are retained; replication is accomplished at the S-phase; transcription is active at the G1-, S, and G2-phases. In endometaphase (endo-mph) and endoanaphase (endo-aph) endochromosomes condense and transcription declines up to minimum; sister chromatid segregation takes place at the endoanaphase. Arrow indicates transformations of one pair of sister endochromosomes in the course of the endomitotic cycle. In polyteny chromosome replication is accomplished in S-phase; cyclic changes of chromosome condensation and transcription take place; chromatid segregation is not observed.

Apart from the classical or "insect-type" endomitosis, the so-called "angiospermal endomitosis" was observed in cells of many higher plants (Tschermak-Woess, 1971; Nagl, 1978). In this case the cyclic chromosome condensation appears to be much lower (rudimentary) than in the insect-type endomitosis. Therefore, it is rather difficult to detect different endomitotic phases as compared to the classic endomitosis.

It is to be specified that endomitotic pictures do not always reflect genome multiplication via endocycle progression. In cells of the testicular follicle of grasshoppers, all endomitotic stages were detected morphologically. Nevertheless, DNA synthesis in these cells was not detected at the stages when the phases of endomitosis can be seen (Kiknadze, Istomina, 1980). By contrast, these cells show intensive transcription by the ^{3}H-uridine labeling. Thus, in such a case, endomitotic chromosome appears to be a specific form of the polyploid nucleus with high transcription activity without genome multiplication (Kiknadze, Istomina, 1980). It can be explained, for example, by the specific differentiation of the testicular follicle cells, in which they lose the DNA replication cycle, but accomplish their tissue-specific function that implies high protein synthesis.

Interestingly, in this case, endometaphase chromosomes resemble the organization of lampbrush chromosomes. ^{3}H-uridine label was concentrated over the loops projected from the central part of endochromosomes (Kiknadze, Istomina, 1980). Such a peculiarity makes endomitotic chromosomes of grasshopper similar to other examples of the classic endomitosis.

To explain the difference between these two "endomitoses" - replicative and non-replicative one, it is of interest to mention that in the snail protein gland, DNA replication was not detected at the terminal stage of differentiation - despite the presence of typical endomitotic figures (Anisimov, 1997a). However, the level of ^{3}H-uridine labeling was decreased significantly as compared to the earlier, "replicative" stages in the lifespan of the cells.

To sum up, endomitosis represents a specific type of cell cycle, in which some degree of chromosome condensation and transcription is maintained throughout the whole endocycle (Fig.1). Therefore, endomitosis may be considered as a specific form of transcriptionally active nucleus (Brodsky, Uryvaeva, 1985). It is strengthened by the similarity of the endomitotic chromosomes with lampbrush chromosomes characteristic of the diplotene of the I meiotic division (Callan, 1986). Lampbrush organization and uncomplete condensation suggest that endomitosis is a way to gain highly specified cell types with high transcriptional activity of tissue-specific chromosome loci; this transcriptional activity may be important for the special function of the cells.

The classic endomitosis may be of doubtless interest due to its occurrence in malignant cells, first of all, in cervical cancer and complete hydatidiform moles (Therman et al., 1982; 1983; 1986).

2.2.2 Polyteny

The most shortened cycle that consists of merely two phases - presynthetic G and synthetic S - is *endoreduplication* that results in *polyteny* and *G2-block* (Pearson, 1974; Nagl, 1978, 1995; Brodsky, Uryvaeva, 1985; Zybina, 1986; Zybina, Zybina, 1996, 2005; Brodsky, Uryvaeva, 1985; Edgar Orr-Weaver, 2001).

According to V. Brodsky and I. Uryvaeva (1985), in G2-block and polyteny the cell cycle is devoid of the whole mitosis; therefore, the pre- and postmitotic phases are united. In this case the sister chromatids do not separate, each chromatid beginning a new round of replication in the new S-phase. As a result of a series of successive endoreduplication cycles, polytene chromosomes are formed.

Control of endoreduplication cycle is not elucidated completely. However, it is certainly associated with cessation of expression of cyclins A and B that are necessary for mitosis progression (Nagl, 1995; Edgar, Orr-Weaver, 2001). Nevertheless, the detailed study of expression of cyclins, cyclin-dependent kinases as well as other proteins regulating endocycle progression prove that endocycle does not imply the complete switching off the components of the mitotic machinery. The switching from mitotic cycle to endocycle itself appears to be impossible without expression of factors regulating transition through mitotic phases. In switching from mitosis to endocycles, cells in the Drosophila embryo downregulate the mitotic regulators Cdk1, Cyclin A, cyclins B and B3 as well as Cdc25/string (Sauer et al., 1995, Edgar, Orr-Weaver, 2001). Meantime, studies on Fzr/Cdh1, a regulator of APC, show that APC activity is required for switch from mitotic cycles to endocycles (Edgar, Orr-Weaver, 2001). A series of investigation proved that initiation of endocycles required expression of E cyclins (Knoblich et al., 1994; Lilly, Spradling, 1996; Su,

O'Farrell, 1998; Edgar, Orr-Weaver, 2001). Besides, it is oscillatory (i.e. cyclic) expression of cyclin E that is required for successive endocycles in Drosophila tissues, i.e.ovarian nurse cells, embryonic gut, and embryonic larval tissues (Lilly, Spradling, 1996; Su, O'Farrell, 1998; Edgar, Orr-Weaver, 2001). In the endopolyploid murine giant trophoblast cells the oscillation of cyclin E expression was not demonstrated; in this case, fluctuation of Cdk2 occurs due to the periodic activity of the S-phase inhibitor $p57^{kip2}$ (Hattori et al., 2000; Hu, Cross, 2010). Therefore, endocycle retains the cyclic expression of several components and regulators of the mitotic cell division machinery.

It seems to be of importance that the degree of polytene structure widely varies, and three main types may be distinguished: (1) classic polyteny with characteristical band structure, for example, in the salivary glands of Diptera (Beermann, 1972; Kiknadze et al., 1976; Zhimulev, 1992); (2) the cell with uncomplete expression of polytene features, for example, in the giant trophoblast cells (Zybina, Zybina, 1996, 2005), in the suspensor of higher plants (Nagl, 1978, 1981), in trophocytes of insect ovaries (Dej, Spradling, 1999), and in various endocycles of Invertebrata (Nagl, 1978); (3) the cells, in which the polytene features are not revealed, and polyteny may be suggested basing on the multifold DNA replication in the absence of mitosis (Brodsky, Uryvaeva, 1985).

At present it is considered that morphological and functional features of the classical polytene chromosomes are accounted for by the following factors. First, the homologous chromosomes are bound due to the somatic conjugation. Therefore, the cells with polytene chromosomes show the haploid chromosome number. Second, in the course of successive endocycles the daughter chromatids stay bound to the initial ones; as a result, accumulation of the bound chromatids leads to thickening of the chromosomes. Third, the chromosomes are characterized by the weakening of the cycle of spiralization-despiralization characteristic of mitotic cycle; the degree of spiralization corresponds to prophase or interphase. It is probably the reason of their significant length that exceeds many times the length of mitotic chromosomes. The tightness of chromatid attachment in the polytene chromosome, most probably, also correlates with the degree of their despiralization and depends on their degree of ploidy (Ashburner, 1972; Kiknadze, 1972, Nagl, 1978).

Non-classic polytene chromosomes are well-studied in the higher plants. They were discovered in the highly polyploid nuclei of the provisory cells important to embryo development: antipods, synergids, cells of suspensor and angiospermal haustorium (Geitler, 1953; Tschermak-Woess, 1971; Hasitschka, 1956, 1957; Hasitschka-Jenschke, 1957, 1959; Nagl, 1969, 1978). Somatic conjugation probably is not obligatory for these chromosomes. As a result, nuclei of suspensor of several plants contain diploid number of chromosomes, in rare cases - the haploid one (Geitler, 1953; Nagl, 1978; Tschermak-Woess, 1971, 1973). In general, polytene chromosomes are composed of loosely attached cable-like structures, their ends being split more or less (Nagl, 1981). Their disc pattern is less regular than in classical polytene chromosomes because of not very tight attachment of chromatids. In many cases, chromatid attachment is not observed at the full length of the chromosome.

The degree of chromatid attachment may widely vary at different lifespan steps and depends on many factors including physiological state of the cell. In particular, it depends on the stage of polytene chromosome formation, i.e., the number of replication rounds. At the initial endocycles, chromatid attachment is restricted by the pericentromeric heterochromatin blocks; in the euchromatic regions, chromatids are separated to a significant distance. Each subsequent endocycle makes polytenic structure more clear-cut, and the "well-developed" polytene chromosomes can be identified precisely, although their separate loci are less distinguishable than in the classical polytene chromosomes (Nagl, 1978).

Besides, the degree of condensation depends on the stages of polytene nucleus cycle. In the highly endopolyploid cells of suspensor at the stage of replication chromonemes decondense and disjoin at a significance distance (Avanzi et al., 1970; Brady, Clutter, 1974). Disjunction of chromatids and their decondensation is observed in euchromatin and β-heterochromatin regions, whereas α-heterochromatin region stays condensed and retains chromatid attachment throughout the whole cycle of polytene nucleus (Brady, Clutter, 1974).

Transition to the endoreduplication (polytene) cycle that may be necessary in some specific cases. Thus, as pointed out by B. Edgar and T. Orr-Weaver, the endocycles, once initiated further mitotic divisions are "ill advised for mechanical reasons". Indeed, polyteny is present in the highly differentiated cells. Besides, polyteny allows cells to increase their mass and metabolic output. Another possible advantage of endoreduplication is that it allows combining fast growth of the tissue with its functioning. In this connection, a very important consideration is that transition to endocycles allows growth without periodic rearrangement of cytoskeletal elements or cell-cell contacts, as happens in mitoses, and it is less disruptive to highly structured tissues than in mitotic proliferation (Edgar, Orr-Weaver, 2001). All this seems to be appropriate to all kinds of endocycles. In this connection, polyteny appears to be the most advantageous to gain the highest possible ploidy levels (Nagl, 1978, 1981). By contrast, the lower ploidy levels are generally achieved via uncompleted mitoses, these cycles being more characteristic of mammalian tissues, i.e. in hepatocytes (Brodsky, Uryvaeva, 1985; Kudryavtsev et al., 1993; Celton-Morizur, 2010), megakaryocytes (Ravid et al., 2002); cardiac myocytes (Pfitzer, 1971; Rumyantsev, 1991; Anatskaya et al., 2001).

Meantime, it seems to be important that, in some cases genome multiplication implies entrance mitosis, in the other cases genome reproduction is achieved without the nuclear envelope disappearance. The biological significance of this difference, in our opinion, is demonstrated by the occurrence of different genome multiplication ways and their mutual transition in the trophoblast of mammalian placenta.

3. Cell cycle modification in trophoblast cell of mammalian placenta

The trophoblast cells of the rodent embryos represent an example that in the functionally different cell populations of the common origin have different ways of genome multiplication. The level of ploidy clearly correlates with the ability of cells to invade endometrium, to lyse and to phagocytose partly its tissues in the course of embryo implantation. Beginning from the onset of differentiation, the primary and secondary giant trophoblast cells undergo a series of endoreduplication cycle reaching very high ploidy level - 512c–1024c in rat and mouse (Zybina, Mosjan, 1967; Barlow, Sherman, 1972 ; Zybina, Zybina, 1996, 2005); 2048c and 16384c in the field vole (Zybina et al., 1975; Zybina et al., 2003; Zybina et al., 2009). The cells have the non-classical polytene chromosomes and can combine cell replication with the invasive and phagocytic activity (Zybina, Zybina, 2005).

3.1 Polytene nucleus cycle in the secondary giant trophoblast cells

Two phases - endointerphase (S) and endoprophase (G) - were determined in the polytene cycle of the secondary giant trophoblast cells in rat placenta by using ^{3}H-thymidine labeling (Zybina, Zybina, 1996, 2005). In endoprophase non-classic polytene chromosomes in a form of bundles of quite condensed chromatids of chromomeric structure are observed (Fig. 2b). The bundles are attached to the nuclear envelope. At the endointerphase nucleus is filled by paired thin Feulgen-positive threads, the "threads" being scattered throughout the caryoplasm and bound to the nuclear envelope (Fig. 2a). The minimal chromosome condensation characteristic of the interphase nucleus is observed at the endointerphase; however, some chromosome regions are visualized at this phase. Thus, parallel chromosome threads with characteristic disc pattern can be observed in the site where chromosomes penetrate nucleolus (Fig. 2a). Later on, three phases of endoreduplication were discerned - G1, S, and G2 - based on the S-phase inhibitor $p57^{kip2}$ (Hattori et al., 2000).

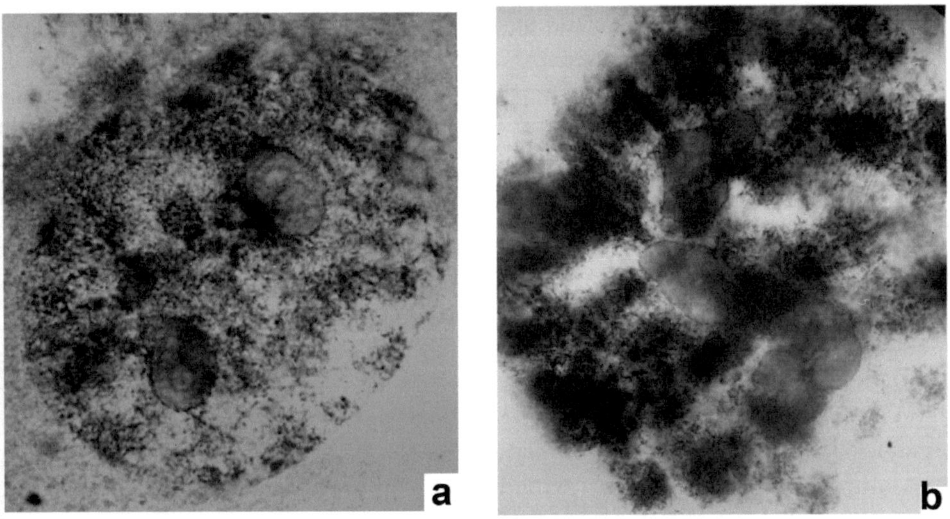

Fig. 2. Polytene chromosomes in the rat secondary giant trophoblast cell. A. endointerphase, b. endoprophase.

Two phases of polytene cycle are also observed in the mouse and rabbit giant trophoblast cells. In endoprophase some nuclei showed lampbrush-like structure (Fig. 3a, b): loops are running from the heterochromatic condenced region. At the phase contrast preparations, polytene chromosomes look like the long threads attached to the nuclear envelope (Fig. 3c).
DNA replication takes place at the endointerphase, as this was demonstrated by using both authoradiography (Zybina, 1986) and cytophotometry (Zybina et al., 1985). The level of ploidy of "meshwork" nuclei (Fig.2a) was 16c–256c, i.e., somewhat lower than in nuclei with chromosome bundles (Zybina, Zybina, 1985;1996). In particular, it may be accounted for by the presence of a number of nuclei, in which polytene chromosome bundles were not yet formed: the clear-cut bundles are observed beginning from 64c. In the group of nuclei of "polytene" type (Fig. 2b) the sharp peaks corresponding to ploidy classes 64c, 128c, 256c, and 512c are observed. By contrast, in the group of "meshwork" nuclei there are many intermediate values that correspond to DNA synthesis. The intermediate nuclei are also characterized by sharp peaks, but ploidy level is lower than in "bundles": the nuclei probably correspond to the process of decondensation of polytene chromosome bundles or the early endocycles when polytene structure is yet underdeveloped. The data confirm that endoreduplication cycle includes the cycle of polytene chromosome condensation, the maximum condensation level being in the endoprophase.

The rate of the polytene cycle proved to be rather high, it is especially high at the implantation period. Using DNA cytometry, it was demonstrated that at the 5-7 day of gestation in mouse some of the trophoblast cells undergo 3 cycles reaching 32c and 64 c. Thereafter, a decrease of polyploidisation is observed with subsequent constant rate of polyploidization: one endoreduplication cycle per day (Barlow, Sherman, 1972; Zybina, 1986); according to autoradiographic data, duration of S-phase in rat trophoblast cells is about 6 h, which is approximately equal to duration of S-phase in diploid cells. However, duration of G-phase upon polyplodidzation increases from 8.3 to 24.9 h for 12-15 days of gestation (Andreeva, 1964). Meantime, there also may be an increase of S-phase duration from 45-h to 6-7-h upon the endoreduplication progression (Zavarzin, 1967).
An increase of endoreduplication cycle duration was also detected in the case of classic polyteny of Drosophila (Rudkin, 1972). In the Drosophila salivary glands S-phase lengthens upon polyploidization from 2^{10}n to 2^{11}n by 20% (Gunderina et al, 1984). However, the highest ploidy levels are mainly achieved via endocycles.

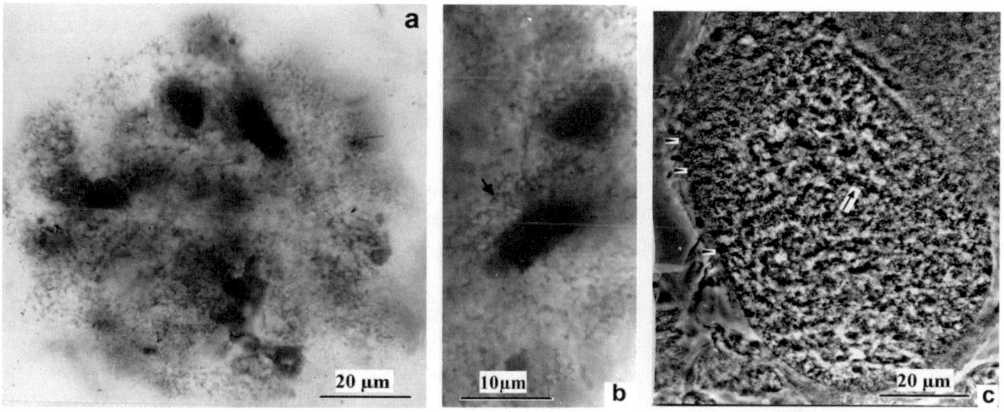

Fig. 3. Polytene chromosomes in the mouse (a, b) and rabbit (c) secondary giant trophoblast cells. (a) - non-classic polytene chromosome bundles; (b) - lampbrush chromosome-like structure: the loops (arrows) run out of the condensed part of the chromosome bundle; c - polytene chromosome bindles seen as parallel chromosome threads (arrow). a, b - acetoorcein staining, c - unstained preparation at phase contrast.

Both endointerphase or endoprophase are characterized by a certain level of transcriptional activity. However, in endoprophase the RNA synthesis is decreased (Zybina, 1963). Therefore, like in endomitosis, transcriptional activity is maintained, but oscillates in the course of the whole endoreduplication cycle. The nucleolus also persists throughout the cycle. According to the electron microscope study, the volume of the granular component that reflects the amount synthesis and accumulation of preribosome particle is higher at endointerphase; at this phase the number of fibrillar center that reflects the number of site of rRNA synthesis is also higher than at endoprophase (Zybina, 1986; Zybina, Zybina, 1996). In the highly differentiated giant trophoblast cells that exits from the cell cycle (the ^{3}H-thymidine labeling is not seen any longer), the polytene chromosome bundles become indiscernible, probably, due to weakening of the sister chromatid attachment. However, in this case, transcriptional activity does persist, and the transcriptionally active nucleolus may be observed (Zybina, 1986; Zybina, Zybina, 1996), although a decrease of granular component and fibrillar center amount prove the attenuation of the preribosome synthesis and processing. In this case, however, two types of nuclei that differ in the degree of chromatin condensation also are observed; they are also different in the transcriptional characteristics of the nucleolus (Zybina, 1986; Zybina, Zybina, 1996). Therefore, in the absence of DNA replication the polytene cycle is maintained, it is reflected, at least, in the variation of the chromosome condensation and transcription activity.

Differentiation of the giant trophoblast cells that involves exit from the regular mitotic cycle and the onset of endoreduplication is under the developmental control. In the differentiation of giant trophoblast cells from the Rcho-1 choriocarcinoma cell line the downregulation of *Id1* and *Id2* occurs, being concomitant with upregulation of the basic helix-loop-helix factor *Hxt* and acquisition of an increased adhesiveness (McAuley et al., 1998) that triggers the onset of invasive capability of the giant trophoblast cells. Cell cycle modification is triggered by switched Cyclin D isophorm expression from D3 to D1. The initiation of the S-phase during endocycles appeared to involve synthesis of cyclins E and A, and termination of the S-phase during endocycles was associated with abrupt loss of cyclins E and A. Both cyclins were absent from the gap-phase during endocycles, which suggests that their degradation may be necessary to allow reinitiation of the endocycle. The arrest of the mitotic cycle at the onset of endoreduplication was associated with a failure to assemble cyclinB/$p34^{cdk1}$ complexes during the first endocycle. In the subsequent endocycles, the cyclin B expression was suppressed. Therefore, at the first endocycle, its regulation retains some traits of mitotic cycle and then switches to the specific endoreduplicative regulation pattern. Interestingly, in the murine giant trophoblast cell population, expression of *cyclin B1* trascripts was found at the transcriptional level both in diploid and in polyploid cells, whereas the B1 protein was detected exclusively in the diploid cells. Therefore, downregulation of Cyclin B is the key event that switches off the mitotic machinery. Meantime, *Cyclin D1* transcripts were found only in giant trophoblast cells, even prior to that of *placental lactogen I* being early marker of giant trophoblast cell differentiation. This pattern of expression probably means that mural trophoblast differentiation and endoreduplication depend on the prolonged G1-phase. The authors state that D-type cyclins are required for endocycle maintenance, keeping in mind that antisence oligonucleotids to Cyclin D3 were found to block endoreduplication in murine megakaryocytes; besides, overexpression of cyclin D3 proved significant increase of endomitosis in the megakaryocytes (Zimmet et al., 1997). The zinc finger transcription factor Snail regulates the "G_2 decision point" whether the trophoblast cells go through mitosis or enter endocycle (Nakayama et al., 1998).

The polytene cycle of the giant trophoblast cells involves periodicity of S-phase during endoreduplication. During the mitotic cell cycle, biochemical events coincident with mitosis lead to the re-setting of the origins of replication (Elledge, 1996). This includes degradation of the protein Geminin that otherwise suppresses the firing of origins of replication (McGarry, Kirschner, 1998). Geminin mutant embryos die during preimplantation development and show ectopic endoreduplication in blastomeres (Gonzales et al., 2006; Hu, Cross, 2010). Another important mechanism to maintain periodicity during the endocycle involves cyclic expression of $p57^{kip2}$, a G1/S Cdk inhibitor (Hattori et al., 2000). During subsequent endocycles, the $p57^{kip2}$ level fluctuates and this identifies two phases: the endo-G2 phase with the $p57^{kip2}$ completion of S-phase and the endo-G1-phase with $p57^{kip2}$ declining several hours before entry into S-phase (Hattori et al., 2000). It is hypothesized that periodic expression of $p57^{kip2}$ protein promotes alternating S and "gap" phases in the endocycle (Hu, Cross, 2010), the "gap" probably corresponding to endoprophase.

3.2 Transition between different modes of genome multiplication

Junctional zone and labyrinth trophoblast in the rat and field vole placenta represents a cell population, in which a high proliferative activity is accompanied by a multidirectional differentiation. These cells do not reach a high ploidy level characteristical of the primary and secondary trophoblast cells, they achieve the ploidy level as high as 16c and 32c (Zybina, Zybina, 2000, 2005). These cell populations are characterized by different ways of genome multiplication in development of one cell line at different stages of ontogenesis. The incidence of this phenomenon among the multicellular organisms is not studied in detail. Nagl (1978) pointed out that the first step of polyploidization was achieved via restitution mitosis. In the rat proliferative trophoblast cell populations the acytokinetic and uncompleted mitosis are characteristic of the first step of polyploidization. The meta- and anaphase restitutions also were often found in these cells (Fig. 4).

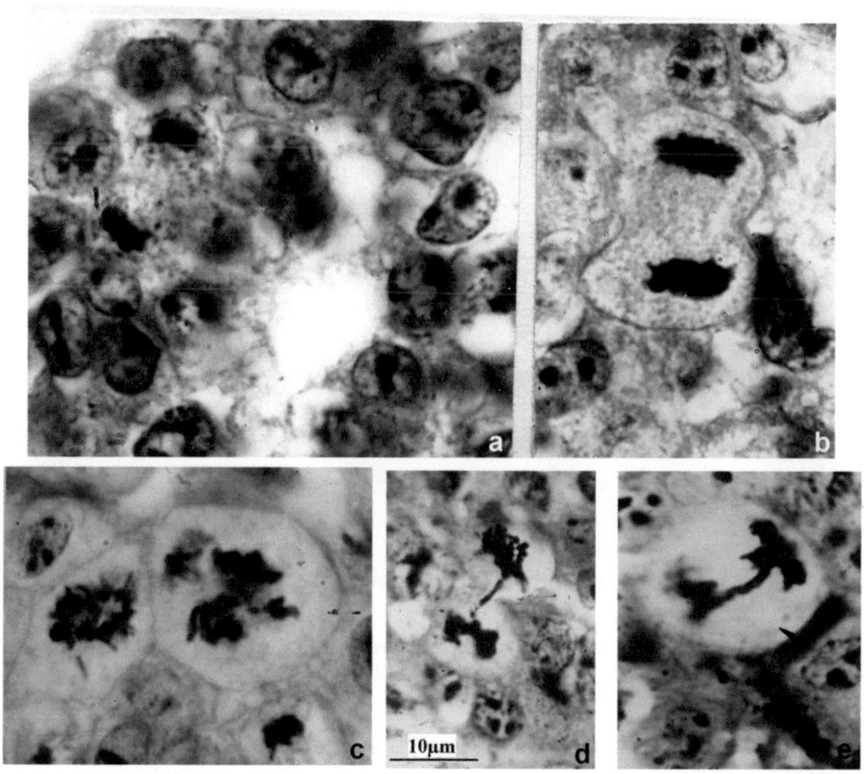

Fig. 4. Restitution mitoses in the junctional zone of the rat placenta. a, b -regular diploid (a) and polyploid (b) anaphases; c – a regular metaphase and metaphase with irregular chromosome alignment; d, e –restitutional anaphase with chromosome bridges.

Cytophotometrically among the mitotic figures of different ploidy (4c, 8c, and 16c), all mitotic stages were found – from prophase to telophase. Hence, mitosis in the junctional zone and labyrinth trophoblast can proceed up to octaploid level. Meantime, there was a noticeable predominance of earlier mitotic stages (pro- and metaphase) over the later ones (ana- and telophases) among the polyploid mitoses (Zybina et al., 2005). Among the polyploid mitotic figures, mostly restitution mitoses were present, very often anaphases with multiple bridges were revealed, so the cells had no chance to segregate. Therefore, upon a rise of the ploidy level, the ability to undergo the complete mitosis falls down. Besides, it is to be emphasized that upon cessation of the mitotic activity their cycles of replication do not stop. The cells continue to uptake ^{3}H-thymidine and reach the ploidy level 32c, sometimes 64c and 128c via endoreduplication (Zybina et al., 2000, 2005).

Transition from the regular mitosis to the uncompleted one and then – to endocycle was described in several tissues of snail (Anisimov, Kirsanova, 2002). In the course of neuron development of the snail *Succinea lauta* in the dorsal bodies and procerebrums besides the usual mitoses there occurred metaphases resembling k-mitoses with chromosome disorientation in metaphase. The chromosome arrangement showed sparseness that made possible to count chromosome number. In anaphase there occurred chromosome lagging and bridges as well as lack of segregation to the poles. All this indicates progression of restitution mitoses. The cycle resulted in the cells 4c, 4c/2n, and 4c/4n, where c is ploidy determined by DNA content, and n – ploidy determined by the chromosome number counting. In the course of differentiation of neurons there occurred transition to the endomitosis cycle that resulted in nuclei 32c-64c and later – 512c and higher (Anisimov, Kirsanova, 2002). The data confirm the regularity found in the trophoblast cell whose initial steps of polyploidization (mainly up to 8c) are achieved by uncompleted (restitutional) mitoses, then switch to endocycles.

It is to be mentioned that the trophoblast cell population that starts their genome multiplication via uncompleted mitoses does not prove invasive properties. As soon as they move to the border with maternal tissues (decidua basalis) or penetrated endometrium, they lose their capability for mitosis and DNA replication and reside inside the semiallogenic tissue in a form of a polyploid cells (Zybina, Zybina, 2005). Arrest of mitosis and complete repression of DNA replication after a series of endoreduplication cycles makes hardly probable the renewal of mitotic activity in the deeply invading tertiary giant trophoblast cells, thereby preventing the possibility of their ectopic expanding in the maternal tissues during the normal pregnancy.

3.3 Genome multiplication in the trophoblast cells of carnivore and ruminants

Trophoblast in the hemochorial placenta of silver fox and mink is also highly invasive. Among the trophoblast cells of fox and mink, polyploid cells prevail, the level of ploidy being mainly 2c-64c, the cells with highly polyploid nuclei 128c and 256c being rare (Zybina et al., 1992, 2001).

The common ways of polyploidization appear to be the same as in the rodent placenta. The nuclei reach 4c-8c via restitution mitoses, whereas the higher ploidy levels are achieved via endoreduplication (Zybina et al., 2001, Zybina, Zybina, 2005).

Ruminants do not have highly invasive trophoblast cells: their placenta is epitheliochorial in which trophoblast cells mostly attach the uterine epithelium and do not penetrate uterine wall. Among the trophoblast cells there is a portion of polyploid cells mostly up to 8c (Klisch et al., 1999). The examples considered in this chapter confirm the regularities obtained in the rodent placenta. The invasive trophoblast cells in Carnivora that come into a close contact with the allogenic tissue reach high ploidy levels via endocycles, whereas the low-invasive trophoblast cells in ruminants reach 4c-8c and some higher via acytokinetic and other uncomplete mitoses.

3.4 Genome multiplication of the extravillous trophoblast cells in the human placenta alongside the invasive pathway

In the human placenta, polyploidization also takes place, though the cells do not reach as high ploidy level as other Mammalia. Meantime, like in other mammals, the highest ploidy level are characteristic of the invasive trophoblast cells.

In human placenta, the differentiation of the trophoblast cells that invade endometrium during pregnancy is accomplished in the cell columns at the tips of encoring villi (Kaufmann, Castellucci, 1997). The invasive pathway includes several steps (Zybina et al., 2002, Fig. 5a): (a) stem cells of cell column (CC) attached to the basal membrane at the apical part of the ancoring villi; they have high mitotic activity and express integrins $\alpha_6\beta_4$ (Kaufmann, Castellucci, 1997); (b) a proximal part of CC composed of a few compact layers of proliferative trophoblast cells, in which mitotic figures are present; (c) a distal part of CC composed of more loosely arranged EVT cells that contain larger nuclei and more abundant cytoplasm; they express integrins $\alpha_5\beta_1$, $\alpha_v\beta_3$, and $\alpha_v\beta_1$ (Kaufmann, Castellucci, 1997); (d) EVT

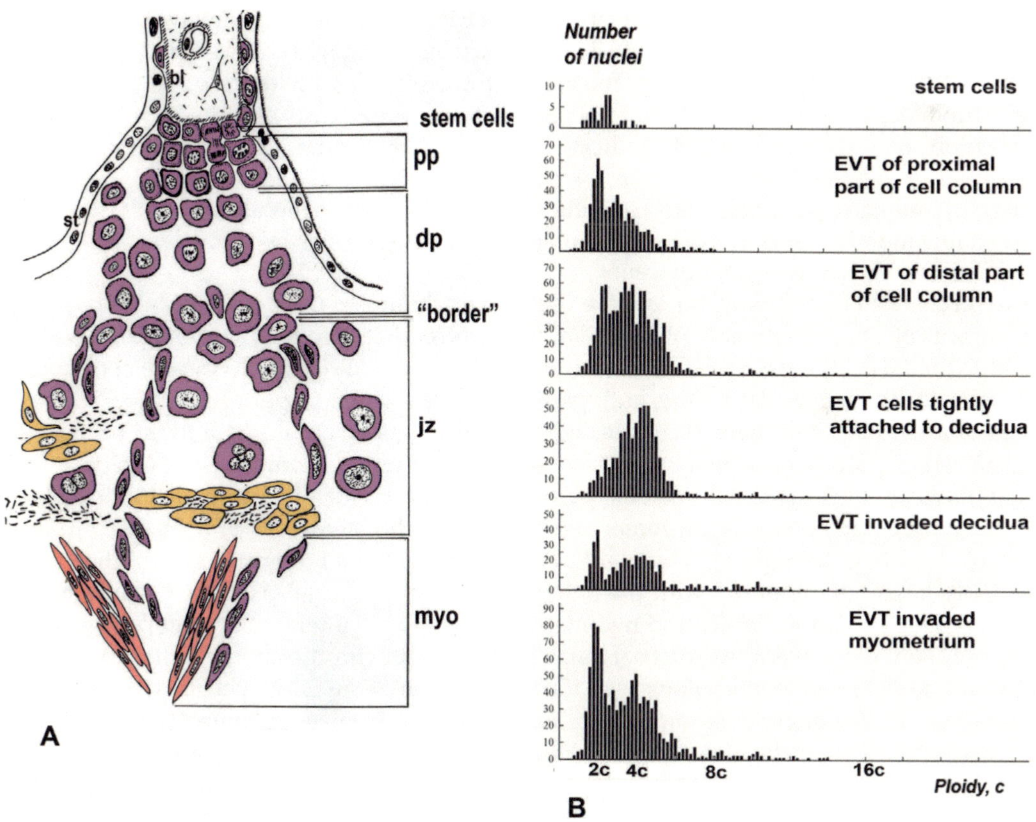

Fig. 5. Invasion of the extravillous trophoblast into the uterine wall in human placenta and its polyploidization. A - the trophoblast cells are proliferative in the zone of stem cells and proximal part (pp) of cell column, in the distal part (dp) they acquire invasive phenotype and migrate into junctional zone (jz), i.e. decidualized endometrium, a proportion of trophoblast cells reach myometrium (myo); B - polyploidization of the human extravillous trophoblast cells in the course of invasive pathway.

of the distal CC part, most closely attached to the basal plate; (e) invasive EVT cells determined by the cytokeratin-7 positivity within the materno-fetal junctional zone; (f) invasive, cytokeratin-7-positive EVT cells within myometrium.

The stem cells were found to be mainly diploid; a small amount of tetraploid cells (13.8 ± 2.3%) could be attributed to G_2-phase. The percentage of polyploid cells rose upon cell differentiation, so that in the distal part of CC the majority of EVT cells became polyploid, the portion of tetraploid cells (58 ± 1.5%) exceeded that of diploid ones (38 ± 1.5%); some amount of octaploid nuclei appeared. In the group of EVT attached to the basal plate, but not invading it, the percentage of tetraploid cells was the highest (74.7 ± 1.7%), and the octaploid cell group rose to 4.9 ± 0.8%. The EVT cells invading the decidualized endometrium also were predominantly polyploid: the fraction of octaploid nuclei increased to 9.7 ± 1.0% and some amount of 16c nuclei appeared (1.4 ± 1.0%), while the percentage of diploid cells rose slightly. This tendency did also take place in the group of invasive EVT cells within myometrium, although polyploid cells prevailed in the majority of the placentas studied (Fig. 5b). The portion of cells of different ploidy levels changed statistically significantly at every stage of differentiation of the EVT and invasive pathway ($P < 0.01$).

Besides, it is reasonable to note the individual variability of ploidy of invasive trophoblast cells, the higher ploidy level being established in the pregnancies with the greater amount of the extravillous trophoblast (Zybina et al., 2002). In the latter case, a higher level of pKi-67 expression was detected, which indicates their higher proliferative activity (data not shown).

Thus, in human placenta, like in other mammals, the trophoblast cells undergo polyploidization in the course of acquirement of invasive properties. However, the ploidy level is not as high as in rodent placenta.

As to mechanism of polyploidization, the uncompleted mitoses most probably do not play a significant role, despite the low ploidy level. The DNA content in the mitotic figures was 4c, i.e., the diploid cells, most probably, are only able to divide mitotically in the cell columns.

Simultaneously, in both the villous and, partly, the extravillous trophoblast cell populations of the human placenta, there occurs a high amount of cells containing a great number of chromocenters, some of which often resemble endomitotic chromosomes (Zybina et al., 2004). Rather numerous small nucleoli were observed to be attached to the chromocenters. The chromocenters/endochromosomes were found in the stem cells and in the proximal part of CC. Not infrequently, some large nuclei contained chromocenters that were markedly larger as compared with the neighbor cells. In the distal part of CC as well as in the EVT invaded endometrium and myometrium nuclei with a relatively uniform, network-like chromatin distribution were observed. The number of chromocenters in the EVT in the Feulgen and DAPI-stained sections was 15-30, the mode being 20-24 per nucleus, which is comparable to the haploid chromosome number in the human genome. The number of chromocenters / endochromosomes did not increase significantly with rise of the ploidy level. These findings indicate that polyplodization do not involve chromatid disjunction; moreover, the haploid number of endochromosomes suggests somatic conjugation characteristic of polyteny. Therefore, it is reasonable to suggest the first step of endoreduplication / polytenization in the extravillous trophoblast cells.

The intracellular localization of Ki-67 in EVT also provides some data on the ways of genome multiplication. In the stem cells and cells of the proximal part of CC, the Ki-67 immunostaining reminded the chromocenters revealed in Feulgen-, DAPI-, and hematoxylin-stained preparations. Besides, 2-5 small MIB1-positive nucleoli were often revealed in the cells of this CC part. By contrast, in the EVT of the distal part of CC the pKI-67 was located mainly in 1-2 large nucleoli, rather than in chromocenters. Such difference in the intranuclear distribution of Ki-67 indicates changes in the cell cycle, when taking into account that different patterns of the Ki-67 localization characterize different stages of the cell cycle (Starborg et al., 1996; Bridger et al., 1998). Thus, in the early G1, pKi-67 is detected in numerous foci of centromeric and telomeric DNA localization scattered throughout the nucleus (Bridger et al., 1998). In the late G1, S, and G2-phase, pKi-67 is found inside the well-formed nucleolus (Verheijen et al., 1989; Kill, 1996), in mitosis this protein is associated with chromosomes (Bridger et al., 1998; Suurmejer, Boon, 1999). Transition to the predominant nucleolar localization of Ki-67 suggests that redistribution of the protein characteristic of the mitotic cycle does not take place. In combination with cycle progression indicated by Ki-67 immunopositivity and lack of mitoses, it is also a proof for transition to the shortened cell cycle - endoreduplication. However, the relatively low ploidy level suggests progression of a few endocycles, afterward the cells leave the cell cycle, and the invasive EVT loose their capability for replication.

Populatios of the non-invasive - villous - trophoblast also contain a number of octaploid cells (Wakuda, Yosida, 1992; Pötgens et al., 2001), although their frequency is not as high as in cells of invasive pathway.

Giant trophoblast cells undergoing endomitosis and non-classic polyteny were found in some cases of normal human pregnancy (at the early stages of embryonic development) as well as in some pathological cases. The giant cells with bundles of parallel chromatin threads are more specific for trophoblast malignant tumors (Sarto et al., 1982; Therman et al., 1983; Kuhn, Therman, 1988). Endomitotic chromosomes were revealed in the human hydatidiform moles (Therman et al.,1983). These chromosomes sometimes weree not detached from each other in the course of consecutive replication cycles and formed clusters of adjacent endochromosomes. Therefore, endocycles (endomitosis and endoreduplication) appear to be characteristic of human trophoblast cells. Meantime, the well-developed non-classic polyteny in the human trophoblast appears to be not numerous, as the cells, most probably, do not undergo many cycles of endopolyploidization.

Regulation of cell polyploidization of the human EVT is not understood completely, although some data suggest similarity and specificity as compared to the rodent trophoblast. Thus, "mitotic" cyclins A and B1 as well as Ki-67 and PCNA were immunolocalized in proximal and distal EVT as well as in the EVT that invaded the upper decidual segments (Korgun et al., 2006). Cell cycle inhibitors p27 and p57 were expressed in all extravillous trophoblast cells (EVT), but p21 was not. The authors state that the set of cell cycle regulators present in the cell column strongly suggests that cells in both proximal and distal part of CC do not acutely proliferate. However, they maintain this ability because they have not left cell cycle, i.e. they express Ki-67 and PCNA as well as mitotic cyclins. We are of opinion that p27 and p57 expression reflect attenuation of proliferative activity in the EVT trophoblast along the invasive pathway. Meantime, a strong expression of p57 may be a feature of the endoreduplication cycle, because p57, being the S-phase inhibitor, proves oscillatory expression in the course of mouse giant trophoblast cell endoreduplication (Hattori et al., 2000; Hu, Cross, 2010). Mitotic cyclin B1 (as judged from the photo, Korgun et al., 2006) also shows downregulation in the invasive pathway. The immunolabelled cells may be found in the CC, but not inside the decidualized endometrium. However, endomitotic polyploidization may involve cyclin B1/cdk2 activity, as this way of cell cycle involves chromatid segregation, in which p34/cdk2 may take part.

Cyclin D1 also was expressed in the human cytotrophoblast compartment, which suggests its cell cycle processes up to the third trimester of pregnancy (De Falco et al., 2004). In fact, Cyclin D expression may be associated with polyploidization.It is confirmed by the data obtained on megakaryocytes. Thus, Cyclin D3 upregulation in response to thrombopoetin in the megacaryocyte lineage and Cyclin D3 overexpression were found to increase the megacaryocyte ploidy (Zimmet et al., 1997). A decrease in the level of Cyclin D3 blocks polyploidization (Wang et al., 1995). In Drosophila, Cyclin/Cdk4 also increases ploidy in endocycling tissues (Datar et al., 2000); therefore, D cyclins appear to be critical for endocycle progression.

Cyclin E may be also involved in transition to endocycles in human extravillous trophoblast endocycle. Thus, Cyclin E was found to express in the EVT, the highest level was found in the CC. In the EVT of CC, expression of Cyclin E started more distal as compared to Ki-67 and was maintained (with less intensity) in the deeper layer of interstitial trophoblast (Bamberger et al., 2003). According to flow cytometry, there is a correlation between p27 and Cyclin E expression in the human cytotrophoblast of normal placenta and hydatidiform moles (Fukunaga, 2004). The role of Cyclin E is supported by the data of the knockout experiment on murine embryos (Parisi et al., 2003). Double knockout mice with targeted genes encoding Cyclins E1 and E2 showed a marked reduction of ploidy of the trophoblast cells. It suggest a specific role of Cyclin E in trophoblast cell endocycle entry, probably in the absence of mitoses.

Anyway, human trophoblast polyploidization needs further investigation.

4. Depolyploidization and genome segregation is a terminal step of the polytene nucleus cycle

4.1 Transition from the polytene nucleus to the polygenomic one

The lifespan of the giant trophoblast cells in most of rodent placentas finishes by disintegration of the polytene nucleus into low-polyploid nuclear fragments, so that the highly polyploid mononuclear cell becomes a polykaryocyte (Zybina, 1986, 1990; Zybina, Zybina, 1996; Zybina et al., 2005). It is to be emphasized that this process is accomplished at the stage of the complete cessation of DNA replication and attenuation of RNA synthesis. It is not quite clear how the redistribution of chromosomes is achieved. However, in some rodent giant trophoblast cells there occurs disintegration of the polytene chromosome bundles into numerous paired endochromosomes. It is the most strongly pronounced in the highly invasive supergiant trophoblast cells in the field vole placenta, which reach very high ploidy level 256c-16384c (Zybina et al., 2009). The degree of chromatid attachment in these cells is weakening, they detach one-by-one from the surface of the chromosome bundle. As a result, the supergiant nucleus appears to be filled with rather decondensed endochromosomes; at the later stage the endochromosomes undergo condensation and look like paired endomitotic chromosomes (Fig. 6). The stage may be considered as a maximal level of chromosome condensation in the polytene nucleus cycle; it cannot be ruled out that it is one of the stages of chromosome rearrangement before depolyploidization.

Polytene chromosome disintegration into endochromosomes was also described in the endocycle of Dipteran cell types, in which classic polyteny occurs at one of the stages of the cell lifespan. Thus, in the nurse cells of ovaries of *Calliphora erythrocephala* polytene chromosomes with the clear-cut disc pattern were seen in the early endocycles. At the later stages, loosening of the disc pattern occurred with simultaneous shortening of chromosomes due to the spiralization of chromatid and their detachment from each other. As a result, the polytene chromosome broke down into endomitotic chromosomes (Wasserlauf et al., 2003; Ananina, Vedernikov, 2003, 2005). DNA hybridization *in situ* with chromosome 3 probe showed that endochromosomes did not spread throughout the nucleus, but form a chromosome territory formed by a multitude of homologous endochromosomes. This process seems to be analogous to the depolytenization in the giant trophoblast cells. In this case the chromosome structure and the activity cycling also take place. Thus, the nucleolar organizer activity varies during the polytene cycle and cell onthogenesis. In the course of polytene chromosome compactization, nucleolus falls into numerous small nucleoli, then they progressively decrease in number. At the stage of endomitotic chromosomes the nucleoli disappear completely (Wasserlauf et al., 2003). The stage functionally corresponds to mitosis. Thus, disaggregation of polytene chromosomes into endomitotic chromosomes occurs at the stage of attenuation of transcription.

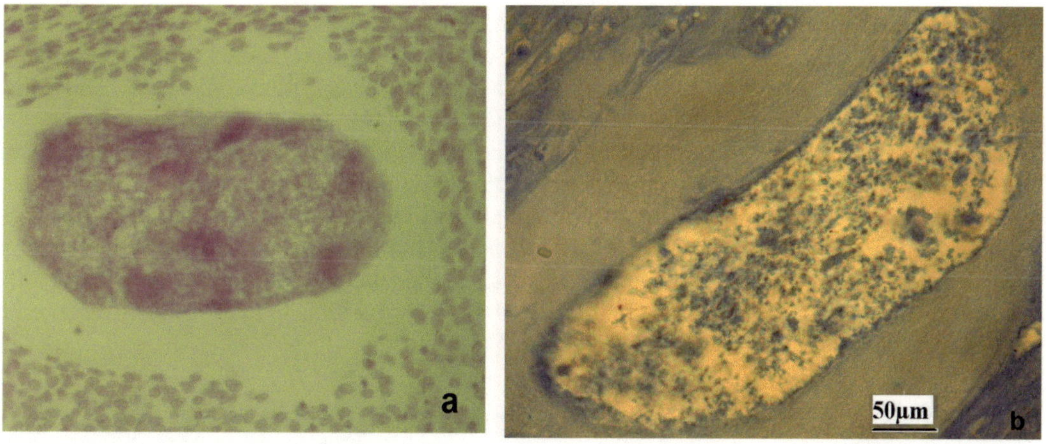

Fig. 6. Supergiant trophoblast cells of *Microtus rossiaemeridionalis*. a - a supergiant nucleus with bundles of non-classic polytene chromosomes; b - desaggregation of polytene chromosomes into endochromosomes.
Staining: a - Feulgen reaction, b - bromphenole blue.

4.2 Fragmentation of the giant trophoblast cells

Genome multiplication in the differentiation of a wide range of tissues in most cases proceeds irreversibly (Brodsky, Uryvaeva, 1985). One property intrinsic to many endocycles is that once they are initiated, further mitotic divisions are ill-advised for mechanical reasons (Edgar, Orr-Weaver, 2001). The mechanism of this phenomenon has not been yet clearly deciphered. These statements are proved, in particular by the examples that illustrate loss of the key components of the mitotic machinery in the cells undergoing endocycles. Thus, in the ovarian trophocytes of Drosophila (Mahowald et al., 1979), on reaching 8c when mitotic divisions decline, the centrioles migrated into oocyte through the intercellular bridges and finally lied adjacent to the oocyte nucleus. Thus, disconnection of chromosome, centrosome, and centriolar cycle and disaggregation of the centriolar complex may be a way of commitment to switching to the irreversible polytene cycle.

The exception is the mammalian trophoblast cell that undergo depolyploidization on reaching high levels of ploidy via a series of endoreduplication rounds (E. Zybina et al.,

1979, 1986). It should be emphasized that fragmentation of the highly endopolyploid nuclei begins after cessation of cycles of DNA replication (Zybina, 1986; Zybina, Zybina, 1996), i.e., at the second half of pregnancy. The non-classic polytene chromosomes are not revealed at this period any longer.

In the course of fragmentation, deep folds of nuclear endvelope (NE) dissect an initial nucleus into nuclei of smaller size (Fig. 7a). In many cases, NE emerges projections at one pole of the nucleus. Later on, small round nuclear fragments are detached from one side of the initial giant nucleus (Fig. 7b). In other cases, the whole nucleus turns out to be segregated into several dozens of small nuclei tightly attached to each other. Sometimes, the both processes take place in the same nucleus, i.e in case of binucleate giant cell; otherwise, initial nucleus first fall down into two giant nuclei, then they undergo fragmentation.

Distribution of chromosomes, most probably, proved to be genome-wise. The DNA cytometry demonstrated that the ploidy level of nuclear fragments corresponded to predominance of 1c, 2c, 4c, 8c (Zybina et al., 1975; Zybina, 1990; Zybina et al., 2005). The natural chromosome markers - nucleoli, Barr bodies (inactivated X-chromosomes) and condensed heterochromatin regions of polytene chromosomes - are distributed into nuclear fragments in accordance with ploidy their level (Zybina, 1986; Zybina, Zybina, 1996). The whole-genome chromosome distribution into the nuclear fragment is confirmed by the use of another natural chromosome marker of the interphase nucleus, i.e., gonosomal chromatin bodies (GCB, Zybina et al., 2003, 2005). Cytophotometrical measurement of DNA content in the nuclei, nuclear fragments, and simultaneously in the gonosomal chromatin bodies was made in the SGTCs of field vole *M. rossiaemeridionalis*. In most cases, 1-2 GCBs were found in the nuclear fragments of different ploidy levels. In the nuclear fragments GCB, the DNA content decreased mostly proportionally to the DNA content in the whole fragments corresponding to 2c, 4c and 8c.

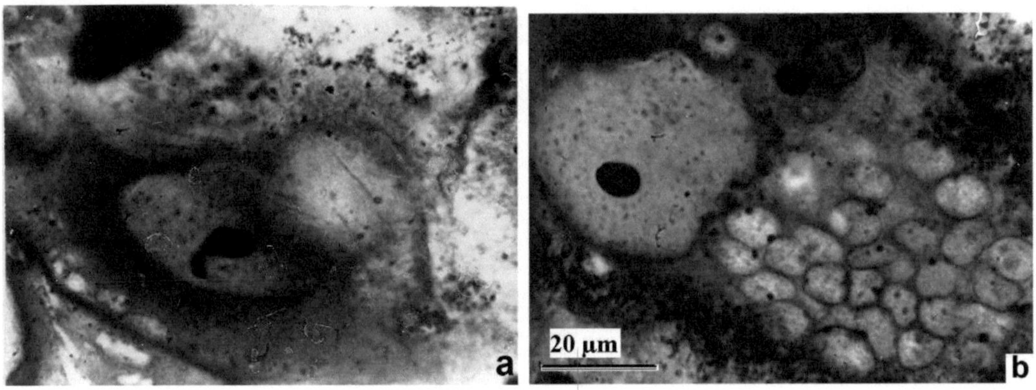

Fig. 7. Fragmentation of the secondary giant trophoblast cells in rat placenta. a - at the beginning of fragmentation the giant nucleus breaks down into two parts that undergo further fragmentation; b – the small nuclear fragments are budding off one side of the initial giant nucleus. Staining: Heidengein hematoxylin.

At the light microscope level it may be observed in rat SGTC that deep folds of the nuclear envelope (NE) dissect the nucleus, these folds separating single nuclei of smaller size (Fig. 7). In many cases the projections lie only at one pole of the nucleus (Fig. 7); in the same cases their localization coincides with the nuclear zone, in which fragmentation begins and fragments start to detach from the initial nucleus (Fig. 7).

Observation of the ultrastructure of the initial giant nuclei during their subdivision into fragments proved NE and its derivatives to play an active role in this process (Zybina, Zybina, 2008). The very deep folds divide the nucleus into several lobes. Apart from NE, a vide range of other NE derivatives may provide a reserve material for the nuclear fragmentation: annulate lamellae (AL), membranous tubules packs of pore complexes, etc. AL represent outgrowth of the inner or outer membrane of nuclear envelope consisting of parallel membranes joined by numerous pore complexes (Kessel, 1992; Zybina, Zybina, 2008). The intranuclear ALs of SGTCs are observed mainly at the periphery of the nucleus, i.e., in the zone of the most extensive NE folding. The areas covered by the double smooth-surfaced membranes were also found in the superficial part of the karyoplasm in the zone of fragmentation.

It is worth mentioning that a significant portion of SGTC undergoing fragmentation does not show any signs of apoptosis; their cytoplasm is reach in ribosomes, the numerous mitochondria, AER channels and cisterns, as well as elements of the Golgi complex. Meantime, some SGTC undergoing fragmentation sometimes show some signs of degeneration (Fig. 8b).

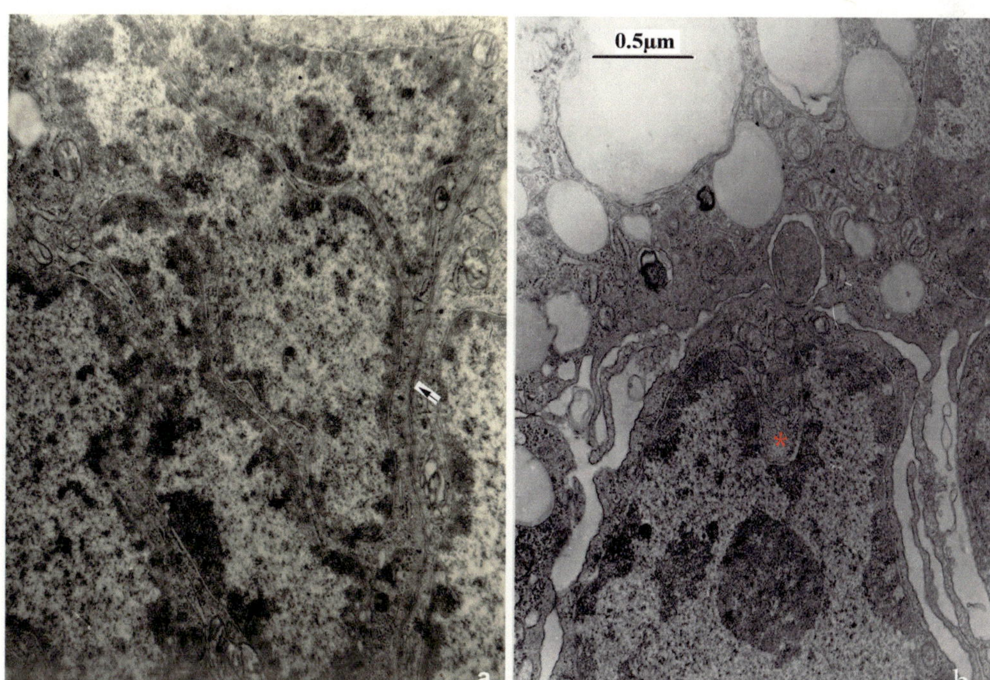

Fig. 8. Ultrastructure of the nuclear fragments. a - nuclear fragments surrounded by narrow cytoplasmic territories are separated by double membrane formed by agranular endoplasmic reticulum; b - cytoplasm shows signs of degeneration; a nuclear fragment shows a transcriptionally active nucleolus; it is isolated from the rest of the giant trophoblast cells by a wide channels of agranular endoplasmic reticulum; a bundle of intermediate filaments is seen inside the double membrane that delimits the nuclear fragment.

Each nuclear fragment is surrounded by the two-membrane NE (Fig.8a) containing numerous pore complexes. Progression of fragmentation is accompanied by the chromatin condensation and inactivation of the nucleolus. In the large fragments with the low-condensed chromatin the nucleolus consists mostly of the fibrillogranular component and the fibrillar centers surrounded by the dense fibrillar component, it indicating their transcriptional activity. The smallest nuclear fragments indicates, most probably, the final step of fragmentation: the chromatin is highly condensed and the nucleoli consist of electron dense fibrils that correspond to the most inactivated nucleolus (Zybina, Zybina, 2008). It indicates a decrease in attenuation of transcription that results, most probably, in apoptosis of the giant trophoblast cell.

Membranous structures were found to play another role in the transformation of giant trophoblast cells (Zybina, Zybina, 2008). At final steps of fragmentation, some nuclear fragments were observed to be surrounded by the cytoplasmic area delimited by the double membrane (Fig.8a, b). Upon compartmentalization of the cytoplasm, the narrow cisterns emerging from the outer membrane of NE pass to the system of the AER channels, which, in turn, participates in formation of the double membranes separating the cytoplasmic zones around individual nuclear fragments or their aggregates inside the trophoblast polykaryocytes (Fig. 8a). Interestingly, the desmosome-like structures appear in flat cisterns of AER that isolate the cytoplasmic area between two fragments (Fig. 8b, (Zybina, Zybina, 2008).). It suggests that the fragments behave, in some aspects, like individual cells. The cytoplamic territories that surround the separate nuclear fragments contain the complete set of viable cytoplasmic organelles – mitochondria, Golgi complex, GER and AER cisterns, numerous polysomes. Signs of degeneration in most cases were not observed in the cell compartments surrounding the nuclear fragments.

Sometimes, the nuclear fragments with the surrounding cell territory appear to be isolated from the rest of the cells, in which signs of degeneration are observed (Fig. 8b). These fragments look viable: they contain active nucleolus, many ribosomes and mitochondria in the narrow layer of the cytoplasm surrounding the nuclear fragment; in this case the cytoplasm territory is isolated from the rest of the cytoplasm by wide cisterns of the agranular endoplasmic reticulum.

A question arises, which structures play the role of the centriolar machinery in the course of fragmentation of the highly endopolyploid nucleus. Glasser (1984) put forward an idea that the centrosome-like bodies consisting of intermediate filaments may play this role. Indeed, at the stage of formation of the cytoplasmic zones around the nuclear fragment bundles, the 6–12-nm intermediate filaments (IF) are observed in the perinuclear zones of the cytoplasm (Zybina, Zybina, 2008).

The decrease of ploidy level is to involve the somatic reduction process, in which genome segregation is achieved in the absence of DNA replication. Non-numerous examples of somatic reduction are described in the literature. Thus, in ileum of the mosquito Culex, nuclei show signs of polyteny. In the course of metamorphosis, polyploid mitoses arise. The mitoses are followed by a series of reductional mitoses that proceed without intervening interphase and result in formation of octa- and tetraploid nuclei (Berger et al., 1938). Similar divisions are also described in ileum of the mosquito *Aedes aegypti* (Risler, 1959). The well-studied example of genome segregation is fragmentation of the highly polyploid nucleus in radiolarian (Raikov, 1982) that results in the breakdown of the primary endopolyploid nucleus into individual genomes.

The above-mentioned processes represent definite steps in differentiation of unicellular and invertebrates, they are less pronounced in vertebrates, by coinciding with completion of cell cycles. Fragmentation, i.e., somatic reduction of the trophoblast endopolyploid nuclei, also represent a definite, specifically terminal, step of the cell lifespan that coincides with cessation of cell cycles. These cells, most probably, are incapable of renewal of mitotic divisions. Therefore, the biological significance of the phenomenon is probably that cessation of functioning of provisory organ, i.e., placenta, makes impossible the renewal of proliferative activity of its cells, especially taking into account their characteristic feature of invasion of maternal tissues. Nevertheless, the possibility of isolation of diploid nuclear fragments with surrounding cell territories anticipates the probability of their transformation into full-value cells. Further studies might possibly throw light on significance of this phenomenon.

5. Reversibility of polyploidization in the lifespan of cells

The processes described above represent certain steps in differentiation of normal animal cells.

Nevertheless, some pathological processes, including carcinogenesis, imply a possibility of progression of polyploidization and depolyploidization cycles, the latter resulting in some cases in formation of the actively proliferating cell clones. Investigation of mechanisms of depolyploidization showed some traits similar to fragmentation of the highly endopolyploid nuclei in the mammalian trophoblast.

A reserve mechanism that allows overcoming the impossibility of cell division under conditions of disorder of the mitotic spindle microtubules was observed in the experiment of irradiation and treatment by a microtubule inhibitor SK&F on the p53 mutated Burkitt lymphoma cell lines (Erenpreisa et al., 2002). Electron microscopy showed large cells with the lobulating, segmenting, and budding nuclei that gave rise to many micronuclei and/or subnuclei. Study of ultrastructure revealed large, endopolyploid cells undergone significant changes, among them envelope-limited chromatin sheets (ELCS) and some other unusual membranous structures including AL and the so-called confronting cisterns (CC). The selective DNA cytometry in these nuclei and their segments showed the most frequently the 2N multiple DNA content. In irradiated cells, single ALs were seen in the close vicinity to ELCS, where they were observed to sequester the cytoplasm around the micronuclei, nuclear segments and buds (Erenpreisa, 2002). The process is similar to cytoplasm compartmentalization around the trophoblast cell nuclear fragments. However, unlike SK&F-treated cells, in trophoblast cells the compartmentalization of the cytoplasm is accomplished by cisterns of AER continuous with the outer nuclear membranes.

In search for a mechanism for genome reduction, acute radiation-induced endopolyploid tumor cells were demonstrated to exit from the mitotic cycle and altered DNA repair. It was found that the 10 Gy dose of photon irradiation (IR) to p53 function-deficient cell lines caused them to undergo extensive changes in the cell cycle progression, so that they transiently form endopolyploid giant cells. After G2-arrest for one to two days, the cells enter aberrant, often bridged mitoses and then either undergo mitotic death or, through "mitotic slippage" or bi-nucleation, become tetraploid. On days 5-6 post irradiation, this phase was switched to depolyploidization and bipolar and multipolar cell divisions occurred. It seems to be important that Aurora B-kinase was expressed in the newly-formed cells. From days 7-9 onwards death of most giant cells can be observed, and cell divisions are seen in the endopolyploid tumor cells. The cells gave rise to small colonies of paradiploid cells (Illidge et al., 2000; Ivanov et al., 2003; Erenpreisa et al., 2005, 2008). It seems to be important that Aurora B-kinase was expressed during segregation of these newly-formed cells suggesting the mitotic mechanism to be involved in this process (Salmina et al., 2010). Interestingly, the β-galactosidase expression changed from positive in the giant cells to negative in the small proliferative cells resulted from reduction division (Puig et al., 2008; Wheatley, 2008). Therefore, restitutive divisions of large (endopolyploid) cells represent a possibility that the tumor can recover post-treatment and start up again (Whetley, 2006).

Upregulation of meiosis-specific genes, such as REC8, MOS, and SPO11, was demonstrated in these cells (Kalejs et al., 2006; Ianzini et al., 2009). Besides, signs of pluripotency and self-renewal stem cell genes NANOG, OCT4, and SOX2 in this polyploidy-dependent survival mechanism were found (Erenpreisa, Cragg, 2010). Therefore, polyploidization and depolyploidization cycles potentially facilitate survival and propagation of the tumor cell population.

Therefore, the recent findings proved that in some cases polyploidy may provide cells a reserve way to survive. The polyploid cells, being more resistant to mutagenic factors and mitotic poisons, can be viable for some time and, moreover, may give rise to a viable diploid progeny with high proliferative potential.

6. Conclusion

Somatic polyploidization characteristic of quite a few tissues in multicellular organisms is achieved by means of various modifications of cell cycle, i.e., uncompleted mitoses including restitution and acytokinetic mitoses followed by polyploidizing mitoses as well as endocycles implying endomitosis and polyteny. These cell cycle modifications are accounted for by reduction of different phases of mitosis or by its almost complete absence. Nevertheless, if in the absence of mitotic division cycle of DNA, replication is retained, it is accompanied by the cyclic changes of transcription activity and chromosome condensation. Progression of the modified cell cycles, like in the regular mitotic cycle, is regulated by the activity of the cyclin-kinase complexes. However, some specific difference in their expression is observed. In particular, in the course of transition of trophoblast cells from mitotic cycles to endocycles a change of cyclin D isophorms – from D3 to D1 – was found. Arrest of mitotic cycle in transition to endoreduplication cycle is accounted for by the lack of assembly of cyclin B/$p34^{cdk1}$-complex in the first endocycle, the subsequent endocycles not involving at all the cyclin B expression.

In the course of uncompleted mitoses the majority of mitotic machinery components and regulation are retained, which favors retaining their ability to undergo mitoses. Thus, Aurora B-kinase, in most cases, proved to retain the mitosis-specific time-table of relocation. By contrast, switching off the expression of several factors that ensure the sequence of mitosis progression ($p34^{cdk1}$, Survivin, etc.) may be accounted for by the lack of kinetochore binding to the spindle and other event that result in chromosome missegregation in ana- and telophase and polyploidization. Unlike the uncompleted mitoses, endocycles are more prone to lose their capability for renewal of mitotic activity.

In the mammalian placenta, various types of cell cycles are characterstic of the functionally different trophoblast cell populations. In this aspect the giant rodent trophoblast cells combine lysis and phagocytosis of allogenic maternal cells with their intensive growth and polyploidization (mostly up to 128c-512c) via endoreduplication, i.e. without disappearance of the nuclear envelope. It allows ruling out contact of genome to the rests of phagocytosed cells that may be mutagenic to the trophoblast cells. By contrast, cells of the placenta junctional zone that partly share the traits of the trophoblast stem cells and undergo polyploidization via uncompleted mitoses do not contact to the allogenic maternal cells that probably favor their genome protection. This example illustrates the significance of different ways of genome multiplication for the tissue-specific functions.

In the rodent giant trophoblast cells, cessation of the DNA replication does not result in the complete cessation of the cyclic changes of transcription activity and chromosome condensation. It cannot be ruled out that the highest level of "cyclicity" is disintegration of polytene chromosomes onto the olygotene chromonemes and/or endochromosomes that may be a prerequisite of the whole-genome depolyploidization of the giant nuclei that result in the polykaryocyte formation. This event represents the terminal step of giant cell lifespan before their apoptosis. However, similar processes described in many pathological processes suggest retaining some reserve mechanisms that allow cells to survive under extreme conditions.

In the human placenta, highly invasive extravillous trophoblast cells also undergo several endocycles before the start of invasion of endometrium. Transition to endomitosis and endoreduplication before the complete cessation of DNA replication favors formation of cells more resistant under condition of their contact with allogenic maternal tissues.

7. Acknowledgements

The authors are grateful to Prof. L.Z. Pevzner for the valuable advices as well as help in editing and translation of the manuscript. The work was supported by the Russian governmental program "Molecular and cell biology".

8. References

Ananina T.V., Vedernikov A.E. (2003). Chromatin spatial organization study in the trophocytes in the course of endomitotic cycle of *Calliphora erythrocephala Tsitologiya;* 45: 848.

Ananina T.V., Vedernikov A.E. (2005). Visualization of chromosome territories in the interphase nuclei of the ovarian trophocytes of Callophora erythrocephala Mg. (Diptera: Calliphoridae). *Genetika;* 41: 1350-1357.

Anatskaya O.V., Vinogradov A.E., Kudryavtsev B.N. (2001). Cardiomyocyte ploidy levels in birds with different growth rates. *J. Exp.Zool.;* 289: 48-58

Andreeva L.F. (1964). DNA synthesis and cell population kinetics study in the giant cells and cellular trophoblast of placenta. In: *Cell Cycle and nucleic acid metabolism in the course of cell differentiation.* Nauka: Moskow.

Anisimov A.P. (2005). Endopolyploidy as a morphogenic factor of development. *Cell Biol. Int.;* 29: 993-1004.

Anisimov A.P. (1997a). A study of genome multiplication mechanisms in the development of albumen gland cells of *Succinea lauta* (Gastropoda, Pulmonata). V. Polyploidizing mitosis and endomitosis. *Tsitologiya;* 39: 218-228.

Anisimov A.P. (1997b). A study of genome multiplication mechanisms in the development of albumen gland cells of *Succinea lauta* (Gastropoda, Pulmonata). VI. Ultrastructural research of the endomitotic cycle. *Tsitologiya;* 39: 229-236

Anisimov A.P. (1997c). A study of genome multiplication mechanisms in the development of albumen gland cells of *Succinea lauta* (Gastropoda, Pulmonata). VII. Transcriptive activity of the nuclei in the endomitotic cycle . *Tsitologiya;* 39: 237-243.

Anisimov A. P. , Kirsanova I.A. (2002). Somatic polyploidy of the gastropod mollusks III. Mitosis and endomitosis in postnatal development of neurons of the succineid snail central nervous system. *Tsitologiya;* 44: 981-987.

Anisimova A.A., Anisimov A.P. (2002) Morpho-functional parameters of nucleoli in the development of polyploidy cells in the protein gland of the *Succinea lauta. Tsitologiya,* 44: 737-746.

Ashburner M. (1972). Puffing patterns in *Drosophila melanogaster* and related species. In: *Developmental studies on giant chromosomes.* (W. Beermann ed.) Springer: Berlin, Heidelberg, New York.

Auer G.U., Backdahl M., Forsslund G.M. Askensten U.G. (1985) Ploidy levels in nonneoplastic and neoplastic thyroid cells. *Anal. Quant. Cytol. Histol.;* 7:97-106.

Avanzi S., Cionini P. G., D'Amato F. 1970. Cytochemical and authoradiographic analysis on the suspensor cells of Phaseolus coccineus. *Caryologia;* 23:605-638.

Bamberger A.M., Aupers S., Milde-Langosch K., Löning T. (2003) Expression pattern of the cell cycle promoter cyclin e in benign extravillous trophoblast and gestational trophoblastic lesions: correlation with expression of Ki-67. *Int. J. Gynecol. Pathol.;* 22(2): 156-161

Barlow P.W., Sherman M.J. (1972). The biochemistry of differentiation of mouse trophoblast: studies on polyploidy. *J. Embryol. Exp. Morphol.;* 27: 447-465

Barlow P. W., Sherman M. J. (1974). Cytological studies on the organization of DNA in giant trophoblast nuclei of the mouse and rat. *Chromosoma;* 47: 119-131.

Beermann, W. (1972). Chromomeres and genes. In: Developmental Studies on Giant Chromosomes. *In: Results and Problems in Cell Differentiation;* 4: 1-33.

Berger C.A. (1938). Multiplication and reduction of somatic chromosome groups as a regular developmental process in the mosquito *Culex pipiens. Carnegie Contrib. Emryol.;* 27: 209-232.

Boivin A., Venderly K., Venderly C. (1948). L'acide desoxyribonucleique de noyau cellulaire depositaire de caractere hereditaire. C.R. Acad. Sci. 226: 1061-1063.

Brady T., Clutter M.E. (1974). Structure and replication of the Phaseolus polytene chromosomes. *Chromosoma;* 45: 63-79.

Bridger J.M., Kill J.R., Lichter P. (1998). Association of pKi-67 with satellite DNA of the human genome in early G1 cells. *Chromosome Res.;* 6: 13

Brodsky V. Ja., Uryvaeva I. V. 1985. *Genome multiplication in growth and development.* Cambridge: Univ. Press. Brodsky V. Ja., Uryvaeva I.V. (1981). *Cell Polyploidy . proliferation and differentiation*. Nauka: Moskow.

Callan H.G. (1986). *"Lampbrush chromosomes"*. Springer-Verlag: Berlin.

Cahill D.P., Lengauer C., Yu J., Riggins G.J., Wilson J.K. Markowitz S.D. et al. (1998). Mutations of mitotic spindle checkpoint genes in human cancers. *Nature;* 392: 300-303.

Celton-Morizur S., Desdoutes C. (2010). Polyploidization of liver cells. Adv. Exp. Med. Biol. 676:123-135.

Compton D. A., Luo C. (1995). Mutation of the predicted p34^{cdc2} phosphorylation sites in NuMa impair the assembly of the mitotic spindle and block mitosis. *J. Cell Sci.;* 108: 621-633.

D'Amato, F. (1989). Polyploidy in cell differentiation. *Caryologia;* 42: 183-211.

Datar S.A., Jacobs H.W., Lehner C.F., Edgar B.A. (2000). The Drosophila cyclin D/Cdk4 complex promotes cellular growth. *EMBO J.;* 19: 4543-4554.

De Falco M., Fedele V., Cobellis L., Mastrogiacomo A., Giraldi D., Leone S., De Luca L., Laforgia V., De Luca A. (2004). Pattern of expression of cyclin D1/cdk4 complex in human placenta during gestation. *Cell Tiss. Res.;* 317: 187-194

Dej K.J., Spradling A.C. (1999). The endocycle controls nurse cell polytene chromosome structure during *Drosophila* oogenesis. *Development;* 126: 293-303.

Edgar B. A., Orr-Weaver T. L. (2001). Endoreduplication cell cycle: more for less. *Cell;* 105: 297-306.

Elledge S.J. (1996). Cell cycle checkpoints: preventing an identity crisis. *Science;* 272: 1664-1672.

Erenpreisa, Je., Ivanov, A., Cragg, M., Selivanova, G., Illidge, T. (2002). Nuclear envelope-limited chromatin sheets are parts of mitotic death. *Histochem. Cell Biol.;* 117, 243–255.

Erenpreisa, J., Ivanov, A., Wheatley, S. P., Kosmacek, E. A., Ianzini, F., Anisimov, A. P., Mackey, M., Davis, P. J., Plakhins, G., and Illidge, T. M. (2008). Endopolyploidy in irradiated p53-deficient tumour cell lines: persistence of cell division activity in giant cells expressing Aurora-B kinase. *Cell Biol Int* 32, 1044-56.

Erenpreisa, J., Kalejs, M., Ianzini, F., Kosmacek, E. A., Mackey, M. A., Emzinsh, D., Cragg, M. S., Ivanov, A., and Illidge, T. M. (2005). Segregation of genomes in polyploidy tumour cells following mitotic catastrophe. *Cell Biol Int* 29: 1005-1011.

Erenpreisa J. , Cragg M.S. (2010). MOS, aneuploidy and the ploidy cycle of cancer cells. *Oncogene*: 1-5.

Fukunaga M. (2004). Immunohistochemical characterization of cyclin E and p27KIP1 expression in early hydatidiform moles. *Int. J. Gynecol. Pathol.;* 23(3): 259-264.

Geitler L. (1953). Endomitose and endomitotische Polyploidizierung. *Protoplasmatologia;* 60:1-89.

Glasser, S.R., Soares, M.J., Julian, J. (1984). Morphological and functional differentiation of rat trophectoderm in vitro: organization of microtubules, expression of cytokeratins and rat placental lactagen in midgestation trophoblast giant cells. *In: Int. Symp. Mammal Reprod. Early Devel.;* Tokyo, August 23–24.

Gonzalez M.A., Tachibana K.E., Adams D.J., Van der Weyden L., Hemberger M., Coleman N., Bradley N., Laskey R.A. (2006). Geminin is essential to prevent endoreduplication and to form pluripotent cells during mammalian development. Genes Dev.; 20: 1880-1884.

Gualberto A., Aldape K., Kozakiewicz K., Tlsty T.D. (1998). An oncogenic form of p53 confers a dominant, gain-of function phenotype that disrupts spindle checkpoint control. *Proc. Natl. Acad. Sci. USA;* 95: 5166-5171.

Gui Y., Gordon H.H., Walsh M.P., Zheng X.L. (2007). Predisposition to tetraploidy in pulmonary vascular smooth muscle cells derived from the Eker rats. *Am. J. Physiol. Lung Cell Mol. Physiol.;* 293: L702-L711

Gunderina L.I., Sherudilo A.I., Mitina R.D. (1984). The replication cycle of DNA during chromosome polytenization in the salivary gland cells in Chironomus thummi. T*sitologiya;* 26: 925-935.

Hancock V. Martin J. F., Lelchuk R. (1993). The relationship between human megakaryocyte nuclear DNA content and gene expression. *Br. J. Haematol.;* 85: 692-697.

Hattori N., Davies T.C., Anson-Cartwright L., Cross J.C. 2000. Periodic expression of the Cdk inhibitor p57Kip2 in trophoblast giant cells defines G2-like gap phase of endocycles. *Mol. Biol. Cell;* 11: 1037-1045.

Heiden F.L, James J. (1975). Polyploidy in the human myometrium. *Z. Mikrosk. Anat. Forsch.;* 89: 18-26.

Hixon M.L., Gualberto A. (2003). Vascular smooth muscle polyploidization. *Cell Cycle;* 2: 105-110.

Howard A., Pelc. S.R. (1953). Synthesis of DNA and its relation to chromosome breakage. *Heredity;* 6: 261-269.

Hu D., Cross J. (2010). Development and function of trophoblast giant cells in the rodent placenta. *Int .J. Dev. Biol.;* 54: 341-354

Holloway S. L., Glotzer M., King R. W., Murray A. W. (1993). Anaphase is initiated by proteolysis rather than by inactivation of maturation promoting factor. *Cell;* 73: 1393-1402.

Ianzini, F., Kosmacek, E. A., Nelson, E. S., Napoli, E., Erenpreisa, J., Kalejs, M., and Mackey, M. A. (2009). Activation of meiosis-specific genes is associated with depolyploidization of human tumor cells following radiation-induced mitotic catastrophe. *Cancer Res.;* 6: 2296-304.

Illidge, T. M., Cragg, M. S., Fringes, B., Olive, P., and Erenpreisa, J. A. (2000). Polyploid giant cells provide a survival mechanism for p53 mutant cells after DNA damage. *Cell Biol Int* 24: 621-33.

Ivanov, A., Cragg, M. S., Erenpreisa, J., Emzinsh, D., Lukman, H., and Illidge, T. M. (2003). Endopolyploid cells produced after severe genotoxic damage have the potential to repair DNA double strand breaks. *J Cell Sci.;* 116, 4095-106.

Kalejs, M., Ivanov, A., Plakhins, G., Cragg, M. S., Emzinsh, D., Illidge, T. M., and Erenpreisa, J. (2006). Upregulation of meiosis-specific genes in lymphoma cell lines following genotoxic insult and induction of mitotic catastrophe. *BMC Cancer* 6: 6.

Kaufmann, P. and Castelucci, M. (1997). Extravillous trophoblast in the human placenta. *Trophoblast Res.;* 10: 21 - 65.

Kessel R. (1992). Annulate lamellae: a last frontier in cellular organelles. Int. Rev. Cytol., 133: 43-120.

Kiknadze I.I. (1972). *Functional organization of chromosomes*. Nauka: Leningrad.

Kiknadze I. I., Istomina A, G. 1980. Endomitosis in grasshopper. 1. Nuclear morphology and synthesis of DNA and RNA in the endopolyploid cells of the inner parietal layer of the testicular follicle. Eur. J. Cell Biol., 21: 122-133.

Kiknadze I.I., Perov N.A., Chentsov Yu. S. 1976. Electron microscopic studies on polytene chromosome salivary glands. Chromosoma. 55: 91-103.

Kill J.R. (1996). Localization of the Ki-67 antigen within the nucleolus. Evidence for a fibrillarin-deficient region of the dense fibrillar component. *J. Cell Science;* 109: 1253-1263.

Klisch K., Pfarrer K., Schuler G., Hoffman B., Leiser R. (1999). Tripolar acytokinetic mitoses and formation of feto-maternal syncytia in the bovine placentome: different modes of the generation of multinuclear cells. *Anat. Embryol.* 200: 229-237.

Korgun E.T., Celik-Ozenci C., Acar N., Cayli S., Desoye G., Demir R. (2006). Location of cell cycle regulators cyclin B1, cyclin A, PCNA, Ki67, and cell cycle inhibitors p21, p27 and p57 in human first trimester placenta and deciduas. *Histochem cell Biol.;*126: 615-624

Knoblich J A., Sauer K., Jones L., Richardson H., Saint R., Lehner C.F. (1994). Cyclin E controls S phase progression and its down-regulation during Drosophila embryogenesis is required for the arrest of cell proliferation. *Cell;* 77:107-120.

Kudryavtsev B. N., Kudryavtseva M. V., Sakuta G. A., Stein G. I. (1993). Human hepatocyte polyploidization kinetics in the course of life cycle. *Virchows Arch. B Cell Patol.;* 64: 387-393.

Kuhn E.M. , Therman E. (1988). The behaviour of heterochromatin in mouse and human nuclei. *Cancer Genet. Cytogenet.;* 34: 143-151.

Lehner C. F., O'Farrell P. H. (1990). The roles of *Drosophila* cyclins A and B in mitotic control. *Cell;* 61: 535-547.

Lee H.O., Davidson J.M., Duronio R. (2009). Endoreplication: polyploidy with purpose. Genes Dev., 23: 2461-2477.

McAuley A., Cross J. C., Werb Z. (1998). Reprogramming the cell cycle for endoreduplication in rodent trophoblast cells. *Molecular Biology of the Cell;* 9: 795-807

McGarry T.J., Kirschner M.W. (1998). Geminin, an inhibitor DNA replication, is degraded during mitosis. *Cell;* 93: 1043-1053.

McCrann D.J., Nguyen H.G., Jones M.R., Ravid K. (2008). Vascular smooth muscle cells polyploidy: an adaptive or misadaptive response? *J. Cell Physiol.;* 215(3); 588-592.

Lilly M.A., Spradling A.C. (1996). The Drosophila endocycle is controlled by cyclin E and lacks of checkpoints ensuring S-phase completion. *Genes Dev.;* 10: 2514-2526.

Nagata Y., Jones M.R., Nguyen H.G., McCrann, Hilaire C. St., Schreiber B., Hashimoto A., Inagaki M., Earnshaw W.C., Todokoro K., Ravid K.(2005) Vascular smooth muscle polyploidization involves changes in chromosome passenger and endomitotic cell cycle. *Exp. Cell Res.;* 305: 277-291.

Nakayama H., Scott I.C., Cross J.C. (1998). The transition to endoreduplication in trophoblast giant cells is regulated by the mSNA zinc finger transcription factor. *Dev. Biol.* 199: 150-163.

Nagl W. (1978). *Endopolyploidy and polyteny in differentiation and evolution. Toward an understanding of quantitative and qualitative variation of nuclear DNA in ontogeny and phylogeny.* North Holland Publishing Company: Amsterdam - N.Y. - Oxford.

Nagl W. (1981). Polytene chromosomes of Plants. *Intern. Rev. Cytol.* 73: 21-53.

Nagl W. (1995). Cdc-2 kinases, cyclins and the switch from proliferation to polyploidization. *Protoplasma;* 188: 143-150.

Nurse P. (1991). How is the cell division cycle regulated? *Philos. Trans. R. Soc. Lond. Biol.;* 33: 271-276.

Ookata K., Hisinaga S.-I., Bulinski J. C., Murofushi H., Aizawa H. et al. (1995). Cyclin B interaction with microtubule associated proteins 4 (MAP4) targets $p34^{cdc2}$ kinase to microtubules and is a potential regulator of M-phase microtubule dynamics. *J. Cell Biol.;* 128: 849-862.

Parisi T., Beck A., Rougier N., McNeil T., Lucian L., Werb Z., Amati B. (2003). Cyclins E1 and E2 are required for endoreduplication in placenta trophoblast cells. *The EMBO Journal;* 22(18): 2794-4803.

Pearson M. J. (1974). Polyteny and the functional significance of the polytene cell cycle. *J. Cell Sci.;* 15: 457-479.

Pfitzer P. (1971). Nuclear DNA content in human myocardial cells. *Curr. Top. Pathol.;* 54: 125-168.

Pötgens A. J. G., Gaus G., Frank H.-G., Kaufmann P.(2001). Characterization of trophoblast cell isolation by modified flow cytometry assay. *Placenta;* 22: 251-255.

Puig P.-E., Guilly M.-N., Boushot A., Drom N., Cathelien D., Bouyer F., et al. (2008). Tumour cells can escape DNA damaging cisplatin through DNA endoreduplication and reversible polyploidy. *Cell Biol. Int.;* 32: 1031-1043.

Raikov I.B. (1982). *The protozoan nucleus. Morphology and evolution.* Springer Verlag: Wien-New-York.

Ravid K., Lu, J., Zimmet J., Jones M. Roads to polyploidy: The megakaryocyte example. *J. Cell Physiol.;* 190: 7-20.

Ribbert D..Chromomeres and puffing in experimentally induced polytene chromosomes of *Calliphora erythrocephala. Chromosoma (Berl.*); 10: 619-653.

Risler H. (1959). Polyplode und somatische Reduction in der Larvenepidermis von Aedes aegypti L. (Culicidae). *Chromosoma;* 10: 184-209.

Rudkin W. (1972). *Replication of polytene chromosomes. In: developmental studies of giant chromosomes.* (W. Beermann ed.) Springer: Berlin-Heidelberg-New York.

Rumyantsev P.P. (1991). *Growth and hyperplasia of cardiac muscle cells.* Harwood Acad Publ.: Chur, Switzerland.

Salmina K., Jankevics E., Huna A., Perminov D., Radovica I., Klymenko T., Ivanov A., Jascenko E., Scherthan H., Mark Cragg M., Jekaterina Erenpreisa E. (2010). Up-regulation of the embryonic self-renewal network through reversible polyploidy in irradiated p53-mutant tumour cells. *Exp. Cell Res.,* 316(13): 209-214.

Sarto G. E., Stubblefield P.A., Therman E. (1982). Endomitosis in human trophoblast. *Human Genetics;* 62: 228-232

Sauer K., Knoblich J.A., Richardson H., Lehner C.F. (1995). Distinct modes of cyclin E cdc2c kinase regulation and S-phase control in mitotic and endoreduplication cycles of *Drosophila* embryogenesis. *Genes Dev.;* 9:1327-1339.

Starborg M., Gell, K., Brundell E., Höög Ch. (1996). The murine Ki-67 cell proliferation antigen accumulates in the nucleolar and heterochromatic regions of interphase cells and at the periphery of the mitotic chromosomes in a process essential for cell cycle progression. *J. Cell Sci.;* 199: 143-153.

Stewart I.J., Clarke J.R. (1993). Ultrastructural study of giant interstitial trophoblast cells in the short-tailed field vole, *Microtus agrestis. Placenta;* 14: A.75.

Su T.T., O'Farrell P.H. (1998). Chromosome association of minichromosome maintenance proteins in *Drosophila* endoreduplication cycles. *J. Cell Biol.;* 140: 451-460.

Suurmeijer A.J.H., Boon M.E. (1999). Pretreatment in a high pressure microwave processor for MIB1 immunostaining of cytological smears and paraffin section to visualize the various phases of the mitotic cycle. *J. Histochem. Cytochem.;* 47: 1015-1020.

Therman E.,Sarto G., Stubbliefield P. (1983). Endomitosis: a reappraisal. *Hum. Genet.;* 63: 13-18.

Therman E., Sarto G.E., Kuhn E.M. (1986). *Cancer Genet. Cytogenet.;* 19: 301-310.

Therman E., Kuhn E. (1989). Mitotic modifications and aberrations in cancer. *CRC Critical reviews in oncogenesis;* 1(3): 293-305.

Tschermak-Woess E. (1971). Endomitose. *In: Zellkern. Hdb. Allg. Pathol.;* 2/2/1.(H.-W. Altmann. Ed.), pp. 569-625. Springer: Berlin, Heidelberg, New York.

Tschermak-Woess E. (1973). Somatische Polyploidie bei Pflantzen. *In: Grundlagen der Cytologie.* Fisher, Stuttgart.

Uryvaeva I.V. (1979). Polyploidizing mitoses and biological significance of polyploidy in the cell of liver. *Tsitologiya;* 21: 1427-1437.

Verheijen R., Kuijpers H.J.K., Schlingenmann R.O., Boehmer A.L.M, van Driel R., Brakenhoff G.J, Ramaekers F.C.S. (1989). Ki-67 detects a nuclear matrix-associated proliferation-related antigen. I. Intranuclear localization during interphase. *J. Cell Sci.;* 92: 123-130

Wakuda K., Yoshida Y. (1992). DNA ploidy and proliferative characteristics of human trophoblasts. *Acta Obstet. Gynecol. Scand.;* 71: 12-16.

Wang Z., Zhang Y., Kamer D., Lees E., Ravid K. (1995). Cyclin D3 is essential for megakaryocytopoesis. *Blood;* 86: 3783-3788.

Warmuza S., Prideau V., Kothary R., Rossant J. (1988). Polytene chromosomes in mouse trophoblast giant cells. *Development;* 102: 127-134.

Wasserlauf I.E., Ananina T.V., Unger M.F., Karamysheva T.V., Melnikova N.N., Rubtsov N.B., Stegnii V.N. (2003). Chromosome organization and differential banding in endomitotic nuclei of nurse cells of *Calliphora erythtocephala.* (Diptera: Calliphoridae). *Genetika;* 39: 1193-1202.

Wheatley D. (2006). Regrowth of tumour cells from supposedly terminal giant cells. *Oncology News; 1(3):2.*

Wheatley D. (2008). Growing evidence of the repopulation of regressed tumours by the division of giant cells. *Cell Biol. Int.;* 32: 1029-1030.

Yang D., McCrann D.J., Nguyen H., St.Hilaire C., DePinho R.A., Jones M.R., Ravid K. (2007). Increased polyploidy in aortic vascular smooth cells during aging is marked by cellular senescence. *Aging Cell;* 6: 257-260.

Zavarzin A.A. (1967). *DNA synthesis and kinetics of cell populations in mammalian onthogenesis.* Nauka: Leningrad.

Zimmet J.M., Ladd D., Jackson C.W., Stenberg P.E., Ravid K. (1997). A role for cyclin D3 in the endomitotic cell cycle . *Mol. Cell Biol.;* 17: 7248-7259.

Zhimulev I.F. 1992. *Polytene chromosomes: morphology and structure.* Nauka, Novosibirsk. 451 p.

Zavarzin A.A. (1967). *DNA synthesis and kinetics of cell populations in mammalian onthogenesis.* Nauka: Leningrad.

Zybina E. V. (1963). Autoradiographic and cytophotometric investigation of nucleic acids (DNA and RNA) in the endomitotic cycle of giant trophoblast cells. *In: Morphology and cytochemistry of cells.* Nauka: Moskow.

Zybina E. V. (1986). *The trophoblast cytology*. Nauka: Leningrad.

Zybina T.G. (1990). DNA in the nuclear fragments that appear in the course of fragmentation of secondary giant trophoblast cells in the field vole. *Tsitologiya;* 32: 806-810.

Zybina E.V., Zybina T.G. (1985). Polyteny and endomitosis in supergiant trophoblast cells of *Microtus subarvalis*. *Tsitologiya;* 27: 402-410.

Zybina, E. V. and Zybina, T. G. (1996). Polytene chromosomes in mammalian cells. *Inter. Rev. Cytol.;* 165: 53-119.

Zybina E.V., Zybina T.G. (2005). Cell reproduction and genome multiplication in the proliferative and invasive trophoblast cell populations of mammalian placenta. *Cell Biol. Intern*. 29, 1071-1083.

Zybina E.V., Zybina T.G. (2008). Modifications of nuclear envelope during differentiation and depolyploidization of rat trophoblast cells. *Micron;* 39: 593-606.

Zybina E. V., Mosjan I.A. (1967). Sex chromatin bodies during endomitotic polyploidization of trophoblast cells. *Tsitologiya;* 9: 265-272.

Zybina E.V., Kudryavtseva M.V., Kudryavtsev B.N. (1975). Polyploidization and endomitosis in giant cells of rabbit trophoblast. *Cell Tiss. Res.;* 160: 525-537.

Zybina E.V., Kudryavtseva M.V., Kudryavtsev B.N. (1979). The distribution of chromosome material during giant nuclear division by fragmentation in the trophoblast of rodents. *Tsitologiya;* 21: 12-20.

Zybina E.V., Zybina T.G., Isakova G.K., Kiknadze I.I., Stein G.I. (1992). Polyploidy and polyteny in the mink trophoblast cells. *Tsitologiya;* 34: 53-57.

Zybina T.G., Zybina E.V., Stein G.I. (1985). Nuclear DNA content in the secondary giant cells of rat trophoblast at different phases of cell cycles of polytene nucleus. *Tsitologiya;* 27: 957-960.

Zybina T. G., Zybina E. V., Kiknadze I. I., Zhelezova A. I. (2001). Polyploidization in the trophoblast and uterine glandular epithelium of the endotheliochorial placenta of silver fox (Vulpes fulvus Desm.), as revealed by the DNA content. *Placenta;* 22: 490-498.

Zybina T.G., Kaufmann P., Frank H.-G., Freed J., Kadyrov M., Biesterfeld S. (2002). Genome multiplication of extravillous trophoblast cells in human placenta in the course of differentiation and invasion into endometrium and myometrium. I. Dynamics of polyploidization. *Tsitologiya;* 44: 1058-1067.

Zybina T.G., Zybina E.V., Bogdanova M.S., Stein G.I. (2003). Quantitative investigation of reproduction of gonosomal condenced chromatin during trophoblast cell polyploidization and endoreduplication in east-European field vole *Microtus rossiaemeridionalis*. *Reprod. Biol. Endocrinol.;* 2003, 1:32, online, doi: 10.1186/1477-7827-1-32.

Zybina T.G., Kaufmann P., Frank H.-G., Freed J., Biesterfeld S. (2004). Genome multiplication of extravillous trophoblast cells in human placenta in the course of differentiation and invasion into endometrium and myometrium. II. Mechanisms of polyploidization. *Tsitologiya;* 46: 640-648

Zybina, E.V., Bogdanova M.S., Stein G.I., Vlasova T.D., Zybina T.G. (2009). Endopolyploidization and the interstitial invasion of the supergiant trophoblast cells of the field vole *Microtus rossiaemeridionalis*. *Tissue and Cell;* 41: 362-366.

12

Injury-Induced DNA Replication and Neural Proliferation in the Adult Mammalian Nervous System

Krzysztof Czaja[1*], Wioletta E. Czaja[2], Maria G. Giacobini-Robecchi[3], Stefano Geuna[3] and Michele Fornaro[3]

[1]*Department of Veterinary and Comparative Anatomy, Pharmacology, and Physiology, College of Veterinary Medicine, Washington State University, Pullman*

[2]*Biochemistry and Biophysics, School of Molecular Biosciences, Washington State University, Pullman*

[3]*Department of Clinical and Biological Sciences, San Luigi Gonzaga School of Medicine, University of Turin*

[1,2]*USA*

[3]*Italy*

1. Introduction

Neurons located in the mammalian central (CNS) and peripheral (PNS) nervous system are, for the most part, a stable post-proliferative population. Indeed, recent evidence indicates that a vast majority of CNS neurons pushed into the cell cycle will die. Thus, understanding the processes of induced DNA replication, neural proliferation and neurogenesis in adult individuals is a major goal of modern neurobiology. Neurogenesis is a process that produces functional neurons from stem/progenitor cells. It is widespread during development, but in the mature mammalian nervous system, under physiological conditions it occurs only in two discrete regions: the subventricular zone of the lateral ventricle (SVZ) and in the subgranular zone (SGZ) of the dentate gyrus (DG) in the hippocampus (Gage 2002; Kempermann et al. 2004). It is believed that in the adult mammalian CNS, neurogenesis outside of these two regions is extremely limited or non-existent. However, some studies of ganglionic nerve centers located outside the CNS revealed DNA replication leading to neural cell division and differentiation into neurons, presenting the possibility of adult neurogenesis in the PNS (Devor and Govrin-Lippmann 1985; Czaja et al. 2008; Silva et al. 2008; Gallaher et al. 2011). In this chapter we will present background knowledge regarding DNA synthesis leading to production of new neurons in the adult mammalian CNS and PNS.

In the CNS, some external factors, such as brain insults, have been reported to trigger adult neurogenesis in regions otherwise considered to be non-neurogenic (Parent 2003). Several studies support the hypothesis of insult-induced neurogenesis in the CNS and show that during development, damage to the adult nervous system induces factors and mechanisms that control neuronal proliferation, migration, differentiation, and connectivity. However, an induction of large-scale neurogenesis that results in addition or replacement of a significant number of neurons has not been reported in adult mammalian brain, although it does occur in some non-mammalian vertebrates. The presence of neural stem cells in the brain offers the potential for neuronal replacement and regeneration after injury. The most broadly-studied is ischemia-induced neurogenesis (Parent et al. 2002). However, the outcome of ischemia-induced neurogenesis is not robust and does not produce large numbers of new neurons. Few of the newborn neurons persist for an extended period of time after the insult, and this population is significantly smaller compared with the substantial increase in proliferating and migrating neuroblasts. There is also little evidence to suggest that those newborn neurons that do survive become functional and integrate into the existing circuitry. On the other hand, the response of the CNS after injury is not limited to the production of neurons. Induced stem cells and neural progenitors may also differentiate into astrocytes and oligodendrocytes. Thus, the increase in CNS progenitor cells in response to injury is not limited to neural progenitors, since glial progenitors increase as well. Radial glia cells function as glia progenitors and provide a cellular source for neurogenesis during development but may also act as neuronal progenitors in the adult CNS by dividing and producing astrocytes and neurons. The aim of this chapter also will be to review the current knowledge related to injury-induced neural proliferation in the CNS.

The situation in the PNS may be significantly different than in the CNS. In the PNS, neural crest cells, which drive the development of many different nerve structures, also may play a role in the post-developmental period. This is because some of the migratory elements persist as a peripheral reserve pool of multipotent stem cells that can undergo a late differentiation into mature glia or neurons (Lagares et al. 2007). The recruitment of this reserve pool may be stimulated by various physiological and pathological conditions in which new cells are needed. We will review the current knowledge regarding neural proliferation in the adult PNS and discuss the possibility that adult neurogenesis is not restricted only to very limited regions of CNS. The alternative to late differentiation of multipotent cells may be the process of dedifferentiation in the PNS. This is the process by which differentiated neural cells revert to a pluripotent or multipotent state. The process of induced reprogramming of cell fate, which is the transforming one cell type into another by exogenous factors, might have enormous potential for medical and research advances. However, this potential of cell fate reprogramming has not been well explored. Therefore, in this chapter we will present the body of knowledge suggesting the possible cellular candidates in the PNS for dedifferentiation after injury. The possibility of induced DNA replication, neural proliferation and adult neurogenesis in the PNS is almost completely unexplored territory. Moreover, the few available studies have resulted in contrasting conclusions. However, the PNS has been reported to utilize neural precursors that proliferate in vitro and can be induced to differentiate into neurons. The possible existence of in vivo damage-induced replacement of neurons destroyed by injury, revealed by several investigators in the CNS, is limited to a few reports in the PNS (Czaja et al. 2008; Gallaher et al. 2011). Therefore, we will review the current literature dealing with DNA synthesis, neural proliferation and neurogenesis in the adult PNS under physiological and pathological conditions, and we will discuss possible mechanisms involved in these phenomena.

The main purpose of this chapter is to highlight the niche for further studies on DNA replication and to direct this powerful and fascinating discipline toward a very exciting but very challenging nervous system. The extremely high need for studies of DNA replication in neural tissue is reflected by Pub Med searches using two different sets of key words. DNA together with synthesis generated about 70,000 hits, while by adding nervous system to this equation we limited the number to about 400. We believe that the conclusion is obvious.

2. Injury to the adult CNS induces neural proliferation: hope for self repair

Despite the fact that neurogenesis was first described in the adult mammalian brain nearly 100 years ago (Allen 1912), adult neurogenesis has been accepted by the scientific community in the last four decades. One year after Ezra Allen's report of neurogenesis in the adult rat brain in 1912, Santiago Ramón y Cajal, arguably the most recognizable name in neuroscience was quoted as saying, "In the adult centers, the nerve paths are something fixed, ended and immutable. Everything may die, nothing may be regenerated." This claim effectively suppressed further investigations of adult neurogenesis for 50 years; until the use of tritiated thymidine by Joseph Altman in the 1960s (Altman 1962; Altman and Das 1965; Altman and Das 1967). Even then, the prevailing belief in the stability of the adult brain was upheld for roughly 30 years after these initial reports. During that time, more and more sensitive techniques were developed to detect cell division (Nowakowski et al. 1989; Nowakowski and Hayes 2001; Wojtowicz and Kee 2006).

Currently, the idea of adult neurogenesis is widely accepted by the scientific community. However, definitive evidence for generation of new and functional neurons in the adult uninjured mammalian CNS has been restricted to the subventricular zone (SVZ) of the lateral ventricle and to the subgranular zone (SGZ) of the dentate gyrus in the hippocampus (Lee and Son 2009; Ehninger and Kempermann 2008; Taupin 2006; Ming and Song 2005; Kempermann et al. 2004; Alvarez-Buylla and Garcia-Verdugo 2002). The discovery of adult neurogenesis has also uncovered the exciting potential for novel approaches to repair the injured brain and spinal cord. Some animals, such as lizards, can regenerate their injured nervous system. The mammalian CNS does not have this capacity; however, it does appear to have a greater regenerative ability than was previously believed. The traditional idea that lineages for neurons and glia become set aside during development has been challenged, and it is now well accepted that progenitors for each cell lineage persist into adulthood (Gage 2000). Moreover, several studies show that neurogenesis is stimulated in the CNS in response to injury (Emery et al. 2003; Parent et al. 2002; Parent and Lowenstein 2002; Parent 2003; Richardson et al. 2007; Shi et al. 2007). Understanding the developmental process and how injury is recapitulating these developmental stages may provide insights into the regenerative capacity of the adult nervous system and speed up the development of strategies to manipulate this neurogenic potential.

Following brain injury, factors that stimulate proliferation of adult neural stem cells and their respective receptors are upregulated (Bambakidis et al. 2005; Yoshimura et al. 2001). Moreover, several studies have suggested that factors and mechanisms regulating neuronal proliferation, migration, differentiation and connectivity during development are reactivated by injury in the adult nervous system (Zhang et al. 2005; Sun et al. 2007). These factors appear to be sufficient to direct neural precursors to migrate toward a lesion area, differentiate into neurons, mature and establish synaptic contacts (Mori et al. 2005; Fricker-Gates et al. 2002). Transition from stem cells to fully differentiated neurons progresses through defined steps, and different classes of neuronal precursors can be distinguished by their morphology, expressed markers, and mitotic activity (Encinas and Enikolopov 2008).

Moreover, several lines of evidence suggest that glia participate in injury-induced neurogenesis, suggesting that they serve as both stem cells and progenitors from which neuroblasts develop (Englund et al. 2005; Gubert et al. 2008; Alonso et al. 2008; Alvarez-Buylla and Lim 2004; Hevner 2006). During CNS development, both the radial glia and astrocytes were reported to undergo proliferation and differentiation toward both the neurons and glia (Costa et al. 2009). Moreover, behaving as post-mitotic cells under physiological conditions, following injury glia may undergo phenotypic and functional changes and dedifferentiate. It has been previously shown that after injury, quiescent astrocytes reveal features of immature stages or phenotypes of stem cells and proliferate (Buffo et al. 2008). These proliferating astrocytes however, undergo symmetric divisions and remain within their cell lineage in vivo, while an altered in vitro environment revealed their self-renewal and multipotency.

Based on the current knowledge, the most probable scenario in post-injury brain repair is recruitment of endogenous progenitors to replace lost neurons. Proliferation of neural progenitors in germinal centers can be induced by delivery of trophic factors, such as FGF-2 (Yoshimura et al. 2003; Yoshimura et al. 2001). Recruitment of endogenous progenitors has also been achieved through release of brain-derived neurotrophic factor (BDNF) and induction of neural differentiation (Chmielnicki et al. 2004; Benraiss et al. 2001). The in vivo induction of massive proliferation, directed migration, and differentiation of neural cells in the forebrain of the adult rat after lesion of the substantia nigra were observed after infusions of transforming growth factor alpha into the forebrain (Fallon et al. 2000). Studies of injury-induced neurogenesis in CNS generate substantial enthusiasm for the recruitment of endogenous progenitors as the therapeutic strategy for CNS repair. However, the successful development of stem cell recruitment therapy depends on the ability to control proliferation, differentiation, and functional integration of induced pluripotent cells. In order to develop therapies that can recruit endogenous progenitors to repair damaged areas of the adult CNS, it is also important to understand how neural environment changes following injury.

While injury-induced neurogenesis in mammals does not lead to complete recovery, we believe it represents the brain's attempt to repair itself. However, in adulthood, CNS has been associated with a very limited regenerative response to injury, compared to embryonic CNS (Fry and Saunders 2000; Nicholls and Saunders 1996; Fawcett 1992). Therefore, an understanding how to induce and control self repair process in the brain to promote recovery from injury or neurodegenerative diseases would be the main challenge in regenerative medicine of the 21st century. Reviewed in subsequent sections of this chapter is recent evidence that after injury, the CNS in adults activates cascades of events and gene expressions that are normally observed during development. We will discuss studies showing that under normal circumstances, damage to the CNS, including stroke and traumatic brain injury (TBI), as well as the experimental use of neurotoxins and other external agents in both the brain and the spinal cord result in an increased cell proliferation and neurogenesis in quiescent regions of the CNS.

2.1 Stroke-induced neural proliferation

Stroke, or cerebrovascular accident, results from the middle cerebral artery occlusion (MCAO) leading to brain infarction, is one of the common causes of death and disability in adulthood. However, improvement of brain functions has been reported following stroke, implying the ability for brain repair (Pascual-Leone et al. 2005). One means by which repair might be achieved is neurogenesis, which occurs in the normal adult brain, and is increased in animal models of brain injury including stroke (Katakowski et al. 2007; Jin et al. 2006; Zhang et al. 2004). Post-stroke neurogenesis is associated with migration of newborn neurons from neurogenic niches to injured regions of the brain (Arvidsson et al. 2002). Neuronal precursors proliferate in the SVZ, and newly formed neurons migrate into the ischemic lesions and differentiate to acquire the phenotype of the neurons which were lost. However, the outcome of ischemia-induced neurogenesis is not robust and does not produce large numbers of new neurons. Few of the newborn neurons survive for an extended period of time after the insult, and this population is significantly smaller when compared to the population of migrating neuroblasts. There is also little evidence to suggest that those newborn neurons that do survive become functional and integrate into the CNS circuitry.

On the other hand, the response of the CNS after injury is not limited to the production of neurons. Induced pluripotent cells may also differentiate into glia. Radial glia function as progenitors and provide a cellular source for neurogenesis during development and may also behave as neural progenitors in the adult CNS by proliferating and generating astrocytes and neurons. Stroke induced by MCAO in adult rodents triggers increased neurogenesis in the SGZ and SVZ (Abrahams et al. 2004; Jin et al. 2006; Katakowski et al. 2007; Liu et al. 2007). The SVZ neuroblasts migrate into the damaged striatal areas and adopt the phenotypes of the projection neurons. Previously published studies show that stroke increases the production of neuroblasts in the SVZ, which express doublecortin and polysialylated neural cell adhesion molecule (Arvidsson et al. 2002; Parent et al. 2002); however, few cells survive to become functional neurons, and this percentage is low compared with the substantial increase in proliferating and migrating neuroblasts (Arvidsson et al. 2002; Parent et al. 2002). It has been also shown that after MCAO, the population of BrdU-positive cells increases in the SVZ, reaching the maximum around a week after ischemia (Arvidsson et al. 2002; Parent et al. 2002). Next, the population of doublecortin-expressing neuroblasts migrates outside the SVZ, as observed during their normal migration along the rostral migratory stream. Stroke-activated neuroblasts may also migrate into the injured striatum (Arvidsson et al. 2002; Parent et al. 2002). These cells become striatal projection neurons and express calbindin, markers of striatal medium spiny neurons (Arvidsson et al. 2002; Parent et al. 2002). Several studies show that cortical lesions produced by MCAO, significantly increase SVZ cell proliferation (Ohab et al. 2006; Gotts and Chesselet 2005). After MCAO cell proliferation also increases in the SGZ, even though this area is not directly affected by the stroke, resulting in the production of new neurons in granular zone of the dentate gyrus (Jin et al. 2001). Together, these studies indicate that mitotically active cells, and not mature cells proliferating in response to injury, comprise the majority of proliferating populations after brain ischemia (Jin et al. 2001).

2.2 Traumatic brain injury and neural plasticity

Traumatic brain injury (TBI) is the most common brain injury in humans (Graham et al. 2000). After such injuries, the brain shows a remarkable ability for functional recovery (Nakabayashi et al. 2007). While, mechanisms responsible for this recovery are mostly unknown, the vast majority of neuroscientists hypothesize that synaptic plasticity is responsible for adaptive changes in the CNS following the injury (Zhang et al. 2011; Falo et al. 2008; Scheff et al. 2005). In the last decades, there has been increasing interest in the ability to provide a continuous renewal of neurons in the adult CNS. This increased interest popularized the alternative mechanism for a recovery following TBI: the injury-induced neurogenesis. In CNS injury in general and TBI in particular, there is little data to suggest how damage to the nervous system may induce the proliferating population to differentiate into functional neurons. The neural environment changes associated with CNS injury are initially related to excitotoxicity associated with glutamate release (Hinzman et al. 2010; Gong et al. 1999; Globus et al. 1995). This is followed by an intense inflammatory response due to activated microglia, macrophages and trophic factors (Khuman et al. 2011; Hellewell et al. 2010). Secondary neuronal damage involves delayed cell death by apoptosis (Kim et al. 2010; Dressler and Vemuganti 2009), and then astrocytes form a scar that acts as a barrier to axonal regrowth.

While processes of synaptic plasticity have been well documented over the last decades, very few experiments have directly addressed the role of newly generated cells in the post-TBI remodeling of the CNS. To test this hypothesis, several groups studied the effects of experimental TBI on hippocampal neurogenesis (Emery et al. 2005; Lu et al. 2011; Kernie and Parent 2010). They detected significant increase in the number of dividing cells in dentate gyrus. Moreover, a significant increase in the number of new cells expressing neuronal markers after appropriate maturation periods has been reported (Sun et al. 2007; Sun et al. 2005). This fact suggests that injury-induced DNA replication and cell proliferation in the adult CNS is primarily neurogenic.

2.3 Neural proliferation after spinal cord and brainstem injury

Spinal cord injury research has greatly expanded in recent years. However, understanding of the mechanisms triggering the functional recovery following the neuronal damage is still incomplete. After spinal cord injury (SCI), tissue damage occurs at the impact site and spreads over time (Tederko et al. 2009). This lesion is accompanied by apoptosis of oligodendrocytes and loss of myelin around surviving axons (Wu and Ren 2009). Axonal demyelinization typically peaks during the few days after injury (Wu and Ren 2009; Salehi et al. 2009). Remyelinization by oligodendrocytes and Schwann cells usually begins by a few weeks after damage to the spinal cord (Sasaki et al. 2007; Dasari et al. 2007). Several studies, however, suggest that mature oligodendrocytes do not proliferate in response to trauma (Keirstead and Blakemore 1997; Amat et al. 1998; Redwine and Armstrong 1998). However, more recent studies show that neurogenesis can be induced in the spinal cord following specific types of injury. A substantial gliosis was previously reported in the lesion area, which resulted in the formation of a glial scar (Fitch and Silver 2008). However, generation of new and functional neurons was not observed after hemisection or lesion of dorsal column (Vessal et al. 2007; Yang et al. 2006). They revealed significant gliogenesis and reported that new born oligodendrocytes remyelinated host axons in the injury site. Therefore, new born glia may contribute to the neural repair following the damage to the spinal cord.

Studies of neural proliferation in the adult brainstem revealed that production of new neurons occurs in vivo within the dorsal vagal complex (DVC) in adult rats (Bauer et al. 2005). They detected within the DVC newly generated BrdU-positive cells which simultaneously expressed markers of immature and mature neurons (DCX, HuC/D, TUC-4, NeuN). It has been also reported that vagotomy (DVC deafferentation) triggered a large increase of BrdU incorporation in the ipsilateral DVC, associated with proliferation of microglia and genesis of neurons and astrocytes (Bauer et al. 2005). Injury-induced plasticity, neural proliferation and neuronal replacement were recently revealed after damage to pre-Bötzinger Complex, a cluster of interneurons in the ventrolateral medulla of the brainstem (Neumueller et al. 2011). Neuronal counts and evaluation of neuronal density revealed up to 65% more neurons within the ventral and lateral medulla compared to control animals. Concluding studies dealing with neural proliferation in the brainstem we can hypothesize that injury activates plasticity and reorganization of brainstem circuits, late differentiation and even neurogenesis. However, more rigorous studies are necessary to definitely prove injury-induced neurogenesis in the adult brainstem.

3. Neural proliferation in the adult PNS: challenging the dogma

Whereas in the CNS the occurrence of DNA replication and neural proliferation in adult mammals has been broadly accepted from the end of the twentieth century (Johansson et al. 1999), in the PNS it was already documented, or at least hypothesized much earlier. The occurrence of adult neurogenesis in the PNS was suggested by Hatai several decades earlier (Hatai 1902). He reported an increase in sensory neuron counts in DRGs from one-month to five-month-old rats. Later, Miura provided the first evidence of an increase in neuron numbers in the autonomic nervous system, namely in Auerbach's plexus of the rat small intestine (Miura 1913). A conformation of the possibility that neurogenesis occurs in the autonomic nervous system was later provided by Benninghoff, who showed that partial stenosis of rat small intestine induced, in the upstream intestinal loops, an increase in Auerbach's plexus ganglion neuron numbers (Benninghoff 1951). Moreover, Filogamo and coworkers demonstrated that in the same experimental model, neurogenesis led to a fourfold increase in the number of Auerbach's plexus ganglion neurons of the loops upstream from the intestinal obstruction (Filogamo and Vigliani 1954). Yet, the occurrence of adult neurogenesis was revealed in other sites of the autonomic nervous system including DRGs in the rat (Devor and Govrin-Lippmann 1985; Devor 1991; Popken and Farel 1997). Studies of neural proliferation in the adult PNS were previously reviewed by Geuna (Geuna et al. 2002).

It should be pointed out that the above-mentioned studies, that were based on neuron counts led authors to the conclusion that, since there was no evidence of mitosis by nerve cells detectable by colchicine blocking, the observed increase in neuron number should be attributed to the persistence of poorly differentiated or undifferentiated cells capable of turning into neurons during adulthood and/or under the influence of exceptional stimuli. The introduction of the techniques for investigating DNA replication, especially 3H-thymidine (and afterwards BrdU) administration, cytophotometry/cytofluorimetry and S-phase markers (e.g. PCNA and Ki67), opened new horizons for interpreting the adult neuron addition. In a series of studies, Giacobini-Robecchi and coworkers showed the presence of DNA replication (by autoradiography after 3H-thymidine administration and PCNA immuno-staining) in myenteric neurons from the small intestine loops upstream from a partial stenosis (Corvetti et al. 2001; Poncino et al. 1990; Giacobini Robecchi et al. 1988). However, cytophotometry after Feulgen staining showed that myenteric neuron DNA replication might not be due to a tetraploid DNA content related to cell division, but instead to unscheduled DNA synthesis that leads to a hyper diploid DNA content (Poncino et al. 1990; Giacobini Robecchi et al. 1988). Electrophoretic analysis of total genomic DNA has also suggested that unscheduled DNA synthesis can be due to DNA amplification (Giacobini Robecchi et al. 1995).

The evidence of DNA replication in the adult sensory ganglia has been also provided in Ciaroni's and Czaja's laboratories (Cecchini et al. 1995; Ciaroni et al. 2000; Czaja et al. 2008; Gallaher et al. 2011; Ryu et al. 2010). However, it should be noted that the occurrence of adult neurogenesis in the PNS has been questioned by several experimental studies that failed to confirm the numerical increase of adult neurons in both the myenteric plexus (Gabella 1984) and DRGs (La Forte et al. 1991; Pover et al. 1994; Bergman and Ulfhake 1998). In this view, cell counting has raised a lively debate over the last years in the neuroscience field, and it appears that in many cases the discrepancy in the results might be due to bias in the counting methods used (Popken and Farel 1997; Geuna 2005). Studies based on unbiased stereological neuronal counts have confirmed again the occurrence of neuron number increases in adult sensory ganglia (Lagares et al. 2007), thus raising a question about the origin of the new neurons. Two possibilities have been tentatively proposed to explain the increase in the number of neurons during adulthood: 1) de novo neurogenesis (i.e., based on DNA replication and cell division); 2) neuron addition (i.e., late differentiation of poorly differentiated neuronal precursors without cell division) (Farel 2001; Farel 2002; Geuna et al. 2000). Although the detection of DNA replication (Ciaroni et al. 2000; Farel 2001; Farel 2002; Geuna et al. 2000; Giacobini Robecchi et al. 1988) is considered a predictor of cell division and thus de novo neurogenesis, it might also be due to selective amplification of a few DNA sequences (Corvetti et al. 2001; Giacobini Robecchi et al. 1995). On the other hand, the possibility that the neuron number increase is due to the late differentiation of slightly immature neurons is partially ruled out by the difficulty in identifying (even with careful electron microscope investigation) the immature neurons in adult DRGs (Geuna, unpublished). Therefore, a third tentative explanation, which falls between the other two options, is being sought, namely the possibility that a neuronal precursor niche from neural crest origin persists all along adulthood in the PNS (Gallaher et al. 2011; Lagares et al. 2007). Although, sensory ganglia have been reported to contain precursor cells (Arora et al. 2007; Lagares et al. 2007; Li et al. 2007) that can proliferate in vitro and can be induced to differentiate into neurons (Liu et al. 2009; Namaka et al. 2001), the possibility of in vivo adult neurogenesis in the adult PNS is almost completely unexplored. Moreover, the few published studies have resulted in contradictory conclusions. For example, age-related increases in the number of dorsal root ganglia (DRG) neurons have been reported in rat by two groups (Popken and Farel 1997; Ciaroni et al. 2000), while other investigators have provided data suggesting that adult neurogenesis does not occur in the adult DRG (Pover et al. 1994; Mohammed and Santer 2001). Thus, there is as yet no consensus regarding the neurogenic potential of the adult PNS sensory ganglia.

3.1 Injury-induced neurogenesis in sensory ganglia

A strong evidence for the potential of PNS cells to produce new neurons arises from Czaja's laboratory. They have examined the sequels to toxin-induced neuronal destruction. Thus, evidence of neuronal replacement following lesions, which has been reported by several investigators in CNS models, (Hou et al. 2008; Lie et al. 2004; Parent 2003), is limited to our recent reports for the PNS (Czaja et al. 2008; Gallaher et al. 2011). Our key observation is that neuronal losses following capsaicin-induced neuronal destruction are not permanent. In fact, following a precipitous post-capsaicin decline, the numbers of neuronal nuclei in nodose ganglion (NG) from capsaicin-treated rats equaled or exceeded the numbers found in control rats by 60 days after capsaicin treatment. Furthermore, we observed that restoration of neuronal numbers after capsaicin was accompanied by BrdU incorporation, which ultimately labeled mature neurons (Czaja et al. 2008). Our observation of apparent neuronal number restoration in NG led us to hypothesize that damage to the primary sensory neurons induces proliferation of endogenous progenitors and/or lineage reprogramming and generation of induced multipotent stem cells (iMSCs), which differentiate into new neurons. The satellite cell population housed in DRG or NG may, under adequate conditions, represent a source of multipotent cells for the new neurons (Li et al. 2007; Singh et al. 2009; Gallaher et al. 2011). Moreover, morphological observations have recently provided further support to this hypothesis and revealed that NG cultures from capsaicin-treated rats contained bipolar neurons, normally found only during development (Gallaher et al. 2011). Furthermore, we observed that restoration of neuronal numbers after capsaicin was accompanied by BrdU incorporation that ultimately labeled mature neurons (Czaja et al. 2008; Gallaher et al. 2011). Our observation of apparent restoration of neuronal numbers in NG led us to hypothesize that damage to the primary sensory neurons induces proliferation of endogenous progenitors and/or lineage reprogramming and generation of induced multipotent stem cells (iMSCs) which differentiate into new neurons. The existence of ganglionic MSCs would suggest that PNS could serve as a source of committed autologous cells that are capable of being stimulated to produce neurons in vivo, thus avoiding an immune rejection. The discovery of neural progenitors and mechanisms involved in the induced neurogenesis in the adult PNS could enable autologous grafting of new neurons into damaged areas of the CNS to replace neurons lost due to injury or disease.

4. Mechanisms involved in post-injury DNA replication and cell proliferation

In the brain, new neurons are formed from neural stem cells (NSCs), which are multipotent and self renewing. Neural stem cells can undergo symmetric or non-neurogenic divisions that produce two neuro-epithelial stem cells and cause horizontal expansion of the proliferative population (Gotz and Huttner 2005). Alternatively, they engage in asymmetric divisions that are associated with the generation of neuronal progenitors (Falk et al. 2008). The DNA synthesis and proliferation of NSCs are critical processes which regulate the size and neurogenic potential of the nervous system. Multiple signaling pathways have been implicated in the regulation of neural stem and progenitor-cell proliferation (Riccio 2010; Suh et al. 2009). Signalling pathways controlling NSCs niche and signaling after brain injury, outside NSCs niche share a significant overlap converging on two canonical pathways, mammalian target of rapamycin (mTOR) and mitogen-activated protein kinase (MAPK) (Robel et al. 2011).

One of the key pathways regulating cell proliferation in the nervous system is WNT (wingless-type MMTV integration site family)/ β-catenin signaling (Wexler et al. 2009) WNT signaling regulates neural plasticity during development and in the adult nervous system. During development, β-catenin signaling regulates proliferation of neuronal stem cells, leading to the correct number of neurons in the developing embryo. WNT also regulates proliferation and preserves pluripotent and multipotent state of NSC and neural progenitors in the adult brain by keeping them in a dividing stage that prevents differentiation (White et al. 2010). WNT signaling operates through autocrine signaling loop among NSCs. NSCs express WNTs ligands and WNT receptor (Wexler et al. 2009).WNTs are glycoprotein morphogens that interact with G-protein-coupled receptors and initiate different signaling pathways, including the canonical pathway involving β-catenin. Binding of WNT to the receptor triggers the β-catenin-LEF/TCF signal transduction and activation of a WNT responsive target gene, such as cycline D1, which promotes cellular proliferation. Over-expression of WNTs or persistent activation of the downstream signaling component b-catenin in the CNS promotes cell-cycle progression and negatively regulates cell-cycle exit, resulting in horizontal expansion of precursor populations (Chenn and Walsh 2002).

4.1 Immune system and regulation of neurogenesis

Brain injury induces an excess of factors that modulate plasticity of various cells and induce neurogenic potential within damaged tissue. Several lines of evidence indicate that various components of the immune system may positively regulate neurogenic processes (Yirmiya and Goshen 2011; Ziv and Schwartz 2008) . Brain damage activates microglia, which rapidly migrate to the injury site and initiate recruitment and activation of macrophages and lymphocytes. These cells release a number of anti- and pro-inflammatory factors creating a positive feedback loop that results in neural damage and causes both detrimental and positive consequences to neurogenesis. It has been demonstrated that upon severe injuries such as hypoxia or stroke, a portion of microglia proliferate. Furthermore, microglia also reveal in vitro stem cell potential with self-renewal and multipotency (Robel et al. 2011).

Several in vitro and in vivo studies have demonstrated that lymphocytes, specifically T cells may promote neurogenesis. T-cells derived cytokines IL-4 or INF-γ activate microglia cells (Ziv and Schwartz 2008). Interestingly, WNT- and β-catenin signal increases in adult proliferating astrocytes and in NG2 glia after traumatic brain injury, suggesting that WNT signaling plays a role in the control of gliogenesis following cortical injury (White et al. 2010). Growth factors including FGF2, EGF and VEGF are released by various cell types after brain injury and activate mTOR or mitogen-activated protein kinase (MAP) pathways. These growth factors also activate ERK and Jun N-terminal kinase (JNK)-dependent MAPK pathways in astrocytes after injury. These signaling pathways act synergistically to phosphorylate the immediate early gene products c-FOS and c-JUN which increase proliferation of astrocytes. Phosphorylation of ERK is specifically detected in reactive astrocytes after injury (Robel et al. 2011).

The activated microglia seemed to exert the neurogenic effect via expression of the anti-inflammatory/neuroprotective cytokine transforming growth factor-beta (TGF-β1), which has a (concentration-dependent) neurogenic effect by acting on the proliferation of neural progenitors (Battista et al. 2006; Ziv and Schwartz 2008). TGF-β1 decreases the expansion of neural stem and precursor cells in a dose-dependent manner (Aigner and Bogdahn 2008). While WNT positively controls expansion of neural stem and progenitor pools, transforming growth factor β (TGF-β) upregulates cell cycle inhibitors and counteracts cell cycle progression. Therefore TGF-β signaling controls the size of specific brain areas by antagonizing canonical WNT signaling and negatively regulating self-renewal of neuroepithelial stem cells. TGF-β has been associated with neuronal differentiation and survival in CNS under physiological conditions (Falk et al. 2008). Post-injury cell renewal, such as precursor cell proliferation in CNS, is positively regulated by microglia-derived TGF-β (Ziv and Schwartz 2008). Three isoforms of TGF-β (TGF-β 1, 2, 3) are expressed in neurons and in glia cells. TGF-β1 isoform is predominantly upregulated and activated after CNS lesions or, in cases of neurodegeneration, TGF-β signals through activation of TGF-β receptor type I and II (Tgfbr1 and Tgfbr2) and phosphorylation of the signaling mediators Smad2 and Smad3 (Aigner and Bogdahn 2008). TGF-β not only activates the Smad signaling

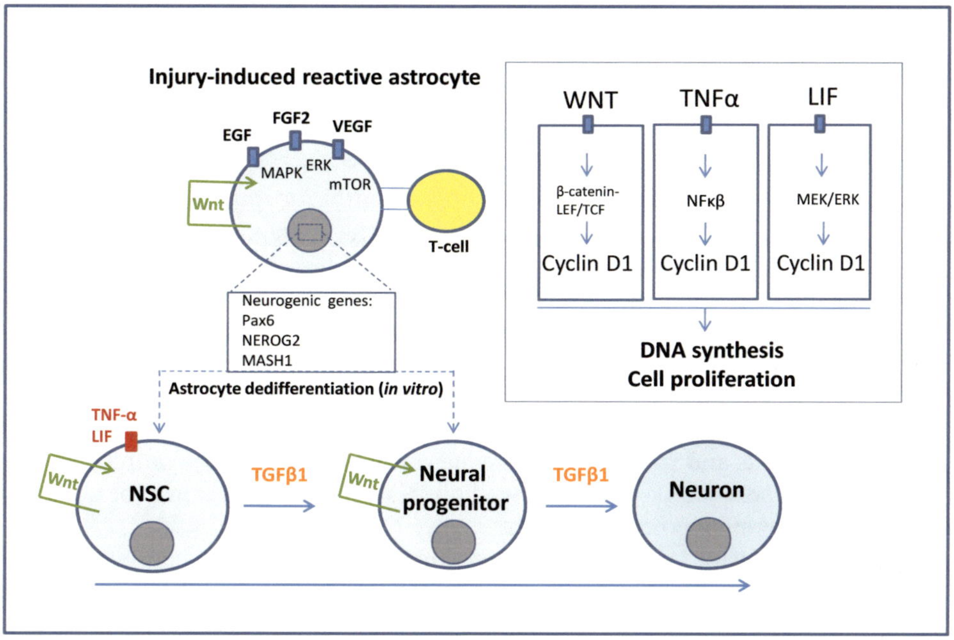

Fig. 1. Mechanism involved in post-injury cell proliferation in CNS

Injury to the brain triggers complex responses between populations of immune cells (yellow circle), microglia, neural stem cells (NSC), neural progenitors and differentiated neurons (all shown as blue circle). The NSC and neural progenitors represent the main precursors of neurons. Two antagonistic signalling pathways WNT and TGF-β regulate proliferation and differentiation in adult neurogenesis. While WNT positively control expansion of neural stem and progenitor pools, TGF-β counteracts cell cycle progression and is associated with neuronal differentiation and survival in CNS. Injury-activated microglia emerges as a new potential source of NSC and neural progenitors. T-cells may promote neurogenesis by interacting with microglia. T-cells derived cytokines (IL-4 or INF-γ) activate microglia cells. The activated microglia seemed to exert the neurogenic effect via expression of the anti-inflammatory/neuroprotective cytokine TGF-β1. Growth factors including FGF2, EGF and VEGF are released by various cell types after injury, bind to receptors (blue bars) expressed at the surface of activated microglia cells and initiate intracellular signal transduction and activate mTOR, ERK and MAPK pathways in astrocytes. These signalling pathways act synergistically to increase proliferation of astrocytes and they are also involved in up regulation of the neurogenic genes (Pax6, NEROG2, MASH1). WNT- and β-catenin signalling also increases in adult proliferating astrocytes after traumatic brain injury. Glia cells were successfully reprogrammed to NSC or neural progenitors in vitro by induced over expression of neurogenic genes. Adult, injury-induced cellular proliferation during neurogenesis is regulated by cytokines (TNF-α, LIF) and morphogens WNTs. Signalling from these molecules has a common target, cycline-D1 which triggers cell cycle entry and DNA synthesis.

pathway, but it may diverge into and modulate other known classical signaling cascades such as RAS/ERK/MAPK. Activation of RAS/ERK/MAPK signaling by TGF-β can induce an autocrine amplification loop of TGF-β1 expression. It has been reported that adult rat dorsal root ganglion (DRG) neurons after injury are able to synthesize TGF β-1 isoform, which is able to elicit Schwann cell proliferation and modulates regeneration processes in the PNS (Rogister et al. 1993).

Immune responses modulate the NSCs. Proliferation of NSCs is regulated by cytokines and immuno-modulating polypeptides (Gonzalez-Perez 2010). TNF-α is one of the crucial inflammation mediators. In the CNS, TNF-α binds to TNF receptors expressed by glia cells and neurons. Pro-inflammatory cytokine TNF-α has been associated with the pro-neurogenic role by increasing proliferation of NSCs through activation of NFκB and TGF-β activated kinase-1 (TAK-1) signaling cascade. NFκB transcriptionally regulates cyclin-D1 in NSCs (Fig.1). The cyclin-D1/CDK4-complex is necessary for NSC cell cycle progression by promoting passage through G1/S restriction point (Widera et al. 2006). Injury to the peripheral nervous system results in the upregulation of TNF-α. TNF-α is released from neurons, Schwann cells and proliferating satellite cells in DRG. The role of the TNF-α in the injury of peripheral nervous system is not well understood; however it may be an important inducer of the proliferative potential of cells.

Leukemia inhibitory factor (LIF) is another cytokine that displays pro-neurogenic effects in the injured adult brain. LIF has been demonstrated as a key signal for injury-induced neurogenesis in adult mouse olfactory epithelium (Bauer and Patterson 2006). LIF appears to promote NSC self-renewal and expansion. LIF stimulates the initiation of DNA synthesis and cell division through a common signaling mechanism that involves MEK/ERK activation as well as STAT1 cytoplasmic nuclear translocation. LIF acts on NSC and maintains them in a loop of symmetric/self-renewing divisions in vivo (Bauer and Patterson 2006). LIF stimulates DNA synthesis through MEK/ERK; this is a direct mechanistic molecular link between tissue damage inflammation and tissue renewal. The ERK cascade is activated by hormones, cytokines, and growth factors that result in either proliferation or growth arrest, depending on the duration and intensity of the ERK activation. This pathway, consisting of Raf, MEK1/2, and ERK1/2, regulates cell proliferation via its impact on cell cycle control. Activation of this mitogen-activated protein kinase pathway promotes the expression of cyclin-D1. These key events result in the activation of the cyclin-dependent protein kinase CDK4/6, which promote cell cycle entry by phosphorylation of the retinoblastoma tumor suppressor (Rb), leading to the release of the transcription factor E2F. This in turn promotes the transcription of cyclins A and E, resulting in the activation of CDK2. Activated CDK2 phosphorylates Rb at additional sites and, thus, enables DNA synthesis and centrosome duplication via further liberation of E2F. Furthermore, sustained expression of p21cip1 has been shown to be responsible for the ERK-mediated proliferation inhibition (Ussar and Voss 2004).

4.2 Mechanisms involved in the neurogenic potential of glia

Brain studies provide increasing evidence that adult glia could be a source of new neurons (Robel et al. 2011). Glia in the adult brain may act as neural progenitors and neural stem cells. Following lesion-induced reactivation, astrocytes dedifferentiate to astrocyte-like stem cells. Several studies suggest that the WNT/β-catenin pathway may be involved in the dedifferentiation process following injury. Interestingly, injury-induced WNT/b-catenin signaling has already been shown to be required for the dedifferention of other cells such as epithelial cells to form hair follicles and Mueller glia to form retinal cells (Osakada et al. 2007). Remarkably, WNT signaling has been associated with peripheral nerve injury. Peripheral nerve lesions induce upregulation of the WNT signaling mediator Ryk on DRG neurons, which may potentially indicate a role of WNT in neuroregeneration and/or neurogenesis (Li et al. 2008).

Pax6 neurogenic transcription factor plays a crucial role in neurogenesis, both during development and in adulthood. It is expressed by NSC. Astrocytes forced to express Pax6 acquired neuronal morphology. PAX6 and other neurogenic factors such as NEUROG2, MASH1 signaling can cause a true glia-to-neuron conversion in vitro. NEUROG2 is epigenetically silenced in postnatal astrocytes. Upregulation of neurogenic genes could be induced following injury in proliferating reactive astrocytes, which would acquire potential to dedifferentiate and be reprogrammed to neurons (Robel et al. 2011). Given that the retroviral vectors used in these studies incorporate only in proliferating cells and that neurons are post mitotic, it seems that the origin of these new neurons is the glia whose proliferation is enhanced after injury. Interestingly, some signals promoting astrocytes dedifferentiation may derive from injured astrocytes themselves, as suggested by scratch wound-injured rat spinal cord astrocytes (Robel et al. 2011).

Sox2 is a member of the SRY-related group of transcription factors that plays a significant role during neural cell development. Sox2 maintains the pluripotency and developmental potential of neural stem cells (Li et al. 1998). It has been shown that expression of Sox2 and the transcription factors Oct4, c-Myc and Klf4 is sufficient to reprogram adult fibroblasts to generate pluripotent stem cells (Chang et al. 2010; Park et al. 2008). The constitutive expression of Sox2 has been shown to inhibit neuronal differentiation, while suppression of Sox2 leads to cell cycle exit and neuronal differentiation (Graham et al. 2003). Sox2 expression is also upregulated following injury to the peripheral nerves. It has been shown that Sox2 expression was elevated in glia cells in Krox20 knockout mice (Le et al. 2005). These results indicate that Sox2 is suppressed, either directly or indirectly, by Krox20. Krox20 and Sox2, like Krox20 and c-Jun, inhibit each other. It has been suggested that c-Jun controls Sox2 levels and that some of the inhibitory effects of c-Jun are channeled by Sox2 (Parkinson et al. 2008). Other studies indicate that Sox2 acts downstream of Notch (Woodhoo et al. 2009). Sox2 expression is essential to specify glia cell fate from neural crest cells.

4.3 The molecular events involved in damage-induced DNA replication and cellular proliferation in PNS

The neurogenic potential of PNS has been recently reported (Gallaher et al. 2011). Formation of new neurons in the adult NG was followed by capsaicin-induced neuronal damage and cell death via apoptosis. Cell proliferation was detected by BrdU incorporation during DNA synthesis, which is a standard marker of dividing cells. The molecular events involved in damage-induced DNA replication and cellular proliferation in PNS are not well understood. However, by analogy to damage-induced neurogenesis in CNS, components of the immune system may play important regulatory roles. This will be under stress and tissue damage condition where components of immune system such as pro-inflammatory cytokines may play a role of molecular triggers affecting cell cycle of differentiated neurons.

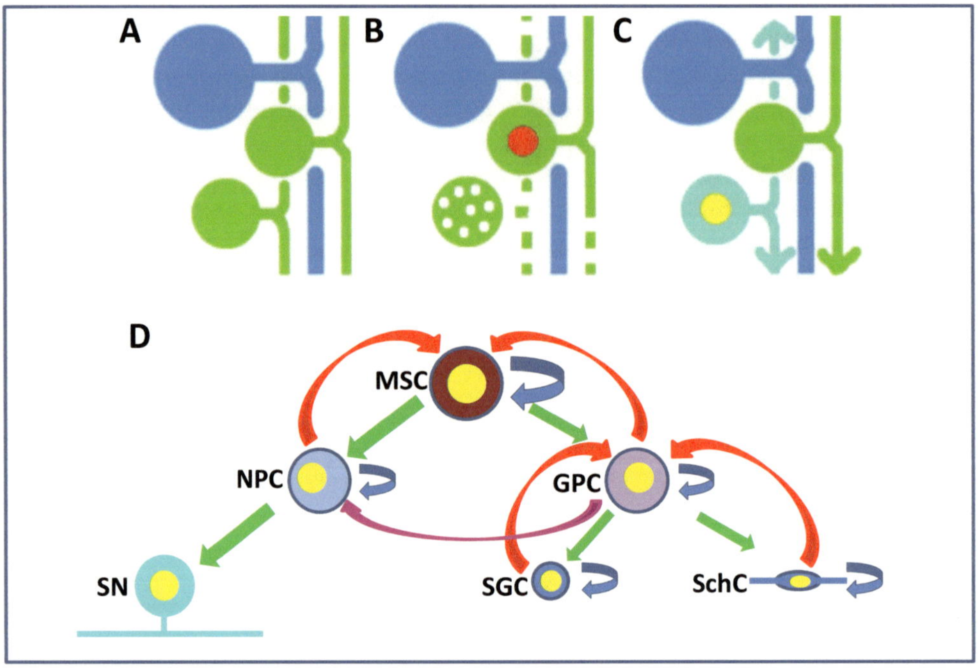

Fig. 2. Post-injury degeneration and regeneration in sensory ganglia

The adult sensory ganglia comprises TRPV-1 expressing (A: green) and non-TRPV-1 expressing neurons (A: blue). Following injury, many neurons will completely degenerate (B: cell body with fragmented nucleus) while others only lose peripheral projections (B: red nucleus). Injury to the NG and loss of neurons will result in the active response from neurons, glia and immune system through upregulation of various cytokines, growth factors and morphogens. These factors may induce DNA synthesis revealed by BrdU incorporation (C, D: yellow) and cell proliferation (D: blue arrows). This cascade of events may change the ganglionic environment and induce dedifferentiation (D: red arrows) of satellite glia cells (SGC), Schwann cells (SchC), glia progenitors (GPC) and neuronal progenitors (NPC) to less-differentiated stage within their own lineage. Dedifferentiated cells may next differentiate (D: green arrows) or transdifferentiate (D: purple arrow) to switch the cell lineage. The mechanisms of differentiation, dedifferentiation and transdifferentiation may be responsible for injury-induced neuronal replacement and generation of sensory neurons (SN) in the ganglia.

It has been well known that adult sensory ganglia are composed of terminally differentiated neurons and glia cells. However, recent studies show that the pool of immature glial precursor cells could be present in the adult sensory ganglia (Gallaher et al. 2011; Lagares et al. 2007). Injury to sensory ganglia triggers an inflammatory response and bursts of pro-inflammatory cytokines, growth factors, and morphogens, which are known to exert their effects through common signaling pathways and modulate neuronal plasticity. Specifically, TNF-α, TGF-β, and WNT have been activated after a peripheral nerve lesion (Li et al. 2008;

Saade et al. 2002). The MAP Kinases pathway (MAPK/ERK/p38) also has been reported to activate in peripheral nerve injury (Agthong et al. 2006). In the sensory ganglia injury initially damages peripheral axons and depending on the damaging factor, some neurons will die and some will survive and regenerate (Fig. 2A-C). Moreover, the cascade of degenerative events may induce molecular signaling triggering proliferation, differentiation and dedifferentiation of ganglion cells, which provide a source of neural progenitors or induced multipotent cells for new neurons (Fig. 2D).

The identity and function of differentiated, post-mitotic cell is no longer a permanent feature. Studies of the last decade suggest that cell identity is determined by transcriptional and/or epigenetic actions and, more importantly, that it is subject to reprogramming by resetting intrinsic programs (Vogel 2010). The ability of a cell to dedifferentiate to a pluripotent state is critically dependent on the ability of that cell to re-enter cell cycle and replicate its genome. The molecular forces triggering change in cellular identity are not well understood. Injury may trigger programs of regeneration, which may involve changes in cell plasticity and identity. This principle may underline the injury-induced plasticity, lineage reprogramming and neurogenesis in the adult PNS. Therefore, studies of injury-induced neurogenesis in the context of neural plasticity will provide new insights into the complexity of DNA replication and cellular identity at the tissue level.

5. Conclusion

The review of the current literature dealing with DNA synthesis, neural proliferation and neurogenesis in the adult nervous system challenges Cajal's dogma that "In the adult centers, the nerve paths are something fixed, ended and immutable. Everything may die, nothing may be regenerated." Moreover, more and more studies show that brain is not the only place in the adult nervous system where new neurons could be generated. The mammalian CNS and PNS appear to have a greater regenerative ability than was previously believed. The factors that regulate proliferation and differentiation in the uninjured adult brain may contribute to increased DNA synthesis and proliferation after injury. In the adult nervous system, development is complete or near complete and new cells are not in high demand. After injury, however, the need and ability for production of new cells in the adult brain radically increases. This demand may recapitulate developmental mechanisms in the injured adult nervous system. Thus, factors that influence NSCs during development may be more likely to contribute to injury-induced neurogenesis than factors regulating NSCs in the uninjured adult brain. Recent advances in regenerative research show that injury may induce cascade of events forcing the pool of endogenous multipotent cells to enter the cell cycle and differentiate toward glia or neurons. What is even more exciting, recent studies strongly support the hypothesis that terminally differentiated cells can be stimulated to go back to less-differentiated stage within their own lineage (dedifferentiation) in response to injury. Dedifferentiation may even go a step further and regress to a point where neural cells may switch lineage (transdifferentiation). However, further studies are necessary to determine the specific intrinsic and micro environmental cues that drive the injured nervous system for adult neurogenesis. Harnessing the mechanisms involved in the induced neurogenesis in the adult nervous system could enable neural replacement therapy as a new approach in the regenerative medicine.

6. Acknowledgments

This research was supported by WSU Startup Funds and George W. Bagby Research Fund. Authors would like to thank Jeanne Jensen for being always ready to "Polish my English"

7. References

Abrahams JM, Gokhan S, Flamm ES, Mehler MF (2004) De novo neurogenesis and acute stroke: are exogenous stem cells really necessary? Neurosurgery 54:150-155

Agthong S, Kaewsema A, Tanomsridejchai N, Chentanez V (2006) Activation of MAPK ERK in peripheral nerve after injury. BMC Neurosci 7:45

Aigner L, Bogdahn U (2008) TGF-beta in neural stem cells and in tumors of the central nervous system. Cell Tissue Res 331:225-241

Allen E (1912) The cessation of mitosis in the central nervous system of the albino rat. J Comp Neurol 22:547-568

Alonso M, Ortega-Perez I, Grubb MS, Bourgeois JP, Charneau P, Lledo PM (2008) Turning astrocytes from the rostral migratory stream into neurons: a role for the olfactory sensory organ. J Neurosci 28:11089-11102

Altman J (1962) Are new neurons formed in the brains of adult mammals? Science 135:1127-1128

Altman J, Das GD (1965) Autoradiographic and histological evidence of postnatal hippocampal neurogenesis in rats. J Comp Neurol 124:319-335

Altman J, Das GD (1967) Postnatal neurogenesis in the guinea-pig. Nature 214:1098-1101

Alvarez-Buylla A, Garcia-Verdugo JM (2002) Neurogenesis in adult subventricular zone. J Neurosci 22:629-634

Alvarez-Buylla A, Lim DA (2004) For the long run: maintaining germinal niches in the adult brain. Neuron 41:683-686

Amat JA, Farooq M, Ishiguro H, Norton WT (1998) Cells of the oligodendrocyte lineage proliferate following cortical stab wounds: an in vitro analysis. Glia 22:64-71

Arora DK, Cosgrave AS, Howard MR, Bubb V, Quinn JP, Thippeswamy T (2007) Evidence of postnatal neurogenesis in dorsal root ganglion: role of nitric oxide and neuronal restrictive silencer transcription factor. J Mol Neurosci 32:97-107

Arvidsson A, Collin T, Kirik D, Kokaia Z, Lindvall O (2002) Neuronal replacement from endogenous precursors in the adult brain after stroke. Nat Med 8:963-970

Bambakidis NC, Theodore N, Nakaji P, Harvey A, Sonntag VK, Preul MC, Miller RH (2005) Endogenous stem cell proliferation after central nervous system injury: alternative therapeutic options. Neurosurg Focus 19:E1

Battista D, Ferrari CC, Gage FH, Pitossi FJ (2006) Neurogenic niche modulation by activated microglia: transforming growth factor beta increases neurogenesis in the adult dentate gyrus. Eur J Neurosci 23:83-93

Bauer S, Hay M, Amilhon B, Jean A, Moyse E (2005) In vivo neurogenesis in the dorsal vagal complex of the adult rat brainstem. Neuroscience 130:75-90

Bauer S, Patterson PH (2006) Leukemia inhibitory factor promotes neural stem cell self-renewal in the adult brain. J Neurosci 26:12089-12099

Benninghoff A (1951) Vemerhung und vergrosserung von nervzellen bei hypertrophie des innervationgebietes. Z Naturforsch38-44

Benraiss A, Chmielnicki E, Lerner K, Roh D, Goldman SA (2001) Adenoviral brain-derived neurotrophic factor induces both neostriatal and olfactory neuronal recruitment from endogenous progenitor cells in the adult forebrain. J Neurosci 21:6718-6731

Bergman E, Ulfhake B (1998) Loss of primary sensory neurons in the very old rat: neuron number estimates using the disector method and confocal optical sectioning. J Comp Neurol 396:211-222

Buffo A, Rite I, Tripathi P, Lepier A, Colak D, Horn AP, Mori T, Gotz M (2008) Origin and progeny of reactive gliosis: A source of multipotent cells in the injured brain. Proc Natl Acad Sci U S A 105:3581-3586

Cecchini T, Cuppini R, Ciaroni S, Barili P, De Matteis R, Del Grande P (1995) Changes in the number of primary sensory neurons in normal and vitamin-E-deficient rats during aging. Somatosens Mot Res 12:317-327

Chang MY, Kim D, Kim CH, Kang HC, Yang E, Moon JI, Ko S, Park J, Park KS, Lee KA, Hwang DY, Chung Y, Lanza R, Kim KS (2010) Direct reprogramming of rat neural precursor cells and fibroblasts into pluripotent stem cells. PLoS ONE 5:e9838

Chenn A, Walsh CA (2002) Regulation of cerebral cortical size by control of cell cycle exit in neural precursors. Science 297:365-369

Chmielnicki E, Benraiss A, Economides AN, Goldman SA (2004) Adenovirally expressed noggin and brain-derived neurotrophic factor cooperate to induce new medium spiny neurons from resident progenitor cells in the adult striatal ventricular zone. J Neurosci 24:2133-2142

Ciaroni S, Cecchini T, Cuppini R, Ferri P, Ambrogini P, Bruno C, Del Grande P (2000) Are there proliferating neuronal precursors in adult rat dorsal root ganglia? Neurosci Lett 281:69-71

Corvetti G, Fornaro M, Geuna S, Poncino A, Giacobini-Robecchi MG (2001) Unscheduled DNA synthesis in rat adult myenteric neurons: an immunohistochemical study. Neuroreport 12:2165-2168

Costa MR, Bucholz O, Schroeder T, Gotz M (2009) Late origin of glia-restricted progenitors in the developing mouse cerebral cortex. Cereb Cortex 19 Suppl 1:i135-i143

Czaja K, Burns GA, Ritter RC (2008) Capsaicin-induced neuronal death and proliferation of the primary sensory neurons located in the nodose ganglia of adult rats. Neuroscience 154:621-630

Dasari VR, Spomar DG, Gondi CS, Sloffer CA, Saving KL, Gujrati M, Rao JS, Dinh DH (2007) Axonal remyelination by cord blood stem cells after spinal cord injury. J Neurotrauma 24:391-410

Devor M (1991) Chronic pain in the aged: possible relation between neurogenesis, involution and pathophysiology in adult sensory ganglia. J Basic Clin Physiol Pharmacol 2:1-15

Devor M, Govrin-Lippmann R (1985) Neurogenesis in adult rat dorsal root ganglia. Neurosci Lett 61:189-194

Dressler J, Vemuganti R (2009) Apoptosis and gene expression after TBI. Leg Med (Tokyo) 11 Suppl 1:S54-S55

Ehninger D, Kempermann G (2008) Neurogenesis in the adult hippocampus. Cell Tissue Res 331:243-250

Emery DL, Fulp CT, Saatman KE, Schutz C, Neugebauer E, McIntosh TK (2005) Newly born granule cells in the dentate gyrus rapidly extend axons into the hippocampal CA3 region following experimental brain injury. J Neurotrauma 22:978-988

Emery DL, Royo NC, Fischer I, Saatman KE, McIntosh TK (2003) Plasticity following injury to the adult central nervous system: is recapitulation of a developmental state worth promoting? J Neurotrauma 20:1271-1292

Encinas JM, Enikolopov G (2008) Identifying and quantitating neural stem and progenitor cells in the adult brain. Methods Cell Biol 85:243-272

Englund C, Fink A, Lau C, Pham D, Daza RA, Bulfone A, Kowalczyk T, Hevner RF (2005) Pax6, Tbr2, and Tbr1 are expressed sequentially by radial glia, intermediate progenitor cells, and postmitotic neurons in developing neocortex. J Neurosci 25:247-251

Falk S, Wurdak H, Ittner LM, Ille F, Sumara G, Schmid MT, Draganova K, Lang KS, Paratore C, Leveen P, Suter U, Karlsson S, Born W, Ricci R, Gotz M, Sommer L (2008) Brain area-specific effect of TGF-beta signaling on Wnt-dependent neural stem cell expansion. Cell Stem Cell 2:472-483

Fallon J, Reid S, Kinyamu R, Opole I, Opole R, Baratta J, Korc M, Endo TL, Duong A, Nguyen G, Karkehabadhi M, Twardzik D, Patel S, Loughlin S (2000) In vivo induction of massive proliferation, directed migration, and differentiation of neural cells in the adult mammalian brain. Proc Natl Acad Sci U S A 97:14686-14691

Falo MC, Reeves TM, Phillips LL (2008) Agrin expression during synaptogenesis induced by traumatic brain injury. J Neurotrauma 25:769-783

Farel PB (2001) Neuron addition and neurogenesis are not interchangeable terms. Anat Rec 265:159-160

Farel PB (2002) Sensory neuron addition in juvenile rat: time course and specificity. J Comp Neurol 449:158-165

Fawcett JW (1992) Intrinsic neuronal determinants of regeneration. Trends Neurosci 15:5-8

Filogamo G, Vigliani F (1954) Ricerche sperimentali sulla correlazione tra estensione del territorio di innervazione e grandezza e numero delle cellule gangliari del plesso mienterico (di Auerbach) nel cane. Riv Patol Nerv Ment1-32

Fitch MT, Silver J (2008) CNS injury, glial scars, and inflammation: Inhibitory extracellular matrices and regeneration failure. Exp Neurol 209:294-301

Fricker-Gates RA, Shin JJ, Tai CC, Catapano LA, Macklis JD (2002) Late-stage immature neocortical neurons reconstruct interhemispheric connections and form synaptic contacts with increased efficiency in adult mouse cortex undergoing targeted neurodegeneration. J Neurosci 22:4045-4056

Fry EJ, Saunders NR (2000) Spinal repair in immature animals: a novel approach using the South American opossum Monodelphis domestica. Clin Exp Pharmacol Physiol 27:542-547

Gabella G (1984) Size of neurons and glial cells in the intramural ganglia of the hypertrophic intestine of the guinea-pig. J Neurocytol 13:73-84

Gage FH (2000) Mammalian neural stem cells. Science 287:1433-1438

Gage FH (2002) Neurogenesis in the adult brain. J Neurosci 22:612-613

Gallaher ZR, Ryu V, Larios RM, Sprunger LK, Czaja K (2011) Neural proliferation and restoration of neurochemical phenotypes and compromised functions following capsaicin-induced neuronal damage in the nodose ganglion of the adult rat. Front Neurosci 5:

Geuna S (2005) The revolution of counting "tops": two decades of the disector principle in morphological research. Microsc Res Tech 66:270-274

Geuna S, Borrione P, Filogamo G (2002) Postnatal histogenesis in the peripheral nervous system. Int J Dev Neurosci 20:475-479

Geuna S, Borrione P, Fornaro M, Giacobini-Robecchi MG (2000) Neurogenesis and stem cells in adult mammalian dorsal root ganglia. Anat Rec 261:139-140

Giacobini Robecchi MG, Borrione P, Canavese M, Geuna S, Paraninfo A, Poncino A, Silengo L (1995) DNA neosynthesis in Auerbach plexus ganglia isolated from the rat hypertrophic gut: an electrophoretic analysis. Int J Dev Neurosci 13:635-637

Giacobini Robecchi MG, Poncino A, Geuna S, Giacometti S, Filogamo G (1988) DNA content in neurons of Auerbach's plexus under experimental conditions in adult rats. Int J Dev Neurosci 6:109-115

Globus MY, Alonso O, Dietrich WD, Busto R, Ginsberg MD (1995) Glutamate release and free radical production following brain injury: effects of posttraumatic hypothermia. J Neurochem 65:1704-1711

Gong QZ, Phillips LL, Lyeth BG (1999) Metabotropic glutamate receptor protein alterations after traumatic brain injury in rats. J Neurotrauma 16:893-902

Gonzalez-Perez O (2010) Immunological regulation of the central nervous system: From physiological to pathological processes. Curr Immunol Rev 6:149

Gotts JE, Chesselet MF (2005) Mechanisms of subventricular zone expansion after focal cortical ischemic injury. J Comp Neurol 488:201-214

Gotz M, Huttner WB (2005) The cell biology of neurogenesis. Nat Rev Mol Cell Biol 6:777-788

Graham DI, McIntosh TK, Maxwell WL, Nicoll JA (2000) Recent advances in neurotrauma. J Neuropathol Exp Neurol 59:641-651

Graham V, Khudyakov J, Ellis P, Pevny L (2003) SOX2 functions to maintain neural progenitor identity. Neuron 39:749-765

Gubert F, Zaverucha-do-Valle C, Pimentel-Coelho PM, Mendez-Otero R, Santiago MF (2008) Radial glia-like cells persist in the adult rat brain. Brain Res

Hatai S, (1902) Number and size of the spinal ganglion cells and dorsal root fibers in the white rat at different ages. J. Comp. Neurol. 12, 107–124.

Hellewell SC, Yan EB, Agyapomaa DA, Bye N, Morganti-Kossmann MC (2010) Post-traumatic hypoxia exacerbates brain tissue damage: analysis of axonal injury and glial responses. J Neurotrauma 27:1997-2010

Hevner RF (2006) From radial glia to pyramidal-projection neuron: transcription factor cascades in cerebral cortex development. Mol Neurobiol 33:33-50

Hinzman JM, Thomas TC, Burmeister JJ, Quintero JE, Huettl P, Pomerleau F, Gerhardt GA, Lifshitz J (2010) Diffuse brain injury elevates tonic glutamate levels and potassium-evoked glutamate release in discrete brain regions at two days post-injury: an enzyme-based microelectrode array study. J Neurotrauma 27:889-899

Hou SW, Wang YQ, Xu M, Shen DH, Wang JJ, Huang F, Yu Z, Sun FY (2008) Functional Integration of Newly Generated Neurons Into Striatum After Cerebral Ischemia in the Adult Rat Brain. Stroke

Jin K, Minami M, Lan JQ, Mao XO, Batteur S, Simon RP, Greenberg DA (2001) Neurogenesis in dentate subgranular zone and rostral subventricular zone after focal cerebral ischemia in the rat. Proc Natl Acad Sci U S A 98:4710-4715

Jin K, Wang X, Xie L, Mao XO, Zhu W, Wang Y, Shen J, Mao Y, Banwait S, Greenberg DA (2006) Evidence for stroke-induced neurogenesis in the human brain. Proc Natl Acad Sci U S A 103:13198-13202

Johansson CB, Momma S, Clarke DL, Risling M, Lendahl U, Frisen J (1999) Identification of a neural stem cell in the adult mammalian central nervous system. Cell 96:25-34

Katakowski M, Chen J, Zhang ZG, Santra M, Wang Y, Chopp M (2007) Stroke-induced subventricular zone proliferation is promoted by tumor necrosis factor-alpha-converting enzyme protease activity. J Cereb Blood Flow Metab 27:669-678

Keirstead HS, Blakemore WF (1997) Identification of post-mitotic oligodendrocytes incapable of remyelination within the demyelinated adult spinal cord. J Neuropathol Exp Neurol 56:1191-1201

Kempermann G, Wiskott L, Gage FH (2004) Functional significance of adult neurogenesis. Curr Opin Neurobiol 14:186-191

Kernie SG, Parent JM (2010) Forebrain neurogenesis after focal Ischemic and traumatic brain injury. Neurobiol Dis 37:267-274

Khuman J, Meehan WP, III, Zhu X, Qiu J, Hoffmann U, Zhang J, Giovannone E, Lo EH, Whalen MJ (2011) Tumor necrosis factor alpha and Fas receptor contribute to cognitive deficits independent of cell death after concussive traumatic brain injury in mice. J Cereb Blood Flow Metab 31:778-789

Kim DH, Ko IG, Kim BK, Kim TW, Kim SE, Shin MS, Kim CJ, Kim H, Kim KM, Baek SS (2010) Treadmill exercise inhibits traumatic brain injury-induced hippocampal apoptosis. Physiol Behav 101:660-665

La Forte RA, Melville S, Chung K, Coggeshall RE (1991) Absence of neurogenesis of adult rat dorsal root ganglion cells. Somatosensory & Motor Research 8:3-7

Lagares A, Li HY, Zhou XF, Avendano C (2007) Primary sensory neuron addition in the adult rat trigeminal ganglion: evidence for neural crest glio-neuronal precursor maturation. J Neurosci 27:7939-7953

Le N, Nagarajan R, Wang JY, Araki T, Schmidt RE, Milbrandt J (2005) Analysis of congenital hypomyelinating Egr2Lo/Lo nerves identifies Sox2 as an inhibitor of Schwann cell differentiation and myelination. Proc Natl Acad Sci U S A 102:2596-2601

Lee E, Son H (2009) Adult hippocampal neurogenesis and related neurotrophic factors. BMB Rep 42:239-244

Li HY, Say EH, Zhou XF (2007) Isolation and characterization of neural crest progenitors from adult dorsal root ganglia. Stem Cells 25:2053-2065

Li M, Pevny L, Lovell-Badge R, Smith A (1998) Generation of purified neural precursors from embryonic stem cells by lineage selection. Curr Biol 8:971-974

Li X, Li YH, Yu S, Liu Y (2008) Upregulation of Ryk expression in rat dorsal root ganglia after peripheral nerve injury. Brain Res Bull 77:178-184

Lie DC, Song H, Colamarino SA, Ming GL, Gage FH (2004) Neurogenesis in the adult brain: new strategies for central nervous system diseases. Annu Rev Pharmacol Toxicol 44:399-421

Liu MT, Kuan YH, Wang J, Hen R, Gershon MD (2009) 5-HT4 receptor-mediated neuroprotection and neurogenesis in the enteric nervous system of adult mice. J Neurosci 29:9683-9699

Liu XS, Zhang ZG, Zhang RL, Gregg S, Morris DC, Wang Y, Chopp M (2007) Stroke induces gene profile changes associated with neurogenesis and angiogenesis in adult subventricular zone progenitor cells. J Cereb Blood Flow Metab 27:564-574

Lu KT, Sun CL, Wo PY, Yen HH, Tang TH, Ng MC, Huang ML, Yang YL (2011) Hippocampal Neurogenesis after Traumatic Brain Injury Is Mediated by Vascular Endothelial Growth Factor Receptor-2 and the Raf/MEK/ERK Cascade. J Neurotrauma 28:441-450

Ming GL, Song H (2005) Adult neurogenesis in the mammalian central nervous system. Annu Rev Neurosci 28:223-250

Miura M (1913) Aus den Notizien Meiner Phisiologischen und Patologischen Forschung. XXVI. Muscularis Mucosae et Muscularis Propria Gastrointestinalis. Naködo-Verlag193-215

Mohammed HA, Santer RM (2001) Total neuronal numbers of rat lumbosacral primary afferent neurons do not change with age. Neurosci Lett 304:149-152

Mori T, Buffo A, Gotz M (2005) The novel roles of glial cells revisited: the contribution of radial glia and astrocytes to neurogenesis. Curr Top Dev Biol 69:67-99

Nakabayashi M, Suzaki S, Tomita H (2007) Neural injury and recovery near cortical contusions: a clinical magnetic resonance spectroscopy study. J Neurosurg 106:370-377

Namaka MP, Sawchuk M, MacDonald SC, Jordan LM, Hochman S (2001) Neurogenesis in postnatal mouse dorsal root ganglia. Exp Neurol 172:60-69

Neumueller S, Hodges MR, Krause K, Marshall B, Bonis J, Qian B, Pan LG, Forster HV (2011) Anatomic changes in multiple brainstem nuclei after incremental, near-complete neurotoxic destruction of the pre-Botzinger Complex in adult goats. Respir Physiol Neurobiol 175:1-11

Nicholls J, Saunders N (1996) Regeneration of immature mammalian spinal cord after injury. Trends Neurosci 19:229-234

Nowakowski RS, Hayes NL (2001) Stem cells: the promises and pitfalls. Neuropsychopharmacology 25:799-804

Nowakowski RS, Lewin SB, Miller MW (1989) Bromodeoxyuridine immunohistochemical determination of the lengths of the cell cycle and the DNA-synthetic phase for an anatomically defined population. J Neurocytol 18:311-318

Ohab JJ, Fleming S, Blesch A, Carmichael ST (2006) A neurovascular niche for neurogenesis after stroke. J Neurosci 26:13007-13016

Osakada F, Ooto S, Akagi T, Mandai M, Akaike A, Takahashi M (2007) Wnt signaling promotes regeneration in the retina of adult mammals. J Neurosci 27:4210-4219

Parent JM (2003) Injury-induced neurogenesis in the adult mammalian brain. Neuroscientist 9:261-272

Parent JM, Lowenstein DH (2002) Seizure-induced neurogenesis: are more new neurons good for an adult brain? Prog Brain Res 135:121-131

Parent JM, Vexler ZS, Gong C, Derugin N, Ferriero DM (2002) Rat forebrain neurogenesis and striatal neuron replacement after focal stroke. Ann Neurol 52:802-813

Park IH, Zhao R, West JA, Yabuuchi A, Huo H, Ince TA, Lerou PH, Lensch MW, Daley GQ (2008) Reprogramming of human somatic cells to pluripotency with defined factors. Nature 451:141-146

Parkinson DB, Bhaskaran A, Arthur-Farraj P, Noon LA, Woodhoo A, Lloyd AC, Feltri ML, Wrabetz L, Behrens A, Mirsky R, Jessen KR (2008) c-Jun is a negative regulator of myelination. J Cell Biol 181:625-637

Pascual-Leone A, Amedi A, Fregni F, Merabet LB (2005) The plastic human brain cortex. Annu Rev Neurosci 28:377-401

Poncino A, Geuna S, Scherini E, Giacobini Robecchi MG, Filogamo G (1990) DNA synthesis experimentally induced in neurons: tetraploidy or hyperdiploidy? Int J Dev Neurosci 8:621-623

Popken GJ, Farel PB (1997) Sensory neuron number in neonatal and adult rats estimated by means of stereologic and profile-based methods. J Comp Neurol 386:8-15

Pover CM, Barnes MC, Coggeshall RE (1994) Do primary afferent cell numbers change in relation to increasing weight and surface area in adult rats? Somatosens Mot Res 11:163-167

Redwine JM, Armstrong RC (1998) In vivo proliferation of oligodendrocyte progenitors expressing PDGFalphaR during early remyelination. J Neurobiol 37:413-428

Riccio A (2010) Dynamic epigenetic regulation in neurons: enzymes, stimuli and signaling pathways. Nat Neurosci 13:1330-1337

Richardson RM, Sun D, Bullock MR (2007) Neurogenesis after traumatic brain injury. Neurosurg Clin N Am 18:169-81, xi

Robel S, Berninger B, Gotz M (2011) The stem cell potential of glia: lessons from reactive gliosis. Nat Rev Neurosci 12:88-104

Rogister B, Delree P, Leprince P, Martin D, Sadzot C, Malgrange B, Munaut C, Rigo JM, Lefebvre PP, Octave JN, . (1993) Transforming growth factor beta as a neuronoglial signal during peripheral nervous system response to injury. J Neurosci Res 34:32-43

Ryu V, Gallaher Z, Czaja K (2010) Plasticity of nodose ganglion neurons after capsaicin- and vagotomy-induced nerve damage in adult rats. Neuroscience 167:1227-1238

Saade NE, Massaad CA, Ochoa-Chaar CI, Jabbur SJ, Safieh-Garabedian B, Atweh SF (2002) Upregulation of proinflammatory cytokines and nerve growth factor by intraplantar injection of capsaicin in rats. J Physiol 545:241-253

Salehi M, Pasbakhsh P, Soleimani M, Abbasi M, Hasanzadeh G, Modaresi MH, Sobhani A (2009) Repair of spinal cord injury by co-transplantation of embryonic stem cell-derived motor neuron and olfactory ensheathing cell. Iran Biomed J 13:125-135

Sasaki M, Li B, Lankford KL, Radtke C, Kocsis JD (2007) Remyelination of the injured spinal cord. Prog Brain Res 161:419-433

Scheff SW, Price DA, Hicks RR, Baldwin SA, Robinson S, Brackney C (2005) Synaptogenesis in the hippocampal CA1 field following traumatic brain injury. J Neurotrauma 22:719-732

Shi J, Miles DK, Orr BA, Massa SM, Kernie SG (2007) Injury-induced neurogenesis in Bax-deficient mice: evidence for regulation by voltage-gated potassium channels. Eur J Neurosci 25:3499-3512

Silva AT, Wardhaugh T, Dolatshad NF, Jones S, Saffrey MJ (2008) Neural progenitors from isolated postnatal rat myenteric ganglia: expansion as neurospheres and differentiation in vitro. Brain Res 1218:47-53

Singh RP, Cheng YH, Nelson P, Zhou FC (2009) Retentive multipotency of adult dorsal root ganglia stem cells. Cell Transplant 18:55-68

Suh H, Deng W, Gage FH (2009) Signaling in adult neurogenesis. Annu Rev Cell Dev Biol 25:253-275

Sun D, Colello RJ, Daugherty WP, Kwon TH, McGinn MJ, Harvey HB, Bullock MR (2005) Cell proliferation and neuronal differentiation in the dentate gyrus in juvenile and adult rats following traumatic brain injury. J Neurotrauma 22:95-105

Sun D, McGinn MJ, Zhou Z, Harvey HB, Bullock MR, Colello RJ (2007) Anatomical integration of newly generated dentate granule neurons following traumatic brain injury in adult rats and its association to cognitive recovery. Exp Neurol 204:264-272

Taupin P (2006) Adult neurogenesis in mammals. Curr Opin Mol Ther 8:345-351

Tederko P, Krasuski M, Kiwerski J, Nyka I, Bialoszewski D (2009) Strategies for neuroprotection following spinal cord injury. Ortop Traumatol Rehabil 11:103-110

Ussar S, Voss T (2004) MEK1 and MEK2, different regulators of the G1/S transition. J Biol Chem 279:43861-43869

Vessal M, Aycock A, Garton MT, Ciferri M, Darian-Smith C (2007) Adult neurogenesis in primate and rodent spinal cord: comparing a cervical dorsal rhizotomy with a dorsal column transection. Eur J Neurosci 26:2777-2794

Vogel G (2010) Cells rewrite their own destiny. Science 330:1618

Wexler EM, Paucer A, Kornblum HI, Palmer TD, Geschwind DH (2009) Endogenous Wnt signaling maintains neural progenitor cell potency. Stem Cells 27:1130-1141

White BD, Nathe RJ, Maris DO, Nguyen NK, Goodson JM, Moon RT, Horner PJ (2010) Beta-catenin signaling increases in proliferating NG2+ progenitors and astrocytes during post-traumatic gliogenesis in the adult brain. Stem Cells 28:297-307

Widera D, Mikenberg I, Elvers M, Kaltschmidt C, Kaltschmidt B (2006) Tumor necrosis factor alpha triggers proliferation of adult neural stem cells via IKK/NF-kappaB signaling. BMC Neurosci 7:64

Wojtowicz JM, Kee N (2006) BrdU assay for neurogenesis in rodents. Nat Protoc 1:1399-1405

Woodhoo A, Alonso MB, Droggiti A, Turmaine M, D'Antonio M, Parkinson DB, Wilton DK, Al-Shawi R, Simons P, Shen J, Guillemot F, Radtke F, Meijer D, Feltri ML, Wrabetz L, Mirsky R, Jessen KR (2009) Notch controls embryonic Schwann cell differentiation, postnatal myelination and adult plasticity. Nat Neurosci 12:839-847

Wu B, Ren X (2009) Promoting axonal myelination for improving neurological recovery in spinal cord injury. J Neurotrauma 26:1847-1856

Yang H, Lu P, McKay HM, Bernot T, Keirstead H, Steward O, Gage FH, Edgerton VR, Tuszynski MH (2006) Endogenous neurogenesis replaces oligodendrocytes and astrocytes after primate spinal cord injury. J Neurosci 26:2157-2166

Yirmiya R, Goshen I (2011) Immune modulation of learning, memory, neural plasticity and neurogenesis. Brain Behav Immun 25:181-213

Yoshimura S, Takagi Y, Harada J, Teramoto T, Thomas SS, Waeber C, Bakowska JC, Breakefield XO, Moskowitz MA (2001) FGF-2 regulation of neurogenesis in adult hippocampus after brain injury. Proc Natl Acad Sci U S A 98:5874-5879

Yoshimura S, Teramoto T, Whalen MJ, Irizarry MC, Takagi Y, Qiu J, Harada J, Waeber C, Breakefield XO, Moskowitz MA (2003) FGF-2 regulates neurogenesis and degeneration in the dentate gyrus after traumatic brain injury in mice. J Clin Invest 112:1202-1210

Zhang B, Chen X, Lin Y, Tan T, Yang Z, Dayao C, Liu L, Jiang R, Zhang J (2011) Impairment of synaptic plasticity in hippocampus is exacerbated by methylprednisolone in a rat model of traumatic brain injury. Brain Res 1382:165-172

Zhang R, Zhang Z, Zhang C, Zhang L, Robin A, Wang Y, Lu M, Chopp M (2004) Stroke transiently increases subventricular zone cell division from asymmetric to symmetric and increases neuronal differentiation in the adult rat. J Neurosci 24:5810-5815

Zhang RL, Zhang ZG, Chopp M (2005) Neurogenesis in the adult ischemic brain: generation, migration, survival, and restorative therapy. Neuroscientist 11:408-416

Ziv Y, Schwartz M (2008) Orchestrating brain-cell renewal: the role of immune cells in adult neurogenesis in health and disease. Trends Mol Med 14:471-478

13

The Absence of the "GATC - Binding Protein SeqA" Affects DNA Replication in *Salmonella enterica* Serovar Typhimurium

Aloui Amine, Kouass Sahbani Saloua, Mihoub Mouadh, El May Alya and Landoulsi Ahmed
Faculty of Sciences of Bizerta, Carthage University
Tunisia

1. Introduction

The aim of this chapter is to show the consequences of *seqA* gene disruption in *Salmonella typhimurium*. Of special interest is the observation that this disruption causes asynchrony of DNA replication. In fact, lack of SeqA protein causes major changes in the lipid profile of the membrane cell which is implicated in the initiation of DNA replication. Moreover, during passage through the small intestine in the host, *Salmonella typhimurium* faces periodic release of bile and due to the absence of SeqA protein the sensitivity to this bile increases. This unknown sensitivity could be due to an altered membrane composition of phospholipids and fatty acids.
Deoxyribonucleic acid (DNA) contains all the information required to build the cells and tissues of a prokaryotic or an eukaryotic organism. The exact replication of this information in any species assures its genetic continuity from generation to generation and is critical to the normal development of an individual. The information stored in DNA is arranged in hereditary units, known as genes, that control identifiable traits of an organism.
Discovery of the structure of DNA and subsequent elucidation of how DNA directs synthesis of RNA, which then directs assembly of proteins-the so-called central dogma-were monumental achievements marking the early days of molecular biology. However, the simplified representation of the central dogma as DNA→RNA→protein does not reflect the role of proteins in the synthesis of nucleic acids. Moreover, proteins are largely responsible for regulating DNA replication and gene expression, the entire process whereby the information encoded in DNA is decoded into the proteins that characterize various cell types. One of these proteins is the DNA-Binding Protein SeqA.

1.1 SeqA: the DNA-binding protein

SeqA was discovered in some prokaryotes as a protein involved in the methylation / hemimethylation cycle of *Escherichia coli* DNA (Lu et al., 1994). SeqA binds to hemimethylated GATC sites formed by DNA replication and regulates activation of the *Escherichia coli* chromosome replication origin (Lu et al. 1994). Proper chromosome segregation also requires SeqA (Bach et al., 2003). Furthermore, SeqA trails the DNA replication fork and may contribute to nucleoid organization in newly replicated DNA (Brendler et al., 2000; Klungsøyr & Skarstad, 2004; Løbner-Olesen et al., 2003; Yamazoe et al.,

2005). Aside from its roles in chromosome replication and nucleoid segregation, SeqA is known to regulate the transcription of certain genes. In bacteriophage lambda, SeqA activates the p_R promoter in a GATC methylation-dependent fashion.
SeqA also acts as a transcriptional coactivator by facilitating binding of the *c*II transcription factor to the lambda p_I and p_{aQ} promoters. Competition between SeqA and the OxyR repressor for hemimethylated GATC sites has been shown to regulate phase variation in the *Escherichia coli* agn43 gene (Prieto et al., 2007). These examples raised the possibility that SeqA binding to critical GATC sites might likewise regulate the expression of prokaryotic genes like in *Salmonella,* which is a member of the *Enterobacteriaceae* family.

1.2 The genus *Salmonella*

Much of recent research is focused on *Salmonella* (figure 1) which causes diseases ranging from food and blood poisoning to typhoid fever and heart disease (Marinus, 1996).

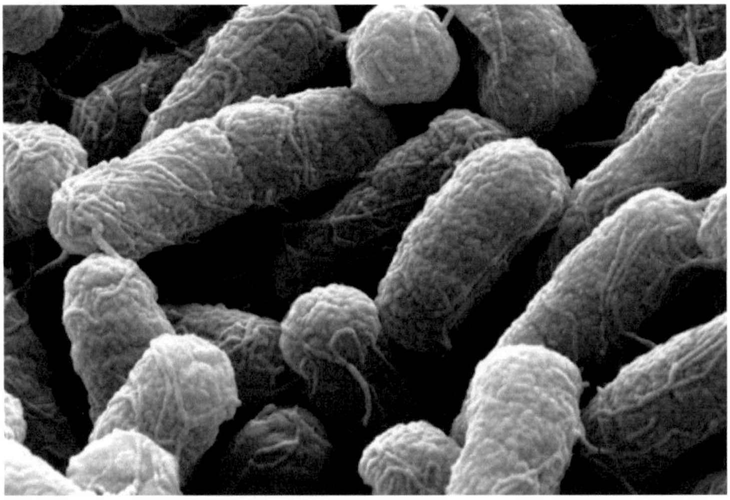

Fig. 1. *Salmonella typhimurium*

Unlike its close relative *Escherichia coli, Salmonella enterica* is never encountered as a commensal in humans but is always associated with disease. Most *Salmonella* serovars capable of infecting humans cause gastro-intestinal disease and are spread via contaminated food and water. The serovar Typhi is unique in that, it is a strict human pathogen which gives rise to a severe systemic disease called typhoid fever. *Salmonella enterica* serovar Typhimurium (which will be referred to as *Salmonella typhimurium* throughout this chapter) causes a systemic disease in certain inbred mouse strains that share many similarities to typhoid fever in humans. The *Salmonella* infection is initiated upon ingestion of the bacteria. A small fraction of the bacteria survive the acidic environment in the stomach and establish an infection in the small intestine, where the *Salmonella* multiply and displace the normal flora bacteria. The bacteria then cross the intestinal epithelium by invading the M cells of the Peyer's patches and enter the blood circulation. Systemic disease in both humans and mice is associated with the capacity of the bacteria to survive and replicate in macrophages and in the late stages of the disease, *Salmonella* can be found in large numbers in the liver and spleen. The murine typhoid fever model has been used extensively to study the interactions between pathogenic bacteria and their host.

Salmonella typhimurium represents a concern with regard to food safety due to its ability to growth in a wide range of adverse environmental conditions. Moreover, *Salmonella typhimurium* which contaminates foods may be derived from environments in which its previous growth occurs at moderate acidic conditions and, consequently, it may develop adaptive responses which enhance its resistance to other stress conditions occurring during food processing (Foster & Hall, 1990; Leyer & Johnson, 1993; Tosun & Gonul, 2003).
One of the most important and intensively studied stress responses in *Salmonella typhimurium* is the acid tolerance response which increases its subsequent ability to survive in high acid foods, as well as in the extreme acid conditions of the gastrointestinal tract, increasing the risk of illness (Greenacre et al., 2003; Leyer & Johnson, 1992; Waterman & Small, 1998; Yuk & Schneider, 2006).

1.3 DNA replication in *Salmonella typhimurium*

In *Salmonella typhimurium*, the initiation of replication of chromosomal DNA is coordinated with cell division. It was demonstrated that DNA replication in bacterial cells is initiated on membranes and the activities of replication proteins are regulated by membrane components (Jacob et al., 1963). Indeed, initiation of DNA replication is precisely regulated in the cell cycles (Messer & Weigel, 1996). The SeqA protein seems to be one of the key proteins in the control of this process (Lu et al., 1994; Wold et al., 1998). It is an inhibitor of the onset of *Escherichia coli* chromosome replication *in vivo* (Boye et al., 1996; Slater et al., 1995) and, at high concentrations, of the replication initiator protein, DnaA *in vitro*, but it may stimulate replication at low DnaA concentrations *in vitro* (Wold et al., 1998). It affects DNA topology and inhibits open complex formation at the replication origin (Kang et al., 2003; Torheim & Skarstad, 1999). It was demonstrated that SeqA limits *in vivo* DnaA activity in replication from the chromosomal origin *oriC* (Von Freiesleben et al., 1994). Moreover, SeqA protein is essential for sequestration, which affects *oriC* in the newly replicated hemimethylated state (Lu et al., 1994; Slater et al., 1995). Disruption of the *seqA* gene of *Salmonella typhimurium* causes filament formation, aberrant nucleoid segregation, induction of the SOS response, envelope instability, and increased sensitivity to membrane-damaging agents like bile salt. These defects are similar to those described in *Escherichia coli*. Recent results (Prieto et al., 2007) indicated that lack of SeqA renders *Salmonella enterica* sensitive to sodium choleate (ox bile extract) but the cause of this sensitivity remains unknown.
In the next sections, we show the importance of DNA sequestration by describing in detail the implication of SeqA in the replication synchrony. Then, we demonstrate the changes in the lipid profile of the membrane cell after *seqA* mutation and we expose explanations of increasing bile sensitivity of *Salmonella typhimurium*, in *seqA* mutant. In final section, we summarize our paper and present the future directions of our research.

2. DNA replication and membrane sequestration

The initiation of chromosomal replication occurs only once during the cell cycle in both prokaryotes and eukaryotes. This initiation is the first and tightly controlled step of a DNA synthesis.
Because much of what is known about the regulation of the initiation of bacterial chromosomal replication comes from studies of *Escherichia coli*, this review focuses mainly on regulatory mechanisms in *Salmonella typhimurium*.

2.1 What is DNA sequestration by SeqA protein?

Replication of the bacterial chromosomal DNA initiates only once, at a specific region known as the origin of chromosomal replication *oriC*, by the initiator protein DnaA. This protein interacts specifically with 9-bp non-palindromic sequences (DnaA boxes) that exists at *oriC*. To ensure that initiation at an origin occurs only once per cell cycle, specific mechanisms exist to control chromosomal replication. In one mechanism, the SeqA protein that is tightly bound to hemimethylated DNA by a mechanism known as sequestration and which recognizes GATC sequences overrepresented within *oriC* and prefers binding to hemimethylated over binding to fully or unmethylated *oriC* (Figure 2).

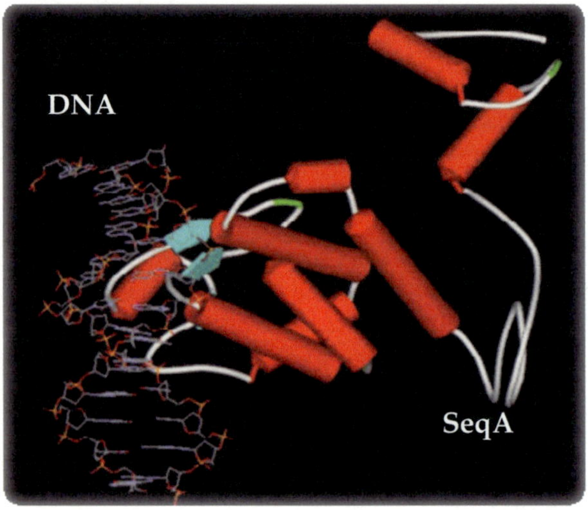

Fig. 2. DNA sequestration by SeqA

The chromosomal DNA is methylated at adenine residues in GATC sequences by Dam methylase. Following passage of the DNA replication fork, GATC sites methylated on the top and bottom strands in a mother cell (denoted as fully methylated) are converted into two hemimethylated DNA duplexes: one methylated on the top strand and nonmethylated on the bottom strand and one methylated on the bottom strand and nonmethylated on the top strand due to semi-conservative replication. Most GATC sites are rapidly remethylated by the enzyme DNA methyltransferase (Dam methylase or Dam) and exist in the hemimethylated state for only a fraction of the cell cycle (Figure 3).

Exceptions are the DNA replication origin of *Salmonella typhimurium*, the dnaA promoter, and possibly additional GATC sites in the chromosome which bind SeqA. SeqA preferentially binds to clusters of two or more hemimethylated GATC sites spaced one to two helical turns apart (Figure 4).

In the case of *oriC*, sequestration delays remethylation and prevents binding of the DnaA protein, which controls the initiation of DNA replication. At other sites, binding of SeqA tetramers to hemimethylated GATC sites may organize nucleoid domains. Notably, the transcription profile of a *Salmonella typhimurium* SeqA$^-$ mutant was found to be similar to that of a Dam overproducer strain. Based on this observation, a model was developed in which Dam and SeqA compete for binding to hemimethylated DNA generated at the replication fork.

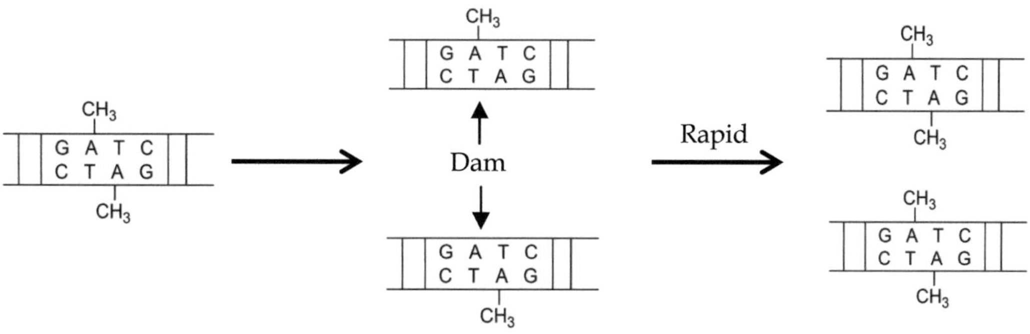

Fig. 3. The vast majority of chromosomal GATC sites are fully methylated until DNA replication generates two hemimethylated species, one methylated on the top strand and one methylated on the bottom strand. Within a short time after replication (less than 5 min), Dam methylates the nonmethylated GATC site, regenerating a fully methylated GATC site.

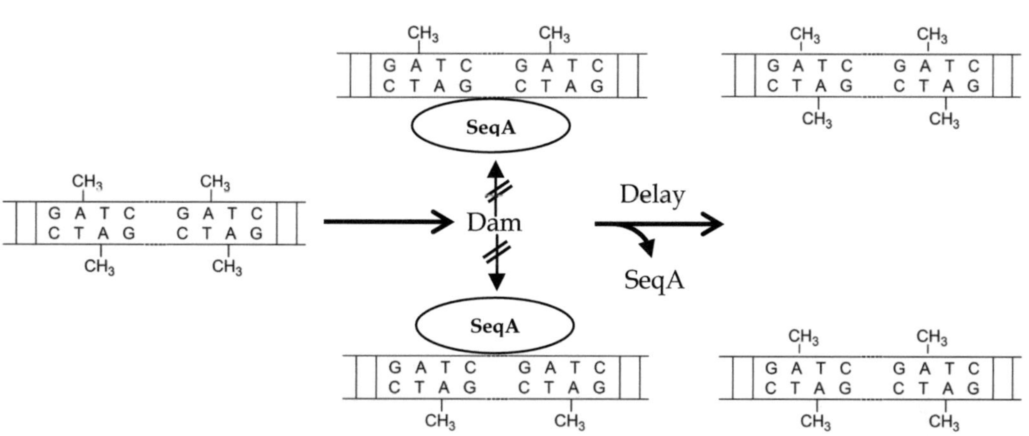

Fig. 4. Two or more helically phased GATC sites can be bound by SeqA when they are in the hemimethylated state. Binding of SeqA inhibits Dam methylation, maintaining the hemimethylated state for a portion of the cell cycle. Dissociation of SeqA allows Dam to methylate the hemimethylated DNAs, generating fully methylated DNA.

2.2 Effects of *seqA* mutation on DNA replication

As we said before, following the replication fork progression and the nascent strand synthesis, the daughter DNA becomes hemimethylated. SeqA protein binds to the hemimethylated GATC sequences (hemi-sites) and performs various roles to control the cell cycle progression. Immediately after the initiation of replication SeqA binds to the replicated *oriC* and sequesters it from remethylation and reinitiation of replication at the replicated *oriC*. SeqA tracks replication forks as a multiprotein complex and contributes to the maintenance of superhelicity and decatenation of daughter chromosomes through the stimulation of topoisomerase IV and results in a synchronous replication.

When rounds of replication are allowed to run to completion, the number of chromosomes per cell is 2n (n = 0, 1, 2, 3, etc). When initiations are asynchronous, as in *dnaA* (Ts) initiation mutants at the permissive temperature and in the Escherichia coli dam mutant (Boye &

Løbner-Olesen, 1990; Skarstad et al., 1988), the presence of a different number of chromosome equivalents (three, five, six, etc.) was detected by flow cytometry. The presence of cells containing a number of chromosomes different from 2n suggests that the seqA mutant has a defect in the synchrony of replication initiation. Wild type and seqA mutant of *Salmonella typhimurium* growing exponentially in glucose-casamino acid medium were treated with rifampicin and cephalexin, which block initiation of replication and cell division respectively. Wild-type cells initiated replication synchronously (number of chromosomes per cell is 2n). The appearance of cells with chromosome numbers other than 2n indicates a moderate asynchrony of initiation. So, flow cytometer analysis of our seqA mutants has shown that replication initiation is asynchronous and can occur throughout the cell cycle, not only at the normal cell age for initiation. The most likely reason for this asynchrony phenotype is that secondary initiations occurred at newly replicated origins in seqA mutants, due to lack of sequestration and inadequate methylation. We showed that initiation synchrony was dependent on intact GATC methylation sites. This loss of synchrony affected culture growth rates and cell size distributions only slightly and suggest that seqA mutants have a slight defect in synchronizing replication initiation. All these results suggest that DNA sequestration plays a role in preventing the occurrence of multiple initiations at a single origin in the same replication cycle. However, using flow cytometry, we found that the asynchrony of initiation, which is one of the phenotypes of the seqA mutation, was returned to almost normal in a seqA null mutant harboring the wild-type *seqA* gene under the control of a tac promoter.

The OFF- to ON-phase rate was reduced in a *seqA* mutant, but much of this effect could be accounted for by a reduction in the Dam/DNA ratio caused by increased asynchronous initiation of DNA replication that occurs in the absence of SeqA, which normally sequesters *oriC* and plays a critical role in timing of DNA replication (Bogan & Helmstetter, 1997).

3. Membrane instability after *seqA* disruption

The origin of replication, *oriC*, is highly enriched in GATC sequences, which are sites for methylation by Dam methylase. Semi-conservative replication of fully methylated DNA generates hemimethylated *oriC* sites.

3.1 Membrane sequestration hemimethylated of *oriC*

Early studies demonstrated that membranes are capable of binding to hemimethylated *oriC* *in vitro* and *in vivo*, but not to fully methylated or unmethylated *oriC* (Ogden et al., 1988). While they are sequestered at the membrane, the recently replicated origins are unavailable for reinitiation and are protected from methylation by Dam methylase for an extended period. The origins remain sequestered until conditions in the cell are no longer in a state supportive for initiation (Figure 5).

Prior to initiation of DNA replication, Dam methylase sites are fully methylated. Immediately following replication, the newly synthesized strand is unmethylated, and the resulting hemimethylated origin is sequestered at the at lipid bilayer of membrane by SeqA. This is not accessible to replicatively active ATP–DnaA. After approximately one-third of the cell cycle, the sequestered origin is released and methylated by Dam methylase. At this point in the cell cycle, the levels of ATP–DnaA are not sufficient to catalyze a new round of replication. As such, sequestration serves as a mechanism to prevent secondary initiations. Subsequent work identified SeqA protein to be an essential factor for *oriC* sequestration.

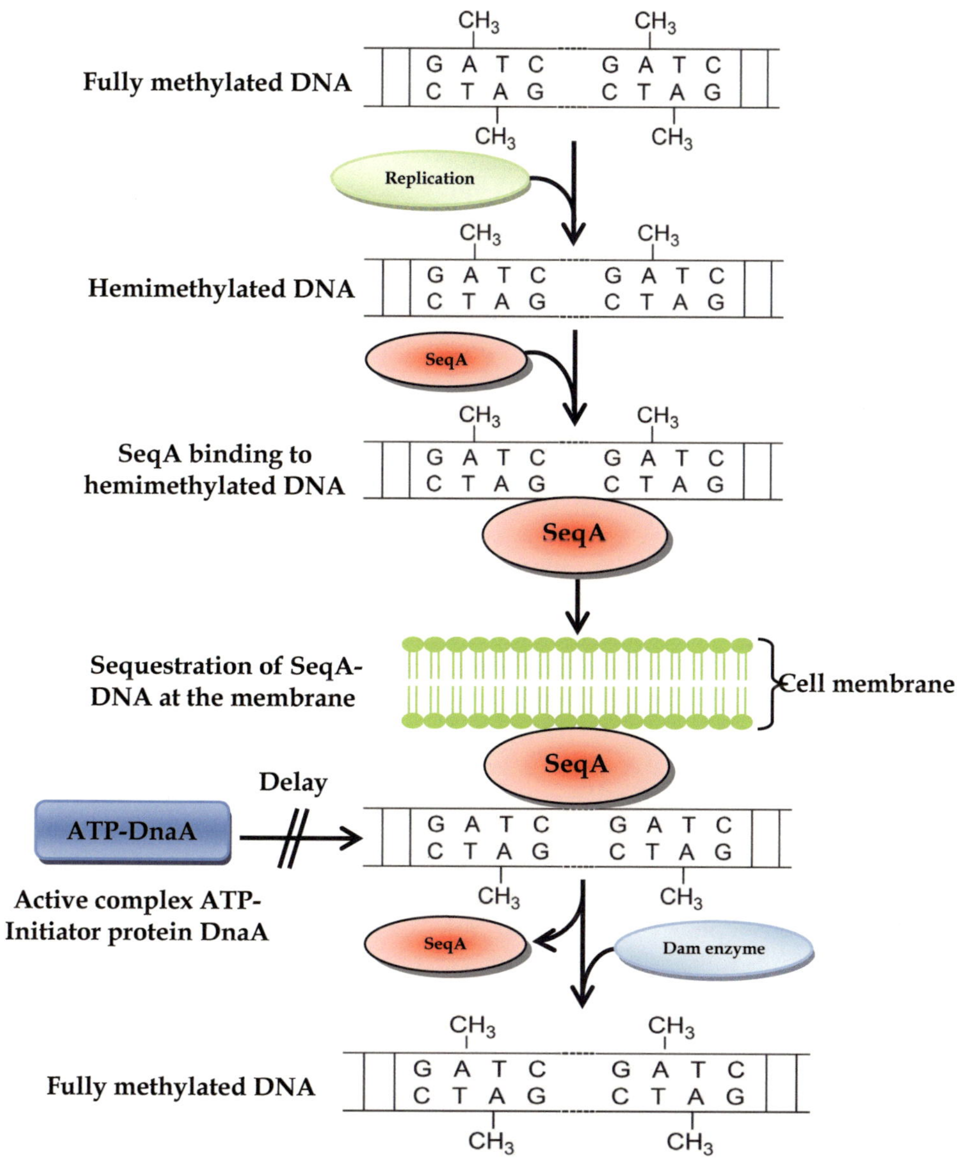

Fig. 5. Membrane sequestration of recently replicated origins.

Even though the first steps of SeqA purificiation involve liberating SeqA from the membrane fraction of cell lysates by treatment with high concentrations of salt and sonication, the primary sequence for SeqA protein does not suggest any obvious membrane-associating domains. This is supported by the crystal structure of the C-terminal DNA-binding domain, and by biochemical studies that show that the N-terminal domain serves in the aggregation of SeqA protein into functional homotetramers (Guarné et al., 2002). Yet, there is some evidence that SeqA has an association with membranes (d'Alencon et al., 1999; Wegrzyn et al., 1999). The original data that newly replicated, hemimethylated origins are

sequestered at the membrane hold true. Whether membrane sequestration of *oriC* occurs directly through the SeqA protein or through an as yet unidentified factor remains unclear.
We speculated that the examination of fatty acids composition and phospholipids fractions in wild type and *seqA* mutants would provide useful information to understand the interaction between SeqA protein and bacterial membrane in *Salmonella typhimurium*.

3.2 Effects of *seqA* mutation on membrane lipids

The coordination of the synchronization of the replication initiation, the activation of the DnaA protein at *oriC*, and the cellular cycle suggested the existence of a very narrow interaction between the bacterial membrane lipids and the SeqA protein (Landoulsi et al., 1990). Acidic phospholipids, such as cardiolipin and phosphatidylglycerol, decrease the affinity of adenine nucleotide for DnaA protein (Mizushima et al., 1997; Sekimizu & Kornberg, 1988). Thus, it has been proposed that phospholipids regulate the activity of DnaA protein in cells and *in vitro* (Makise et al., 2002; Sekimizu & Kornberg, 1988). It has been demonstrated that the *seqA* mutation can overcome the incompatibility phenotype observed between the chromosomal *oriC* and minichromosomal *oriC* copies in the *dam* mutant strain (Lobner-Olesen & Von Freiesleben, 1996). The mutation in the *seqA* gene allows efficient transformation of fully methylated minichromosomes into *dam* mutant cells (Lu et al., 1994; Von Freiesleben et al., 1994). We can suggest a possible interaction between the activities of SeqA protein and membrane lipids.
We analyzed the phospholipids and the fatty acids composition of the bacterial membrane with the aim of correlating the membrane structure variation in this lipids with *seqA* gene mutation.
The Phospholipids extracted from the bacterial membrane were separated and identified by thin layer chromatography. The content of each phospholipid was calculated from the fatty acids contents measured by the capillary gas chromatography method and is reported in the following section. The phospholipids found were phosphatidylethanolamine, phosphatidylglycerol, and cardiolipin on the basis of the following criteria:

- Identity of chromatographic behavior in thin layer chromatography with synthetic and purified commercial phospholipids from various sources;
- The flow rate is the same as that of commercial phospholipids; and
- The phospholipids are the same as those reported by several authors and works (Ames, 1968).
- *Phospholipids composition of Salmonella typhimurium wild type membrane*
  The major phospholipids present in *Salmonella typhimurium* wild type strain membrane were phosphatidylethanolamine, accounting for about 75.2%, followed by phosphatidylglycerol and cardiolipin (19.4% and 5.3%, respectively) (Figure 6.a). These phospholipids distributions agreed very closely to those reported in the literature for *Salmonella typhimurium* (Ames, 1968).
- *Phospholipids composition of the Salmonella typhimurium seqA mutant membrane*
  Phosphatidylethanolamine, phosphatidylglycerol, and cardiolipin proportions were affected by the *seqA* mutation while comparing them with the wild type strain. In the *seqA* mutant, the zwitterionic phosphatidylethanolamine fraction decreased from 75.2% to 20.53%. However, the acidic phospholipid fractions (phosphatidylglycerol and cardiolipin) becomes a majority of total phospholipids with 79.47%, distributed in 70.6% of phosphatidylglycerol and 8.8% of cardiolipin (Figure 6.b).

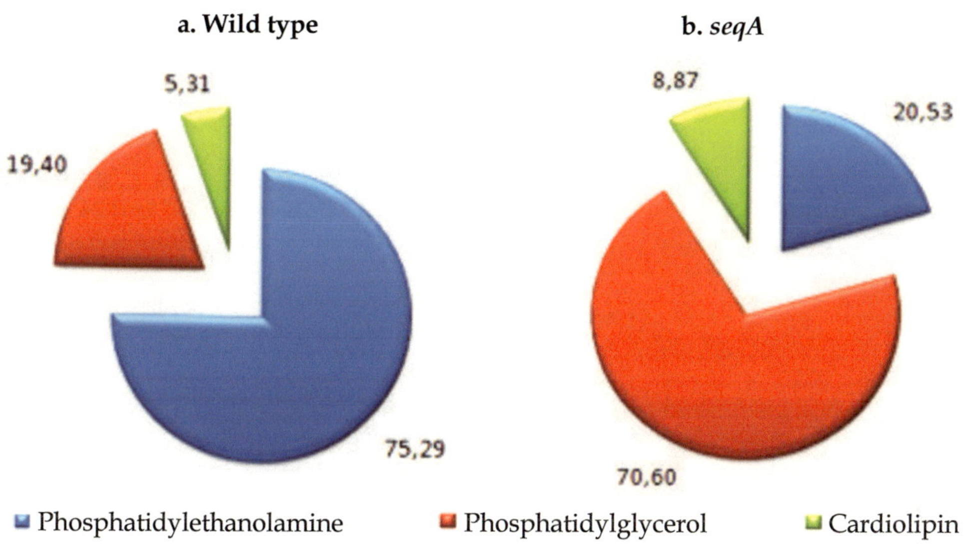

Fig. 6. Comparative analysis of percentage of phospholipids levels in wild type (a) and *seqA* (b) *Salmonella typhimurium* strains. Their contents were calculated from the fatty acid contents measured by the capillary gas chromatography method. Average values of triplicates were given, and the deviation was less than 5% of each value (significance was assessed using the Student's *t*-test).

The membrane fatty acid composition of the *Salmonella typhimurium* wild type strain was determined by the capillary gas chromatography method. Many fatty acids were found and seven main peaks were identified by comparing their retention times with those of known standards. Three saturated fatty acids were tetradecanoic (myristic) acid ($C_{14:0}$), hexadecanoic (palmitic) acid ($C_{16:0}$), and octadecanoic (stearic) acid ($C_{18:0}$), two monounsaturated fatty acids were hexadecenoic (palmitoleic) acid ($C_{16:1w7}$) and octadecenoic (oleic or vaccenic) acid ($C_{18:1w9}$), and two cyclic fatty acids were the cis-9,10-methylenehexadecanoic acid (cyc_{17}) and the cis-9,10-methyleneoctadecanoic (lactobacillic) acid (cyc_{19}). Their relative percentages were between 2% and 46% corresponding to more than 96% of all fatty acids observed. Some other minor fatty acids were also detected at lower relative concentrations: $C_{17:0}$, $C_{18:2w6}$, $C_{18:3w6}$, $C_{18:3w3}$, $C_{19:0}$, and $C_{20:0}$.

- *Fatty acid composition of Salmonella typhimurium wild type membrane*
  In the wild type strain, $C_{16:0}$, $C_{16:1w7}$, and $C_{18:0}$ were the main constituents, representing about 60% of total fatty acids. The proportion of total lipid cyclic fatty acids obtained was about 25.79%. However, minimum cyclic fatty acids levels were observed for phosphatidylethanolamine and Cardiolipin (6.43% and 5.08%, respectively) and higher one for phosphatidylglycerol (38.35%). The unsaturated to saturated fatty acids ratio was in the majority with respect to between the phospholipid fractions (table 1).

Fatty acids	*Total lipids*	*Phosphatidylethanolamine*	*Phosphatidylglycerol*	*Cardiolipin*
$C_{14:0}$	4.20 ± 0.09	4.75 ± 0.1	4.2 ± 0.005	11.27 ± 0.13
$C_{16:0}$	46.61 ± 0.22	53.16 ± 0.26	35.68 ± 0.61	65.2 ± 1.04
$C_{16:1\ w7}$	7.16 ± 0.47	8.54 ± 0.31	5.43 ± 0.77	7.04 ± 0.06
cyc_{17}	7.53 ± 0.6	6.43 ± 0.24	10.70 ± 0.21	2 ± 0.51
$C_{18:0}$	8.51 ± 0.91	1.13 ± 0.04	8.80 ± 0.08	5.90 ± 0.09
$C_{18:1\ w9}$	2.07 ± 0.01	2.45 ± 0.21	3.28 ± 0.31	2.24 ± 0.04
cyc_{19}	18.26 ± 0.38	19.17 ± 0.63	27.65 ± 0.59	3.08 ± 0.82
MUFA	5.66	4.37	4.26	3.27
∑SFA	59.32	59.04	48.68	82.37
∑UFA	9.23	10.99	8.71	9.28
∑CFA	25.79	25.6	38.35	5.08
UFA/SFA	0.155	0.186	0.179	0.113

Table 1. Membrane fatty acid composition (molar percent) in total lipids and different phospholipid classes in the *Salmonella typhimurium* wild type strain (**MUFA**: Monounsaturated fatty acids; **SFA**: Saturated fatty acids; **UFA**: Unsaturated fatty acids; **CFA**: Cyclic fatty acids; **UFA/SFA**: Unsaturated to saturated ratio).

- *Fatty acid composition of the Salmonella typhimurium seqA mutant membrane*
  To determine whether the mutation in the *seqA* gene affected membrane lipid components, fatty acid composition was quantified. Our results indicated that the fatty acid composition of the total lipids appeared to be unaffected by the *seqA* mutation (table 2). The loss of cardiolipin and phosphatidylethanolamine was accompanied with a decrease in the proportion of $C_{14:0}$, $C_{16:0}$, and $C_{16:1w7}$ and an increase in the proportion of $C_{18:0}$ especially for the cardiolipin phospholipid (from 5.9% to 41.93%). Compared with the isogenic wild type strain, cardiolipin and phosphatidylethanolamine phospholipids showed an increase in the percentages of cyc_{19} and a decrease in their $C_{18:1w9}$, which resulted in low level of acyl chain unsaturation of fatty acids (table 2). The phosphatidylglycerol fraction showed a great increase of both $C_{16:0}$ and cyc_{17} and a decrease in $C_{16:1w7}$, which resulted in a low unsaturated to saturated fatty acids ratio (table 2).

Various physiological and biochemical changes took place as a consequence of many gene mutations, which can lead to numerous damages in the structure and function of the membrane cells (Shibuya et al., 1985; Taylor & Cronan, 1976). The purpose of the work presented in this section was to investigate a possible connection between both the *seqA* gene (coding for the sequestration protein SeqA) and some membrane components in *Salmonella typhimurium*. The phospholipids and fatty acids were the object of attention because the membrane delimiting the cell, and presumably playing a key role in DNA replication, is supposed to be constituted largely of lipids. Interactions of SeqA protein with cellular membranes have been previously reported. However, although regulation of the activities of this protein by membranes or their components was reported (Oshima et al., 2002) or suggested (Slater et al., 1995; Wegrzyn et al., 1999), little is known about the influence of SeqA on the composition of *Salmonella typhimurium* cell membranes. So, we suggest that in addition to its direct role in the sequestration of *oriC* region of the chromosome on the membrane, SeqA could activate or impair the expression of some genes (e.g., STM1329: putative inner membrane protein and *yijP*: putative integral membrane protein, respectively) that interact with lipid metabolism and regulate acidic phospholipids synthesis.

Fatty acids	*Total lipids*	*Phosphatidylethanolamine*	*Phosphatidylglycerol*	*Cardiolipin*
$C_{14:0}$	3.74 ± 0.18	4.19 ± 0.25	2.77 ± 0.21	4.85 ± 0.87
$C_{16:0}$	42.81 ± 0.14	45.8 ± 0.32	54.25 ± 0.13	36.38 ± 0.38
$C_{16:1\ w7}$	4.24 ± 0.37	2.53 ± 0.57	1.38 ± 0.02	4.13 ± 0.24
cyc_{17}	11.6 ± 0.11	20.63 ± 0.13	13.70 ± 0.08	0.35 ± 0.05
$C_{18:0}$	12.96 ± 1.06	1.15 ± 0.17	4.08 ± 0.89	41.93 ± 0.01
$C_{18:1\ w9}$	1.5 ± 0.12	0.40 ± 0.18	0.45 ± 0.07	0.000
cyc_{19}	20.7 ± 0.27	24.11 ± 1.06	22.42 ± 0.98	9.77 ± 0.49
MUFA	2.45	1.19	0.95	2.59
∑SFA	59.51	51.14	61.10	83.16
∑UFA	5.74	2.93	1.83	4.13
∑CFA	32.30	44.74	36.12	10.12
UFA/SFA	0.096	0.057	0.030	0.050

Table 2. Membrane fatty acid composition (molar percent) in total lipids and different phospholipid classes in the *Salmonella typhimurium seqA* mutant strain.

4. Increased sensitivity of membrane to bile salt after *seqA* disruption

The overall purpose of this last section was to study the modifications of the cell membrane compounds of *Salmonella typhimurium* during the growth in the presence of ox bile doses. The results obtained evidenced that the tested substances induced noticeable modifications of the phospholipids and fatty acids composition of cell membrane during bacterial growth.

4.1 Phospholipids composition of bile treated *seqA* mutants

Exposed to the ox bile, and compared with the non treated cells, our results indicated that the phospholipids composition of the bile treated wild type strain was in the majority with respect to the non treated wild type strain. So it appeared to be unaffected by the ox bile stress. The acidic phospholipid fractions (phosphatidylglycerol and Cardiolipin) account for 25.4% of total Phls distributed in 20.7% of phosphatidylglycerol and 4.7% of Cardiolipin. A non significant decrease in the phosphatidylethanolamine fraction (74.6%) was observed.
To evaluate the combined effects of the *seqA* mutation and the ox bile stress on the bacterial membrane integrity, we compared the phospholipids composition of the exposed *seqA* mutant with the non exposed *seqA* and wild type strains. Compared with these tow *Salmonella typhimurium* strains, the acidic phospholipids (phosphatidylglycerol and Cardiolipin) showed a great increase with 81.7% and 14.1%, respectively. However, the phosphatidylethanolamine proportion decreased dramatically to 4.2% (Figure 7).

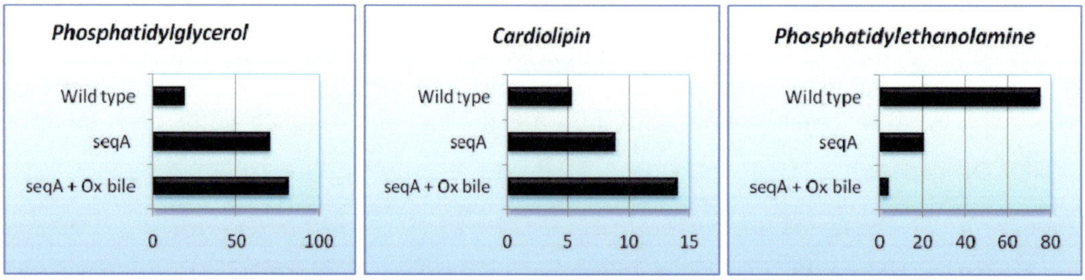

Fig. 7. Comparative analysis of phospholipid levels in *Salmonella typhimurium* wild type and *seqA* strains (control and exposed to ox bile). Exponentially growing wild type strain was incubated at 37°C with ox bile extract at a concentration of one percent. Their contents were also calculated from the fatty acids contents. Average values of triplicates were given, and the deviation was less than 5% of each value (significance was assessed using the Student's *t*-test).

4.2 Effect of the ox bile combined to the *seqA* mutation on membrane fatty acids composition of *Salmonella typhimurium*

The membrane fatty acids composition (molar percent) of the wild type and seqA mutant strains exposed to ox bile is shown in table 3.

- *Membrane fatty acids composition of the wild type strains exposed to the ox bile.*
  For the wild type strain cultured with the ox bile, no significant changes were observed in both total lipids and phospholipids (cardiolipin, phosphatidylglycerol, and phosphatidylethanolamine). The fatty acids composition appeared to be unaffected by the ox bile stress with an unsaturated to saturated ratio, in the majority, with respect to that of wild type control strain.
- *Membrane fatty acids composition of the seqA mutant strains exposed to the ox bile.*
  To determine whether the mutation in the *seqA* gene added to the ox bile stress affected membrane lipid components, fatty acids composition was quantified. The membrane fatty acids composition of the total lipids was highly affected by the ox bile stress (table 3).

The fatty acids were characterized by low level of cyclic fatty acids, representing about 22.06% of total content, and high level of unsaturated fatty acids, representing about 15.74% (25.79% / 9.23% and 32.30% / 5.74%, respectively, for the wild type and the *seqA* mutant strains). These changes were due to a decrease in the cyclopropane derivatives C_{17}- and C_{19}-cyclic fatty acids and a concomitant increase in the unsaturated fatty acids ($C_{16:1w7}$ and $C_{18:1w9}$) and resulted in a high unsaturated to saturated ratio (table 3). The accumulation of the cardiolipin fraction was accompanied with an increase in the $C_{18:1w9}$ composition, which rise up from 0.0% to 3.0% (table 3). In the phosphatidylglycerol fraction, data confirmed that also $C_{18:1w9}$ becomes a prominent species accounting for about 4.25% (3.28% and 0.45% respectively for the wild type and *seqA* phosphatidylglycerol fractions). Finally, we noticed that the phosphatidylethanolamine phospholipids were characterized by a reduction in cyclic fatty acids (cyc_{17} and cyc_{19}) to the profile of their unsaturated fatty acids derivatives ($C_{16:1w7}$ and $C_{18:1w9}$). These phospholipids changes resulted in a high unsaturated to saturated ratio (table 3).

It has been proposed that intracellular pathogens like *Salmonella* are exposed to several stressing agents such as bile during the infection process. Stress conditions which pathogenic pathogen encounter during infection course can affect membrane components.

Fatty acids	*Total lipids*	*Phosphatidylethanolamine*	*Phosphatidylglycerol*	*Cardiolipin*
$C_{14:0}$	4.78 ± 0.04	5.15 ± 0.90	2.80 ± 0.21	5.42 ± 0.06
$C_{16:0}$	44.31 ± 0.56	46.38 ± 0.22	56.01 ± 0.03	37.38 ± 0.03
$C_{16:1\ w7}$	9.89 ± 0.09	4.36 ± 0.07	3.18 ± 0.42	6.13 ± 0.24
cyc_{17}	5.96 ± 0.44	17.03 ± 0.06	11.16 ± 0.18	0.09 ± 0.83
$C_{18:0}$	13.11 ± 0.03	2.84 ± 0.83	4.38 ± 0.61	42 ± 0.01
$C_{18:1\ w9}$	5.85 ± 0.52	4.20 ± 0.03	4.25 ± 0.07	3 ± 0.54
cyc_{19}	16.1 ± 0.07	20.04 ± 0.36	18.22 ± 0.46	5.98 ± 0.07
MUFA	3.06	2.74	1.75	3.43
∑SFA	62.2	54.37	63.19	84.8
∑UFA	15.74	8.56	7.43	9.13
∑CFA	22.06	37.07	29.38	6.07
UFA/SFA	0.253	0.157	0.117	0.107

Table 3. Membrane fatty acid composition (molar percent) in total lipids and different phospholipid classes in the *Salmonella typhimurium seqA* mutant strain exposed to ox bile.

The environmental control of regulatory mechanisms is mediated by complex processes. *Salmonella* comes in contact with bile salts in the intestine and it is able to resist the action of bile and respond to escalating bile concentrations by increasing mechanisms of resistance. Previous studies showed that bacteria with enhanced tolerance to acid, bile and blood serum survive (Morgan et al., 1986, Wilmes-Riesenberg et al., 1996) and cause disease (Foster & Hall, 1990; Rowbury et al., 1989) better than sensitive bacteria and showed that *in vitro* acid adapted *Salmonella* were more resistant towards bile (Velkinburg & Gunn, 1999) and acids (Foster & Hall, 1990) in comparison to non-adapted cells.

Results obtained in this study show that the ox bile stress added to the *seqA* mutation is an important factor affecting *Salmonella typhimurium* resistance and could contribute to find new strategies based on intelligent combinations of hurdles, which could prevent the development or survival of *Salmonella spp.* in gastrointestinal tract. *Salmonella typhimurium* cells have developed efficient protection systems to cope with a variety of physicochemical unfavorable conditions and to adapt to the environmental stresses. In particular, fundamental for the microbial cells is to maintain membrane integrity and functionality in response to environmental stresses encountered during infection. In response to stresses, the phospholipids can alter their acyl chain structure by changing the ratio of saturation to unsaturation, *cis* to *trans* unsaturation, branched to unbranched structure and type of branching and acyl chain length (Russel, 1984). Different modulation mechanisms can be used in relation to the physiological state of the cells (Rock & Cronan, 1996).

In a previous work Prieto et al., (2007) have shown that the *seqA* mutation renders *Salmonella enterica* sensitive to agents known to be antimicrobially active in the host like sodium choleate (ox bile extract) but the cause of this sensitivity remains unknown. In the present study we tried to explain the reasons and to investigate a possible connection between both the *seqA* gene (coding for the sequestration protein SeqA) and some membrane components and the sensitivity to the ox bile observed in *Salmonella typhimurium*.

In *Escherichia coli, seqA* mutants show altered membrane permeability (Wegrzyn et al., 1999) and abnormal phospholipids composition, which may explain their increased sensitivity to a number of dyes. The observation that the envelope of *Salmonella enterica seqA* mutants is likewise unstable (Aloui et al., 2010) can be tentatively correlated with bile sensitivity, because unconjugated bile salts can enter the cell by diffusion (Thanassi et al., 1997). Thus, a structural role of SeqA in envelope stability cannot be discounted (Wegrzyn et al., 1999). An alternative explanation is that SeqA might regulate the expression of genes involved in the stability and the integrity of the cell membrane against bile salts during infection process, a possibility also considered in *Escherichia coli* (Strzelczyk et al., 2003).

In summary, *Salmonella typhimurium* SeqA protein is required for maintenance of membrane integrity against the ox bile. Mutation in the *seqA* gene causes envelope defects and enhances sensitivity to the ox bile which together may contribute to the attenuation of virulence and may induce strong immune responses in infected animals. Recently, it has been demonstrated that *Salmonella typhimurium* lacking *seqA* gene exhibit a decrease of virulence in mice perhaps due to the bile sensitivity during the infection process. So we suggest that this mutant may be applied to the design of a live vaccine.

5. Conclusion

In the *Salmonella typhimurium* cell, DNA sequestration modulates a variety of processes such as DNA replication and transcription of certain genes. Deletion of the *seqA* gene produces a variety of phenotypes ranging from replication asynchrony to virulence attenuation, indicating multiple functions for the GATC-binding protein in modulating gene expression, proper chromosome segregation, initiation of chromosome replication, and nucleoid stabilization. Given these multiple roles, it is not surprising that *seqA* mutation is highly pleiotropic. However, the lack of SeqA protein does not impair viability. *Salmonella typhimurium seqA*- strain described here lacks binding of SeqA to GATC sequences and is more sensitive to this mutation than the wild type which shows the inverse. In addition, no great difference between the *seqA* mutant of *Salmonella typhimurium* and those of some enterobacterial species such as *Escherichia coli* was observed with replication asynchrony or alteration membrane. In conclusion, the role of SeqA in the prokaryotic cellular processes such as the DNA replication and lipids membrane metabolism is clear. So it may rely on its capacity as a global regulator of the gene expression during bacterial life, *in vitro*, in a similar manner as it does *in vivo*.

6. Future research

Our knowledge on the effects of SeqA protein in *Salmonella typhimurium* has considerably improved in the last decade. This fundamental research has several implications that will

prove to be useful for the development of novel therapeutic approaches. But, to date, therapeutic applications are still in their early experimental phases, but several recent studies provide promising results for future clinical developments. Over the last few years, many studies have demonstrated that *Salmonella typhimurium seqA* mutants exhibit asynchronous DNA replication and are highly attenuated for virulence in mice and have been proposed as live vaccines. These results prove that GATC-binding sites might have a role in regulating virulence of *Salmonella typhimurium* and perhaps in other related bacteria.
In addition, future research must focus on the study of the decreasing virulence and the proteomic and enzymatic activities of a *seqA* mutant strain. So this perspectives can be useful to more fully understand the significance of the results obtained above. Of special interests are: firstly, the growing list of genes governed by DNA sequestration in bacterial pathogens ; secondly, the finding of novel genes regulated by SeqA protein using high throughput analysis, and, thirdly, the evidence that this protein may regulate the expression of many unidentified genes involved in DNA replication and membrane metabolism.
Finally, the way in which SeqA participates clearly in the DNA replication and in the membrane integrity is a critical question that deserves further investigation in the near future, and may be research studies will have to identify explanations.

7. Acknowledgment

The work presented in this chapter was supported by the Tunisian Ministry of Higher Education, Scientific Research, and Technology. It has been performed at the biochemistry and molecular biology laboratory which belongs to the Faculty of Sciences of Bizerta. Many people have in different ways supported me in my work and contributed to the completion of this study. I would especially like to extend my gratitude to:

- Dr. Francisco Ramos-Morales (Departamento de Genética, Facultad de Biologia, Universidad de Sevilla, Spain) for the generous donation of the *Salmonella typhimurium* wild type and *seqA* disrupted strain.
- Mr Bchini Zin for proofreading and correcting this manuscript.

8. References

Aloui, A., Mihoub, M., Sethom, M.M., Chatti, A., Feki, M., Kaabachi, N. & Landoulsi, A. (2010). Effects of *dam* and/or *seqA* Mutations on the Fatty Acid and Phospholipid Membrane Composition of *Salmonella enterica* Serovar Typhimurium. *Foodborne Pathog. Dis.*, Vol 7, N°5, pp. (573-583).

Ames, G.F. (1968). Lipids of *Salmonella typhimurium* and *Escherichia coli*: structure and Metabolism. *J. Bacteriol.*, 95, pp. (833–843).

Bach, T., Krekling, M.A. & Skarstad, K. (2003). Excess SeqA prolongs sequestration of *oriC* and delays nucleoid segregation and cell division. *EMBO J.*, 22, pp. (315–323).

Bogan, J.A. & Helmstetter, C.E. (1997). DNA sequestration and transcription in the *oriC* region of *Escherichia coli*. *Mol. Microbiol.*, 26, pp. (889–896).

Boye, E. & Løbner-Olesen, A. (1990). The role of dam methyltransferase in the control of DNA replication in *E. coli*. *Cell*, 62, pp. (981–989).

Boye, E., Stokke, T., Kleckner, N. & Skarstad, K. (1996). Coordinating DNA replication initiation with cell growth: differential roles for DnaA and SeqA proteins. *Proc. Natl. Acad. Sci.* USA, 93, pp. (12206–12211).

Brendler, T., Sawitzke, J., Seerguev, K. & Austin, S. (2000). A case for sliding SeqA tracts at anchored replication forks during *Escherichia coli* chromosome replication and segregation. *EMBO J.*, 19, pp. (6249–6258).

d'Alencon, E., Taghbalout, A., Kern, R., & Kohiyama, M. (1999). Replication cycle dependent association of SeqA to the outer membrane fraction of *E. coli*. *Biochimie*, 81, pp. (841-846).

Foster, J.W. & Hall, H.K. (1990). Adaptive acidification tolerance response of *Salmonella typhimunum*. *J. Bacteriol.*, 172, pp. (771–778).

Greenacre, E.J., Brocklehurst, T.F., Waspe, C.R., Wilson, D.R. & Wilson, P.D.G. (2003). *Salmonella enterica* serovar Typhimurium and *Listeria monocytogenes* acid tolerance response induced by organic acids at 20°C: optimization and modeling. *Appl. Environ. Microbiol.*, 69, pp. (3945–3951).

Guarné, A., Zhao, Q., Ghirlando, R. & Yang, W. (2002). Insights into negative modulation of *E. coli* replication initiation from the structure of SeqA-hemimethylated DNA complex. *Nat. Struct. Biol.*, 9, pp. (839-843).

Jacob, F., Brenner, S. & Cuzin, F. (1963). On the regulation of DNA replication in bacteria. *Cold. Spring. Harb. Symp. Quant. Biol.*, 28, pp. (329–348).

Kang, S., Han, J.S., Park, J.H., Skarstad, K. & Hwang, D.S. (2003). SeqA protein stimulates the relaxing and decatenating activities of topoisomerase IV. *J. Biol. Chem.*, 278, pp. (48779–48785).

Klungsøyr, H.K. & Skarstad, K. (2004). Positive supercoiling is generated in the presence of *Escherichia coli* SeqA protein. *Mol. Microbiol.*, 54, pp. (123–131).

Landoulsi, A., Malki, A., Kern, R., Kohiyama, M. & Hughes, P.(1990). The *E. coli* cell surface specifically prevents the initiation of DNA replication at *oriC* on hemimethylated DNA templates. *Cell*, 63, pp. (1053–1060).

Leyer, G.J. & Johnson, E.A. (1992). Acid adaptation promotes survival of *Salmonella spp.* in cheese. *Appl. Environ. Microbiol.*, 58, pp. (2075–2080).

Leyer, G.J. & Johnson, E.A. (1993). Acid adaptation induces cross-protection against environmental stresses in *Salmonella typhimurium*. *Appl. Environ. Microbiol.*, 59, pp. (1842–1847).

Løbner-Olesen, A., Marinus, M.G. & Hanssen, F.G. (2003). Role of SeqA and Dam in *Escherichia coli* gene expression: a global/microarray analysis. Proc. Natl. Acad. Sci. USA., 100, pp. (4672–4677).

Løbner-Olesen, A. & Von Freiesleben, U. (1996). Chromosomal replication incompatibility in Dam methyltransferase deficient *Escherichia coli* cells. *EMBO J.*, 15, pp. (5999–6008).

Lu, M., Campbell, J.L., Boye, E. & Kleckner, N. (1994). SeqA: a negative modulator of replication initiation in *E.coli*. Cell, 77, pp. (413–426).

Makise, M., Mima, S., Katsu, T., Tsuchiya, T. & Mizushima, T. (2002). Acidic phospholipids inhibit the DNA-binding activity of DnaA protein, the initiator of chromosomal DNA replication in *Escherichia coli*. *Mol. Microbiol.*, 46, pp. (245–256).

Marinus, M.G. (1996). Methylation of DNA in *Escherichia coli* and *Salmonella Typhimurium*, In: *Cellular and Molecular biology*, eds. Neidhardt, F.C., Ingraham, J.L., Brooks, L.K., Magasanik, B., Schaechter, M. & Umbarger, H.E., pp. (782–791), DC: American Society for Microbiology Press, Washington.

Messer, W. & Weigel, C. (1996). Initiation of chromosome replication in *Escherichia coli* and *Salmonella*, In: *Cellular and Molecular Biology*. Neidhardt, F.C., Ingraham, J.L.,

Brooks, L.K., Magasanik, B., Schaechter, M. & Umbarger, H.E., pp. (1579–1601), DC: American Society for Microbiology Press, Washington.

Mizushima, T., Nishida, S., Kurokawa, K., Katayama, T., Miki, T. & Sekimizu, K. (1997). Negative control of DNA replication by hydrolysis of ATP bound to DnaA protein, the initiator of chromosomal DNA replication in *Escherichia coli*. *EMBO J.*, 16, pp. (3724–3730).

Morgan, R.W., Christman, M.F., Jacobson, F.S., Storz, G., & Ames, B.N. (1986). Hydrogen peroxide-inducible proteins in *Salmonella typhimurium* overlap with heat shock and other stress proteins. *Proc. Natl. Acad. Sci. USA.*, 83, pp. (8059–8063).

Ogden, G.B., Pratt, M.J. & Schaechter, M. (1988). The replicative origin of the *E. coli* chromosome binds to cell membranes only when hemimethylated. *Cell*, 54, pp. (127-135).

Oshima, T., Wada, C., Kawagoe, Y., Ara, T., Maeda, M., Masuda, Y., Hiraga, S. & Mori, H. (2002). Genome-wide analysis of deoxyadenosine methyltransferase-mediated control of gene expression in *Escherichia coli*. *Mol. Microbiol.*, 45, pp. (673–695).

Prieto, A.I., Jakomin, M., Segura, I., Pucciarelli, M.G., Ramos-Morales, F., del Portillo, F.G. & Casadesus, J. (2007). The GATC-binding protein SeqA is required for bile resistance and virulence in *Salmonella enterica* Serovar Typhimurium. *J. Bacteriol.*, 189, pp. (8496–8502).

Rock, C.O. & Cronan, J.E. (1996). *Escherichia coli* as a model for the regulation of dissociable (type II) fatty acid biosynthesis. *Biochimica & Biophysica Acta*, 1302, pp. (1–16).

Rowbury, R.J., Goadson, M. & Whiting, G.C. (1989). Habilithation of *E. coli* to acid and alkaline pH and its relevance to bacterial survival in chemically-polluted natural waters. *Chem. Industry.*, 22, pp. (685–686).

Russel, N.J. (1984). Mechanisms of thermal adaptation in bacteria: blue prints for survival. *Trends in Biochemical Science*, 9, pp. (108–112).

Sekimizu, K. & Kornberg, A. (1988). Cardiolipin activation of DnaA protein, the initiation protein of replication in *Escherichia coli*. *J. Biol. Chem.*, 263, pp. (7131–7135).

Shibuya, I., Miyazaki, C. & Ohta, A. (1985). Alteration of phospholipid composition by combined defects in phosphatidylserine and cardiolipin synthases and physiological consequences in *Escherichia coli*. *J. Bacteriol.*, 16, pp. (1086–1092).

Skarstad, K., von Meyenburg, K., Hansen, F.G. & Boye, E. (1988). Coordination of chromosome replication initiation in *Escherichia coli*: effects of different *dnaA* alleles. *J. Bacteriol.*, 170, pp. (852–858).

Slater, S., Wold, S., Lu, M., Boye, E., Skarstad, K. & Kleckner, N. (1995). *Escherichia coli* SeqA protein binds *oriC* in two different methylmodulated reactions appropriate to its roles in DNA replication initiation and origin sequestration. *Cell*, 82, pp. (927-936).

Strzelczyk, B., Slominska-Wojewodzka, M., Wegrzyn, M.G. & Wegrzyn, A. (2003). Non-random distribution of GATC sequences in regions of promoters stimulated by the SeqA protein of *Escherichia coli*. *Acta. Biochim. Pol.*, 50, pp. (941–945).

Taylor, F. & Cronan, J.E. (1976). Selection and properties of *Escherichia coli* mutants defective in the synthesis of cyclopropane fatty acids. *J. Bacteriol.*, 125, pp. (518–523).

Thanassi, D.G, Cheng, L.W. & Nikaido, H. (1997). Active efflux of bile salts by *Escherichia coli*. *J. Bacteriol.*, 179, pp. (2512–2518).

Torheim, N.K. & Skarstad, K. (1999). *Escherichia coli* SeqA protein affects DNA topology and inhibits open complex formation of *oriC*. *EMBO J.*, 18, pp. (4882–4888).

Tosun, H. & Gonul, S.A. (2003). Acid adaptation protects *Salmonella typhimurium* from environmental stresses. *Turk. J. Biol.*, 27, pp. (31-36).

Velkinburg, J.C. & Gunn, J.S. (1999). PhoP-PhoQ-regulated loci are regulated for enhanced bile resistance in *Salmonella spp. Infect. Immun.*, 67, pp. (1614-1622).

Von Freiesleben, U., Rasmussen, K.V. & Schaechter, M. (1994). SeqA limits DnaA activity in replication from *oriC* in *Escherichia coli. Mol. Microbiol.*, 14, pp. (763-772).

Waterman, S.R. & Small, P.L.C. (1998). Acid-sensitive enteric pathogens are protected from killing under extremely acidic conditions of pH 2.5 when they are inoculated onto certain solid food sources. *Appl. Environ. Microbiol.*, 64, pp. (3882-3886).

Wegrzyn, A., Wrobel, B. & Wegrzyn, G. (1999). Altered biological properties of cell membranes in *Escherichia coli dnaA* and *seqA* mutants. *Mol. Gen. Genet.*, 261, pp; (762-769).

Wilmes-Riesenberg, M.R., Bearson, B., Foster, J.W. & Curtiss, R. (1996). Role of acid tolerance response in virulence of *Salmonella typhimurium. Infect. Immun.*, 64, pp. (1085-1092).

Wold, S., Boye, E., Slater, S., Kleckner, N. & Skarstad, K. (1998). Effects of purified SeqA protein on *oriC*-dependent DNA replication *in vitro. EMBO J.*, 17, pp. (4158-4165).

Yamazoe, M.S., Adachi, S., Kanava, K.O. & Hiraga, S. (2005). Sequential binding of SeqA protein to nascent DNA segments at replication forks in synchronized cultures of *E. coli. Mol. Microbiol.*, 55, pp, (289-298).

Yuk, H.G. & Schneider, K.R. (2006). Adaptation of *Salmonella spp.* in juice stored under refrigerated and room temperature enhances acid resistance to simulated gastric fluid. *Food Microbiol.*, 23, pp. (694-700).